Recent Advances in Anesthesiology

(*Volume 2*)

Anesthesia: A Topical Update - *Thoracic, Cardiac, Neuro, ICU*, and *Interesting Cases*

Edited by

Amballur D. John

Department of Anesthesiology and Critical Care Medicine, Johns Hopkins University School of Medicine Baltimore, MD, USA

General:

1. Any dispute or claim arising out of or in connection with this License Agreement or the Work (including non-contractual disputes or claims) will be governed by and construed in accordance with the laws of the U.A.E. as applied in the Emirate of Dubai. Each party agrees that the courts of the Emirate of Dubai shall have exclusive jurisdiction to settle any dispute or claim arising out of or in connection with this License Agreement or the Work (including non-contractual disputes or claims).
2. Your rights under this License Agreement will automatically terminate without notice and without the need for a court order if at any point you breach any terms of this License Agreement. In no event will any delay or failure by Bentham Science Publishers in enforcing your compliance with this License Agreement constitute a waiver of any of its rights.
3. You acknowledge that you have read this License Agreement, and agree to be bound by its terms and conditions. To the extent that any other terms and conditions presented on any website of Bentham Science Publishers conflict with, or are inconsistent with, the terms and conditions set out in this License Agreement, you acknowledge that the terms and conditions set out in this License Agreement shall prevail.

Bentham Science Publishers Ltd.
Executive Suite Y - 2
PO Box 7917, Saif Zone
Sharjah, U.A.E.
Email: subscriptions@benthamscience.org

BENTHAM SCIENCE

CONTENTS

PREFACE

The purpose of this work is to provide a quick update for practitioners on the major topics in Anesthesia. Medicine is a rapidly changing field. In this series:

VOLUME 1 deals with specific anesthetic issues such as regional anesthesia.

Recent Advances in Anesthesiology Vol 1: ANESTHESIA: Essential Clinical Updates for Practitioners – Regional, Ultrasound, Coagulation, Obstetrics and Pediatrics

VOLUME 2 deals with major systems.

Recent Advances in Anesthesiology Vol 2: ANESTHESIA: A Topical Update – Thoracic, Cardiac, Neuro, ICU and Interesting Cases

Despite one's best effort and the efforts of various professional societies, it is often difficult to keep abreast in all aspects of anesthesia. Over time, every practitioner settles into a daily practice and keeps current in that area. However, the nature of modern anesthetic practice requires flexibility to fill various staffing needs. This often necessitates practitioners to do cases that they are not always facile with. There are a variety of resources available to acquire the requisite knowledge from detailed tomes to introductory manuals. The goal of this work is to provide practitioners with current updates on key aspects of anesthesia with a quick read of 15-20 minutes per topic so that a practitioner will be able to rapidly refresh their knowledge and skills. The chapters contained herein are written by outstanding specialist clinicians who are excellent teachers at the foremost anesthesia training programs. My deepest gratitude and sincere thanks to the authors who have taken the time and effort to do this onerous work, and apologizes for the inordinate delays incumbent in the publication process.

My sincere gratitude to the following individuals for their guidance and direction over the years. Dr. Eugenie Heitmiller: Genie is the epitome of excellence and positivity. As a young resident; I was fortunate to have had the opportunity and privilege of working with Genie. Dr. James Schauble who taught me to intubate and do anesthesia. Dr. William Merritt – who always took the time to teach and ensure that I was fed and watered no matter how horrid the day. Dr. Frederick Sieber: Fritz is my boss and friend. Special thanks to Warren Zapol M.D., Chairman Emeritus the Massachusetts General Hospital Harvard Medical School, and Edward Miller Jr. M.D., Emeritus Dean and CEO of Johns Hopkins Medicine, for their kindness and for hiring me.

ACKNOWLEDGEMENTS

My profound gratitude to the outstanding contributors who took time and effort to share thei knowledge by writing the chapters on their areas of expertise, and to Fariya Zulfiqar and Shehzad Naqvi, project managers at Bentham. Thanks to Javita Jenkins and Audra Beard for their help with typing the manuscript. I am grateful to Jessica Terzigni who was able to work with all involved. The opportunity of working with Norm Myers – the illustrator, has been an enlightening educational experience.

A.D. John, M.D.
Department of Anesthesiology and Critical Care Medicine
Johns Hopkins University School of Medicine
Baltimore, MD, USA
E-mail: ajohn1@jhmi.edu

DEDICATION

This book is dedicated to my amazing and supportive parents, David and Lily John.

List of Contributors

Adair Q. Locke	Wake Forest School of Medicine, Winston Salem, North Carolina, USA
Amballur D. John	Johns Hopkins Medical Institutions, Baltimore, Maryland, USA
Chandrika R. Garner	Wake Forest School of Medicine, Winston Salem, North Carolina, USA
Edward A. Bittner	Massachusetts General Hospital, Harvard Medical School, Boston, Massachusetts, USA
Jeffrey Dodd-o	Johns Hopkins Medical Institutions, Baltimore, Maryland, USA
Jonathan E. Sevransky	Emory University School of Medicine, Atlanta, Georgia, USA
Mahmood Jaberi	Johns Hopkins Medical Institutions, Baltimore, Maryland, USA University Hospital Cleveland, Cleveland, Ohio, USA
Matthew L. Kashima	Johns Hopkins Medical Institutions, Baltimore, Maryland, USA
Michael S. Lava	Emory University School of Medicine, Atlanta, Georgia, USA
Nathaniel McQuay	Johns Hopkins Medical Institutions, Baltimore, Maryland, USA University Hospital Cleveland, Cleveland, Ohio, USA
Paul J. Hoehner	Johns Hopkins Medical Institutions, Baltimore, Maryland, USA
Punita Tripathi	Johns Hopkins Medical Institutions, Baltimore, Maryland, USA
Russell D. Dolan	Emory University School of Medicine, Atlanta, Georgia, USA
Sheri Berg	Massachusetts General Hospital, Harvard Medical School, Boston, Massachusetts, USA
Thomas F. Slaughter	Wake Forest School of Medicine, Winston Salem, North Carolina, USA

Recent Advances in Anesthesiology

Volume # 2

Anesthesia: A Topical Update – Thoracic, Cardiac, Neuro, ICU, and Interesting Cases

Editor: Amballur D. John

ISSN (Online): 2589-9392

ISSN (Print): 2589-9384

ISBN (Online): 978-1-68108-723-8

ISBN (Print): 978-1-68108-724-5

CHAPTER 1

Anesthetic Considerations for Otolaryngology and Neck Surgery

Matthew L. Kashima[*]

Johns Hopkins Medical Institutions, Baltimore, Maryland, USA

Abstract: Otolaryngology procedures involve the airway either directly or take place in close proximity to the airway which necessitate the sharing of the airway by the surgical and anesthesia teams. Close co-operation, open communication, clear delineation of the plan as well as backup contingencies for intubation and airway care between the surgical and anesthesia teams are required for successful patient care. Care should be taken in paralyzing a patient with a potentially difficult airway until the ability to mask the patient has been confirmed. Laryngeal disorders can be infectious, benign or malignant growths. Head and neck surgery is complex and muscle relaxation is often contraindicated by the need to monitor nerve function. Pediatrics, epiglottitis, and the aspiration of foreign bodies emphasize this need for close cooperation and communication between all involved in the patient care – surgical staff, anesthesia staff, and nursing staff, for the best results and in order to ensure patient safety.

Keywords: Airway Foreign Body, Airway, Difficult Airway, Epiglottis, Head and Neck Surgery, Larynogectomy, Laryngospasm, Myringotomy, Operating Room Fires, Otolaryngology, Parotidectomy, Thyroidectomy, Tonsillectomy, Tracheostomy, Tympanoplasty.

INTRODUCTION

Anesthesia is needed for most surgical procedures. Otolaryngologic surgery poses some unique circumstances for anesthesiologists. Anesthesiologists are generally considered to be experts in managing the airway. Many otolaryngology procedures involve the airway directly or take place in close proximity to the airway. This necessitates that the surgical and anesthesia teams share the airway (Fig. **1 - 2**).

Preoperative evaluation and planning are crucial for many otolaryngology surgeries. The nature of the disease process and the location of the intervention may require   techniques that are not   needed by   other surgical specialties.

[*] **Corresponding author Matthew L. Kashima:** Johns Hopkins Medical Institutions, Baltimore, Maryland, USA; Tel: 410-550-0460; Fax: 410-550-2870; E-mail: mkashim1@jhmi.edu

Amballur D. John (Ed.)

Anesthesiologists must be able to reach into their entire arsenal of skill and techniques to best care for these patients. Patients presenting for upper airway surgical procedures may require mask ventilation, oral intubation, nasal intubation, apneic techniques, jet ventilation, surgical airways or several of the above in a single operation. The level of anesthesia can vary from none to local to sedation to general anesthesia with or without paralysis. Again combinations of the level of anesthesia needed may vary depending on the portion of the procedure. Open communication about the type of airway needed and the depth of anesthesia required between the operating surgeon and the anesthesiologist prior to the procedure will lead to the best outcomes. This conversation may need to be continued during extended procedures as team members change and different portions of the procedure are performed.

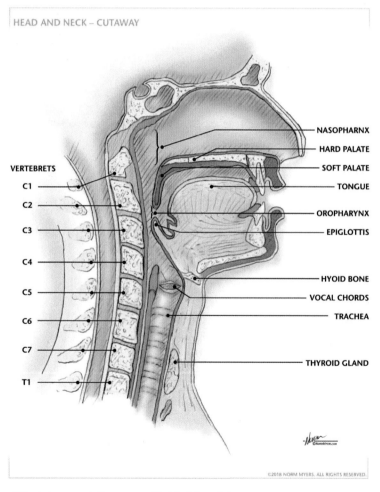

Fig. (1). Head and Neck (cutaway). Image provided by Norm Myers.

LARYNX

Fig. (2). Larynx. Image provided by Norm Myers.

Positioning of the patient during Otolaryngologic procedures frequently separates the anesthesiologist from the patient's head. This requires close communication and cooperation between the surgical and anesthesia teams. Close attention to the patient *via* monitors may also be needed during these cases since the patient is not right in front of the anesthesiologist.

AIRWAY

Anesthesiologists are thought of as airway experts. Similarly, Otolaryngologists are considered to be airway experts. Both specialties are often involved in caring for patients with difficult airways. Again, communication is key to avoiding conflict and complications. **Delineation of the plan for intubation with several contingencies including who is responsible for each intervention can be instrumental in these challenging cases.** This planning is only possible if there is a known airway issue, although planning can be done if there is a high suspicion of difficulty. Various techniques may need to be employed to secure the airway safely. An early decision point is whether to attempt a standard intubation or an awake intubation.

Care should be taken in paralyzing a potential difficult airway until the ability to mask the patient has been confirmed. See Table **1**, Indicators of potential difficult airway.

Various tool and techniques are available to assist in difficult airway situations. Most have advantages in certain situations and disadvantages in others. Competence with multiple techniques and familiarity with the available equipment will allow for more robust planning options. A comprehensive discussion of them is beyond the scope of this chapter. Use of video systems (*e.g.* Fiberoptic bronchoscopes, Glidescope, *etc.*) can communicate valuable information to other people in the room during an intubation that allows for more timely participation and assistance [1].

Anesthetizing the upper airway prior to instrumentation in an awake patient can make the procedure more comfortable and less stressful for everyone involved. Topical application of topical anesthetics can be helpful. These can be sprayed, nebulized, applied in gel or ointment or applied directly on a moistened sponge. Attention must be given to the potential for giving too much local anesthetic. The toxic dose for lidocaine is 5 mg/kg. Topical benzocaine is known to cause methemoglobinemia. The methemoglobin causes the blood to become darker and pulse oximetry can be affected and the patient may appear cyanotic. Treatment consists of obtaining a blood gas and giving methylene blue intravenously 2 mg/kg. Nerve blocks can be done including glossopharyngeal and superior laryngeal nerve blocks [2].

Table 1. Indicators of Potential Difficult Airway.

Indicators of Potential Difficult Airwaynesthesia (hours)*
Indicators of potential difficult airway
History of difficult airway
Head and neck trauma
Prior Head and neck Surgery
Prior Head and neck radiation
Trismus
Limited Cervical mobility
Dysphagia
Hoarseness or stridor
Obesity

Fires in the operating room frequently involve the head and neck region. It has been reported that 65% of surgical fires are either in the airway or located in the head, neck and upper chest region. Airway fires can occur when there is a fuel source, oxygen and ignition source. Oxygen is in air but when supplemental oxygen is given, it can collect in low lying areas as it is denser than air. Drapes, sponges, and the endotracheal tubes are combustible and can serve as fuels in airway fires. Lasers and electrocautery can ignite the fuels when opportunity presents itself. Awareness and preparation are key to avoiding airway fires. When oxygen is being used, care needs to be taken when using an ignition source. Suction should be used to scavenge oxygen and drapes should be positioned to prevent areas where oxygen can collect. Towels and sponges in or near the surgical field should be moistened. Water should be available on the field should a fire start.The fire should be immediately dowsed, including flushing water down the ETT if it is burning. Oxygen and NO_2 should be shut off. The ETT is removed and the airway is examined and the patient is reintubated if needed. Steroid administration should be considered [3].

Post obstructive pulmonary edema can occur following the removal of an airway obstruction. It can present rapidly after intubation of children who are intubated for airway obstruction due to upper airway swelling such as epiglottitis or coup. It can also be seen following surgery for obstructive sleep apnea. It presents with frothy pink sputum and accompanied hypoxemia. Chest x-ray will demonstrate findings consistent with pulmonary edema. Treatment is supportive with supplemental oxygen and positive end expiratory pressure with intubation if needed in severe cases. Diuretics can be used as well [4].

Tracheostomy

A **tracheostomy** is a surgical creation of an epithelialized tract connecting the trachea to the skin. It can be created to temporarily bypass the upper airway for an extensive procedure or as a more permanent tract for ventilation or pulmonary toilet. These procedures usually take 20 minutes but can be performed more rapidly if the circumstances dictate.

The majority of tracheostomies are scheduled elective cases often performed to facilitate prolonged ventilator support. These patients have other medical issues that may need to be addressed perioperatively. The patients are generally positioned supine with a shoulder roll to extend the neck. The neck is prepped and draped. The endotracheal tube should be loosened to facilitate removal during the procedure. The dissection is performed and the trachea exposed. Effort should be made to lower the inspired oxygen to the lowest tolerable level in preparation for the airway being entered. Until the trachea is entered, there is a low risk of fire and cautery may be used. Once the trachea is opened, it is not advisable to use cautery due to the risk of igniting an airway fire. Just prior to entering the airway the surgeon may request that the cuff be deflated to prevent damage and to take the patient off the ventilator to prevent splashing. The endotracheal tube will then need to be withdrawn by the anesthesia team, while the tip is visualized through the tracheostomy. It should not be totally withdrawn. (The endotracheal tube should be left just superior to the tracheostomy in the event that it needs to be advanced to ventilate the patient). Once the tracheostomy tube is inserted into the trachea it can be connect to the anesthesia circuit and ventilation resumed. A jolly tube (short flexible connector) is helpful to connect the circuit. Placement of the tracheostomy tube is confirmed by the presence of CO_2, normal airway pressures, chest rise and bilateral breath sounds. Direct visualization of the placement can be performed using a fiberoptic bronchoscope. Once placement is confirmed and ventilation is restored, the endotracheal tube can be removed.

Complications of tracheostomy can present immediately. Bleeding from anterior jugular veins and pretracheal soft tissue is usually easily controlled during dissection. Care should be taken to have a dry field prior to entering the trachea, as the use of cautery after entry can cause a fire. The dissection can cause a pneumothorax. This can impair ventilation and if large enough will require chest tube placement. Placing the tracheostomy tube outside of the trachea will cause a false passage to develop. If this occurs, there will be no carbon dioxide on capnography. It can lead to pneumomediastinum with cardiovascular collapse if not noted and corrected. The tracheostomy tube can be occluded with secretions and blood shortly after placement. This can lead to high airway pressures and poor ventilation. Suctioning through the endotracheal tube can relieve this issue. Mechanical obstruction due to the tip of the tracheostomy tube hitting the posterior tracheal wall or due to tracheomalacia. This can be confirmed with fiberoptic bronchoscopy through the tracheostomy. Correction may require use of a different tracheostomy tube, a proximal or distal extra-long tracheostomy or an adjustable tracheostomy tube [5, 6].

Occasionally, patients will present in extremus and require a surgical airway either a tracheostomy or a cricothyrotomy. This may be due to mechanical obstruction of the airway by a foreign object, or swelling due to a mass or infection. In these instances, the procedure is often done with an awake patient and local infiltration of anesthetic with conversion to general anesthesia, once the airway has been secured. The complication rate is higher in these cases compared to elective tracheostomies [7]. Depending on the acuity of the situation, some sedation may be used. Due to the emergent nature of presentations, these procedures can occur outside of the operating suite.

Some patients will present for **awake tracheostomy** due to need to access the upper airway and mouth unhindered by an endotracheal tube or due to a mass lesion preventing routine intubation. Preoperative planning is essential in these cases. Supplemental oxygen is used as needed with care taken to limit risk of fire. The patient should be positioned supine with a shoulder roll. The patient may need to have their head elevated. Local anesthesia is used and can be supplemented with sedation as tolerated by the patient. The surgical steps then follow as above ending with securing the tracheostomy tube and connecting to the anesthesia circuit.

There are various types of tracheostomy tubes. In general, tracheostomy tubes are cuffed or uncuffed, single lumen or with an inner cannula, fenestrated or solid, fixed length or adjustable. Some tracheostomy tubes are designed to connect with the anesthesia circuit directly while others require an inner cannula to attach securely to ventilator tubing. Patients presenting to the operating room with tracheostomy tubes can be induced using the trach. If it is a cuffed tube the cuff should be inflated. If it is uncuffed, expect some leakage around the trach, bagging may be difficult. A cuffed trach will be fine for most procedures. If it interferes with the surgical field, it can be replaced by and endotracheal tube and secured to the chest wall. The endotracheal tube should be inserted into the tracheostomy until the cuff cannot be seen and then inflated. Further advancement of the tube increases the chance of mainstem intubation. Presence of a tracheostomy does not preclude transoral or transnasal intubation unless there is a known obstructing mass or stenosis. The tracheostomy tube can be removed and the patient intubated from above. Care should be taken to ensure the cuff is beyond the tracheostomy to prevent leakage of oxygen and anesthetic gasses.

Tracheostomy Types

Tracheostomy Types Fig. (**3**): Portex #6 Cuffed Tracheostomy Tube and inner cannula. Note tracheostomy tube can connect with ventilator tubing without inner cannula. Fig. (**4**): #10 Metal Jackson Tracheostomy Tube with inner cannula and obturator. Will not connect to ventilator tubing with or without inner cannula. Fig. (**5**): Shiley #6 uncuffed distal XLT Tracheostomy Tube and #6 proximal cuffed XLT Tracheostomy Tube. Shown without inner cannula. Will not connect with ventilator tubing without inner cannula. Fig. (**6**): Custom #6 Single Lumen hyperflex tracheostomy tube with obturator. Images provided by Matthew Kashima, M.D., Johns Hopkins.

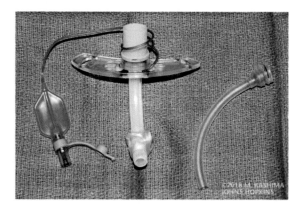

Fig. (3). Portex #6 Cuffed Tracheostomy Tube and inner cannula. Image provided by Matthew Kashima, M.D., Johns Hopkins.

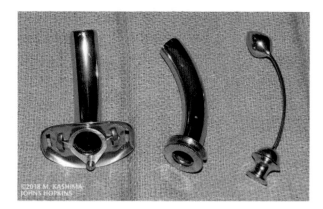

Fig. (4). #10 Metal Jackson Tracheostomy Tube with inner cannula and obturator. Image provided by Matthew Kashima, M.D., Johns Hopkins.

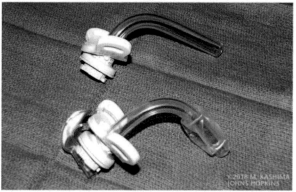

Fig. (5). Shiley #6 uncuffed distal XLT Tracheostomy Tube and #6 proximal cuffed XLTTracheostomyTube. Shown without inner cannula. Image provided by Matthew Kashima, M.D., Johns Hopkins.

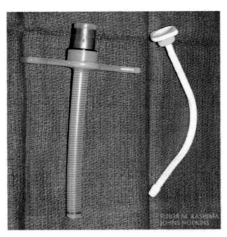

Fig. (6). Custom #6 Single Lumen hyperflex tracheostomy tube with obturator. Image provided by Matthew Kashima, M.D., Johns Hopkins.

LARYNGOLOGY

Laryngeal disorders can be infectious, benign or malignant growths. Laryngeal procedures can be diagnostic therapeutic or both. The majority of these cases last less than 90 minutes, but extended procedures are possible. Discussion of case length prior to induction can help with anesthetic planning. Preoperative preparation is paramount in these cases. The otolaryngologist has seen and examined the patient preoperatively and has visualized the area of concern. Dialog as to the extent and location of the lesion can help with anesthetic planning. Appropriate sizing of the endotracheal tube should be discussed and in certain circumstances, the otolaryngologist may prefer to intubate the patient. This is best accomplished as part of planned course of events rather than a last minute intervention.

Direct laryngoscopy requires deep anesthesia and often muscle relaxation. The patient is usually turned 90 from the anesthesiologist. The endotracheal tube is taped to the lower lip on the left. This allows the right-handed surgeon to most easily instrument the oral cavity. The tube will need to be untaped during the procedure if removal of the tube is needed for exposure. Despite the depth of anesthesia needed, the procedure can be brief and there the surgeon can do is little "closing" that during emergence. Because of the location of the surgery at the glottis, alternate types of ventilation may be needed. Jet ventilation or apneic techniques are often employed during this procedure. Again, close cooperation and communication are required for a successful operation. Care must be taken to maintain oxygen saturation with these techniques. Lasers can be used in these procedures and laser safe tubes should be used if possible. Care must be taken to protect the patient from potential injury from the laser. The eyes need to be covered preferably with a moistened sponge or towel over taped eyes. The face and exposed skin should be covered with moist towels. Personnel in the room should wear laser safe eye protection as indicated by the type of laser employed. The team should be prepared for airway fire and have water on the field as discussed earlier.

Some laryngology cases require that the patient be awake and able to phonate. Patients undergoing vocal cord injections and medializations need to be able to speak. Local anesthetic infiltration and sedation can be used in these cases.

Some surgeons will apply topical anesthetics to the larynx during and at the end of laryngoscopic procedures. This provides local pain control and can assist in hemostasis as well. 4% cocaine is often used due to its analgesic and vasoconstrictive properties. It is absorbed well across mucous membranes. It can have systemic effects such as tachycardia and hypertension. Cocaine can even cause coronary vasospasm, myocardial ischemia and arrhythmias. Anesthesiologist should be made aware if cocaine will be used during the case and notified when it is applied [1].

Professional voice patients (*e.g.* **singers, politicians, actors, teachers,** *etc.*) **merit special considerations.** These professions rely on their voices for their livelihood and are particularly sensitive to anything that might jeopardize their voice. Care should be exercised when obtaining anesthesia consents and setting expectations prior to procedures. Patients should understand that sore throat, hoarseness, vocal breaks, globus sensation, and throat clearing can be expected following intubation. These symptoms generally resolve after 72 hours following short-term intubations. Risks can be minimized by use of laryngeal mask airway (when possible), smaller endotracheal tubes, low cuff pressure, acid reflux prophylaxis, and corticosteroid administration. Despite the vocal professional's concerns regarding the risks of anesthesia, treatment decisions should not deviate significantly from usual anesthesia practice [1, 8, 9].

HEAD AND NECK

Head and Neck anatomy is complex and surgery in this region can involve soft tissue manipulation or resection, intraoperative nerve monitoring, reconstruction (local, region or free tissue transfer) and entry into the aerodigestive tract. Large blood vessels present the risk of significant blood loss. Anesthesia for these cases is driven by the need for meticulous dissection around vital structures. Muscle relaxation is often contraindicated by the need to monitor nerve function.

Parotid surgery. Removal of benign or malignant lesion of the parotid gland is done under general anesthesia. The procedure generally takes from 2-4 hours depending on the size and location of the lesion. The location of the lesion can determine the extent of dissection needed. <u>A posterior superficial lesion</u> may require identification of the main branch of the facial nerve and only one or two divisions. <u>An anterior superior lesion</u> may require identification and dissection of all branches of the facial nerve and a lesion deep to the nerve can require identification and mobilization of all branches of the nerve. Due to the course of the facial nerve through the gland, intraoperative nerve monitoring is frequently done. <u>In order to safely monitor the facial nerve, the dissection needs to be done without muscle paralysis.</u> The face on the side of the lesion is prepped into the surgical field to facilitate observing facial movement. Jaw opening should be assessed for trismus due to the lesion. The endotracheal tube is generally taped to the opposite corner of the mouth. The eye is exposed as well. This can be accomplished by use of a transparent occlusive covering or lightly taping half of the eyelid to ensure closure but not inhibit motion. A smooth emergence without bucking helps to prevent postoperative hematomas [10].

Thyroidectomy can be performed for benign or malignant disease. Large thyroid lesions can distort the airway and make intubation more challenging. Reviewing imaging and discussing the airway with the surgeon is imperative for planning intubation. In order to monitor the recurrent laryngeal nerve, an endotracheal tube with built in electrodes is employed. (*e.g.* NIM TriVantage EMG Endotracheal Tube, Medtronic Xomed Corporation, Figure **7**) The tube has exposed electrodes, which are paced in contact with the vocal folds. Some surgeons prefer to confirm the placement of the electrodes by direct laryngoscopy prior to incision. <u>These tubes are larger diameter than regular endotracheal tubes, so using a tube one size smaller is recommended</u> (*e.g.* #6 NIM tube for women and #7 NIM tube for men). Malignant lesions can affect the recurrent laryngeal nerve causing paralysis, which can narrow the glottic airway. Dissection requires identification and tracing the recurrent laryngeal nerve. At the end of the procedure a smooth emergence lessens the chance of hematoma formation. Attention should be directed to the airway following extubation to assess for vocal fold weakness or paralysis. <u>Stridor indicates a narrowed airway that may require intervention ranging from support to reintubation and placement of a tracheostomy</u> [5].

NIM TriVantage EMG Endotracheal Tube, Medtronic Xomed Corporation

Surgeries for resection of **malignant tumors** of the head and neck region vary according to location and extent of disease. Cases range from minor simple excisions that can be done under local anesthesia to composite resections with large defects requiring free tissue transfer. Removal of the cervical lymph nodes (neck dissections) can include removal of the sternocleidomastoid muscle, internal jugular vein and spinal accessory nerve, radical neck dissection, or any of these structures may be preserved. If the intent is preservation of the spinal accessory nerve, paralysis cannot be used during the neck dissection portion of the procedure to allow for nerve monitoring. Other nerves can be injured during the operation but are not directly monitored. Injury to the vagus nerve can paralysis of the ipsilateral larynx and pharynx as well as loss of sensation at the level of the true vocal fold. This can result in a narrowed airway upon extubation and dysphagia an inability to protect the airway. Injury to the phrenic nerve can affect the diaphragm. A smooth emergence without bucking helps to prevent postoperative hematomas [11].

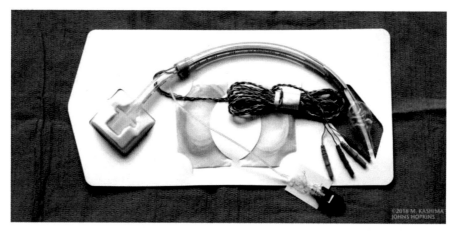

Fig. (7). NIM TriVantage EMG Endotracheal Tube, Medtronic Xomed Corporation. Image provided by Matthew Kashima, M.D., Johns Hopkins.

Laryngectomy and laryngopharyngectomy, removal of the voice box and voice box and portions of the pharynx, will result in complete separation of the airway and alimentary tract. The airway will be part of the surgical field during this procedure and it is often necessary to remove the endotracheal tube at times during the procedure. The surgical team typically does this. Work is done without the patient being intubated. Close communication is important to ensure the patient does not have extensive periods of hypoxia. A smooth emergence without bucking helps to prevent postoperative hematomas.

Free flap reconstructions can add to the length of cases. The donor site is chosen based on surgeon experience, size of defect and type of tissue needed, however, the size of the defect is often not definitively known until the resection is complete. Attention must be paid to the surgical planning to prevent accidental line placement in the donor site, especially for radial forearm donor sites. The surgical team in the preoperative area generally marks these sites, but if there is a question of what is being used for reconstruction, a conversation can prevent a potential complication. Each reconstructive surgeon has a protocol that they want followed regarding timing and dosing of medications (*e.g.* heparin, aspirin), range for hematocrit, and target blood pressures. Most surgeons prefer to avoid vasopressors during the entire case to prevent excessive vasoconstriction of vessels in the free flap that may compromise perfusion and lead to flap failure.

Patients who come to the operating room following a laryngectomy will have permanent stoma. The airway has been permanently separated from the alimentary tract including the mouth, therefore they cannot be masked or given supplemental oxygen *via* the nose or mouth. They can be masked by placing a small mask over the stoma and supplemental oxygen can be given this way too. A mature stoma does not always need a tube in it to maintain patency. Intubating a laryngostome is simply putting a cuffed tube into the opening. The cuff should be visible to prevent mainstem intubation. The tube can be taped or sutured to the chest. Once the patient is breathing at the end of the case, the tube can simply be withdrawn. Obstruction should not occur and there is no chance for aspiration.

OTOLOGY

Otologic surgery varies from minor procedures to large resections. Many of the patients undergoing otologic surgery have hearing deficits in one or both ears, which may impair their ability to communicate verbally during induction and emergence as well as during the case if it is done without general anesthesia. The simplest procedure is Pressure Equalization Tube placement is discussed later. Some procedures are done under sedation and require that the patient be able to communicate with the surgeon during the procedure. Patents must be kept comfortable but too sedated that they become inhibited and move or be unable to reliably answer questions. Adequate use of local anesthesia is important for these cases. Other cases are more extended and will require general anesthesia.

N_2O can be used at the beginning of tympanoplasty procedures but should be discontinued at least 20 minutes prior to placing the graft to prevent gas from dislodging the graft. Paralysis is to be avoided in cases where the facial nerve may be exposed. Facial nerve monitoring is used with electrodes monitoring the orbicularis oris and orbicularis oculi [12].

Many otologic procedures are dressed with a mastoid dressing. These dressings can take five to ten minutes to place on the patient. The dressing is easier to apply if the patient is asleep. Application of the dressing requires some manipulation of the head and can stimulate a patient if they are not in a deep enough plane of anesthesia. As with many Otolaryngologic procedures, smooth emergence is key. In case where the ossicular chain has been reconstructed, smooth emergence prevents dislocation of the prosthesis. Many surgeons want to test the facial nerve during or shortly after emergence to ensure integrity of the facial nerve [12].

Special attention should be paid to control of nausea and emesis. Manipulation of the ear can cause nausea. Use of antacids, antiemetics and steroids can help prevent postoperative nausea and vomiting. Intractable nausea and vomiting in the immediate post-operative setting warrant an evaluation by the operating surgeon [13].

RHINOLOGY

Nasal and sinus procedures can be rather short or prolonged. Extended endoscopic procedures can last for several hours. The patient is generally positioned with the head away from anesthesia. The surgeon is on the right side of the patient. Oral intubation with the tube secured to the left side of the mouth is preferred. The eyes, which are included in the surgical field to be able to assess for orbital injury during the case, should be lubricated. The head is turned slightly toward the surgeon and may be elevated. Local and topical agents are used to help with intraoperative and post-operative pain. Oxymetazoline, epinephrine and cocaine are also used for vasoconstrictive effects. Each of these can have systemic effects too [1]. The patient may have their nose packed at the end of the case to limit postoperative oozing. The packing may be absorbable or may need to be removed in the future. In either case, awareness of the packing including the possibility that it may become dislodged, is important during emergence [12, 14].

Epistaxis can occur as a result of surgical intervention or spontaneously. It is usually minimal but at times can be significant and even life threatening. Intervention can range from direct pressure to open procedures for vessel ligation and embolization. Patients who require posterior nasal packing can have respiratory compromise from the packing directly or from activation of the nasopulmonary reflex. It has been suggested that patients with a history of cardiac or pulmonary disease be admitted to a monitored setting following bilateral posterior nasal packing [14, 15].

At the end of the case, secretions and blood may need to be suctioned from the oral cavity and pharynx prior to extubation. Smooth emergence is important. For many nasal procedures, raw mucosal edges are left that are predisposed to oozing. Clots that have formed at the end of the procedure can be dislodged if the patient is coughing and bucking during emergence. This could cause the need for the patient to be deepened for further intervention.

PEDIATRICS

Providing anesthesia to children requires and understanding of pediatric anatomy and physiology as well as understanding the psychological issues children have coming to the operating room. A skilled anesthesiologist also understands that they must address the concerns and fears of the parents or care givers too. Premedication can be given to help sedate patients prior to coming to the operating room. Oral midazolam (0.5 mg/kg) needs to be given at least 20 minutes before coming to the operating room. Children who are premedicated will often have a delayed emergence at the end of the case particularly for short operations. It is advisable to have at least two people provide anesthesia to children. Depending on the cooperation of the child, a mask induction may be needed before starting an IV. During induction, having two providers allows one person to focus on the airway while the second can be focused on obtaining venous access.

Laryngospasm is the closure of the vocal cords leading to airway obstruction. It presents with lack of airflow in the presence of respiratory effort. Retractions can be seen. Initial attempts at mask ventilation are unsuccessful despite a good mask seal and appropriate positioning. It often occurs during emergence when secretions or instrumentation stimulates the larynx. It is more commonly seen in children. It can lead to hypoxemia. **Treatment** consists of positive pressure airway support. Clearing secretions can prevent further stimulation of the larynx. If the spasm cannot be broken with positive pressure, muscle relaxant (Succinylcholine) can be given to break the spasm [4, 16].

EPIGLOTTITIS

Epiglottitis is an acute infection affecting the supraglottis caused by Haemophilus influenza B as well as other organisms. The epidemiology of epiglottitis has changed over time due to the routine HIB vaccination. A recent review by Shah and Stocks showed a decrease in admissions from 1996 to 2006 overall and specifically among patients 18 and younger. There was an increase in cases of epiglottitis in patients 45 to 64 and in patients over 85. The mortality rate of 0.89% was seen during the study period. The study found patients less than one and older than 85 to be most vulnerable [17].

Children with epiglottitis present with fever, odynophagia, and sore throat. They will often be unable to handle their secretions (drooling) and will be sitting forward on their hands with their mouth open ("**tripod position**"). Their voice may be muffled the "hot potato voice." They may present with hypoxia and stridor indicating airway obstruction. Soft tissue neck x-rays can be taken and can show a swollen epiglottis, the thumbprint sign, in patients with epiglottitis. Some discretion is advised with lateral soft tissue neck films. If the image is rotated the epiglottis can look swollen and lead to an erroneous diagnosis. Adults tend to present with less acuity than young children. Stable patients without signs of airway compromise can have a fiberoptic laryngeal exam performed to assess the airway in the emergency room or on the floor. If the patient is felt to be unstable, securing the airway is paramount. Care should be taken in securing the airway. Preparations should be made to visualize the larynx in a controlled setting where the patient can be intubated or have a surgical airway performed.

A coordinated airway plan should be decided upon between the anesthesiologist and otolaryngologist before any intervention undertaken. Young patients are often taken to the OR before any interventions are performed in order to lessen the agitation of the child which could cause crying and increase airflow. The increased turbulent airflow could cause dynamic airway collapse leading to complete obstruction. If the patient is calm and it is felt to be clinically appropriate, an IV can be started and IV steroids (*e.g.* 0.6 mg/kg of dexamethasone) and antibiotics given. Racemic epinephrine can be given *via* nebulizer. Pulse oximetry, blood pressure cuff and EKG leads can be placed if it will not unduly upset the patient. Prior to arrival in the OR, the anesthesiologist and the otolaryngologist need to discuss the plan to secure the airway including several methods to be employed serially if the first method is unsuccessful. The plan typically includes inhalational induction with direct laryngoscopy with endotracheal intubation followed by rigid bronchoscopy and if this fails, a surgical airway. A variety of ETTs should be available including tubes smaller than the anticipated size based on the patients age and size due to swelling in the airway. Because the obstruction is at the level of supraglottis and glottis, LMA's and positive pressure bagging are usually not able to sustain the airway. Because the supraglottic structures are edematous and erythematous, the normal appearance of the larynx can be considerably distorted. In the most extreme cases, spontaneous ventilation may yield the only hint of the location of the airway by bubbles in secretions [18].

UPPER AIRWAY FOREIGN BODY

Airway foreign bodies present challenges for airway management. Complete acute obstruction of the airway is rarely seen in the hospital setting as these patients either clear the obstruction or expire before presenting to the hospital. The foreign bodies seen in the hospital are more frequently partially obstructing. This allows for some thought and preparation in managing the airway. Knowing the location and type of foreign body can help guide the plan for managing the airway. Plain films of the neck and chest can localize the foreign object. Fiberoptic examination can identify and confirm the location of the object. Care should be taken to avoid converting a partial obstruction to a complete obstruction. Collaboration between the anesthesiologist and otolaryngologist is key for this situation as they will be sharing the airway [19].

Prior to induction, if the clinical situation allows, an albuterol nebulizer can be given to improve ventilation in the setting of airway edema and bronchospasm. Steroids and antibiotics may be given intravenously. Anxiolytics should be given with caution, understanding that sedatives may exacerbate the obstruction. Atropine or glycopyrolate may be given to help reduce secretions [20].

The type of anesthesia for a given case may depend on the location and severity of the obstruction as well as the experience and preference of the surgeon and anesthesiologist. Maintaining spontaneous ventilation may help to sustain ventilation. Positive pressure ventilation may convert a partial obstruction to a complete obstruction. Spontaneous ventilation with negative pressure ventilation may allow for air to get by a partial obstruction. If the foreign object ball valves, it can lead to air trapping and may lead to inability to ventilate or a pneumothorax. Not giving a muscle relaxant makes it possible that the patient may react to stimulation of the airway with bucking and coughing that may move a foreign body deeper into the airway or convert a partial to complete obstruction. The patient's NPO status merits consideration. Rapid sequence induction may be performed in cases where a full stomach is suspected and the stomach needs to be evacuated.

Preparation for multiple methods of securing the airway should be set up prior to bringing the patient into the OR. Various options include MacIntosh and Miller laryngoscope blades, Hollinger and Dedo Laryngoscopes, rigid and flexible bronchoscopes, and tracheostomy sets. If the foreign body is above the glottis preparation for a tracheostomy can be beneficial. If the object is below the glottis a tracheostomy may not be distal to the obstruction and therefore not be beneficial. If the object is high, direct laryngoscopy may allow visualization and removal without intubation. Trying to intubate with a foreign object located above the glottis may result in worsening or even complete obstruction. A tracheal foreign object that is obstructing can be pushed into a mainstem bronchi to allow single lung ventilation if needed and then removed when the patient is more stable [21].

After removal of the foreign body the expectation should be to extubate the patient. The type of object can affect the airway. Organic material may swell leading to injury of the airway. Oils from nuts can cause a local inflammatory response. Hard objects may cause lacerations or puncture the airway with an associated inflammatory response. Swelling needs to be anticipated at extubation and the patient observed for a period of time to ensure reintubation is not needed.

Nasal Foreign Body Removal

Nasal foreign bodies can present to the operating room if they cannot be removed in the Emergency Department or Clinic. These patients, <u>usually young children,</u> can be brought to the operating suite. They are often agitated from prior attempts at removal and may have some nasal bleeding. Care must be taken during induction not to dislodge the foreign object further into the airway where it could be aspirated or swallowed. Communication with the surgeon as to the laterality and location as well as the surgical plan can help inform the anesthetic plan as well. After removal of the object in question, a complete nasal examination should be performed to rule out additional objects presence prior to waking the patient [22].

Pressure Equalization Tube Placement

<u>Pressure equalization tube (myringotomy tube) placement is a common otolaryngologic procedure.</u> In adults it is frequently done in the office with local anesthesia. Young children will not hold still for this to be done in the office and a general anesthetic is needed. The procedure can be very quick taking only a few minutes for an experienced surgeon. A mask anesthetic is often used for this procedure. Care needs to be taken to hold the head still during the procedure to facilitate safe placement of the tubes. Occasionally, the surgeon may request N_2O be used to inflate the middle ear and lift a retracted tympanic membrane allow easier tube placement.

Tonsillectomy

<u>Adenotonsillectomy, removal of the palatine and pharyngeal tonsils, is a commonly performed procedure in children.</u> It is most commonly performed for recurrent/chronic infections, history of peritonsillar abscess or obstructive sleep apnea. It generally takes 30 minutes to perform the procedure. Once general anesthesia is established and the patient intubated, the endotracheal tube should be secured in the midline to the lower lip. This allows for the mouth gag to be placed and hold the endotracheal tube. Care should be exercised to ensure that the ETT is not kinked when the patient is suspended with the mouth gag. Unexpected high airway pressures may indicate that the tube is kinked. Attention to the airway during placement, removal, and manipulation of the mouth gag are important to recognize any inadvertent dislodgment of the endotracheal tube. Blood loss during tonsillectomy is usually less than 50 ml, however, there is a possibility of larger blood loss. The patient's oral cavity and stomach should be suctioned at the end of the procedure to help prevent laryngeal stimulation and possible laryngospasm and postoperative nausea and vomiting. An analysis of respiratory complications following awake *versus* deep extubation in children following adenotonsillectomy

did not see a clinically significant difference in rates [23].

Post tonsillectomy hemorrhage occurs in ~4% of cases. Primary hemorrhage occurs in the first 24 hours and secondary hemorrhage after that. Secondary bleeding usually occurs five to nine days after surgery. No definitive risk factors have been identified for post-tonsil hemorrhage. A small percentage of patients who present with bleeding following tonsillectomy will have an undiagnosed coagulopathy [24]. A small percentage of these patients will need to return to the operating room. Any patient who returns to the OR with bleeding following tonsillectomy should be considered to have a full stomach due to the potential for swallowing blood. A rapid sequence induction should be performed. Suction needs to be available during induction. While most patients will not be bleeding or only slightly oozing on arrival to the OR, active bleeding can start at any time. Clots can be knocked off by a cough or upon mouth opening during laryngoscopy. Patients who are actively bleeding may require direct pressure with a finger or packing during intubation. Once the airway is secured the field is turned to the surgeon who will control the bleeding. The stomach should be evacuated at the start of the case to help ascertain the amount of blood loss and prevent postoperative nausea and emesis.

Deep Neck Infections

Neck infections can be challenging to manage, infections in the neck can cause distortions of anatomy, limit positioning, narrow the oral, pharyngeal and /or glottic airway. Inflammation caused by the infection can lead to trismus inhibiting mouth opening. The airway may need to be secured to facilitate operative drainage of the infection or to protect the airway. IF the patient is stable evaluation should include a contrasted CT scan of the neck. An isolated abscess may be identified. In other cases, no discrete collection may be seen. Many cases are odontogenic.

Ludwig's angina is an infection of the floor of mouth. Due to communication of fascial planes an infection in this area may not present with a discrete abscess but rather with diffuse swelling of the floor of mouth. This results in swelling of the tongue with a firm floor of mouth pushing the tongue posteriorly and affecting the airway. Despite the fact that there is often no discrete abscess, Ludwig's angina requires aggressive treatment with surgical drainage. Retropharyngeal abscesses can narrow the airway and cause muscle spasm making transoral intubation difficult. It can also limit the effectiveness of bagging, LMA and oral airways.

Communication between the anesthesia team and the surgical team is of paramount importance. Discussion of what the sequence of methods used to secure the airway should be had before arriving in the OR if possible. Evaluation of the airway should include physical exam including fiberoptic laryngoscopy if possible as well as review of any imaging available. Transoral intubation, direct or fiberoptic can be entertained if the anatomy is favorable. Transnasal fiberoptic intubation may also be used. Surgical airway may be a last resort or planned if it is deemed the safest way to proceed. Experience of the teams may help inform the method chosen to secure the airway. <u>Swelling and trismus may limit the transoral approach</u>. When the patient is relaxed some trismus may improve allowing for attempts at laryngoscopy. Care should be exercised to prevent inadvertent injury to the upper airway leading to worsening swelling, bleeding or rupture of the abscess into the airway. <u>Preparation for a surgical airway is often done before attempts are made for transoral or transnasal intubation in the event that the airway is lost</u>. The surgical team should have the site prepped and infiltrated with local anesthetic and be gowned with the surgical set up ready [25, 26].

CONCLUSION

Providing anesthesia for Otolaryngology Head and Neck Surgery cases is a demanding and varied practice. It requires communication and preparation on the part of the surgical, anesthesia and nursing teams. The unique location of the surgeries and obstacles to be overcome lends itself to collaboration and creativity to provide the best care for patients.

CONSENT FOR PUBLICATION

Not applicable.

CONFLICT OF INTEREST

The author declares no conflict of interest, financial or otherwise.

ACKNOWLEDGEMENT

Declared none.

REFERENCES

[1]   Lobo E, Pelegrini F, Pusceddu E. Complications in Head and Neck Surgery. 2nd ed. Philadelphia: Mosby 2009; pp. 3-27.
       [http://dx.doi.org/10.1016/B978-141604220-4.50005-5]

[2]   Doyle DJ. Airway anesthesia: theory and practice. Anesthesiol Clin 2015; 33(2): 291-304.
       [http://dx.doi.org/10.1016/j.anclin.2015.02.013] [PMID: 25999003]

[3]   Bruley M. Head and Neck Surgical Fires in Eisele,D, Smith,R Complications in Head and Neck Surgery. 2nd ed. Philadelphia: Mosby 2009; pp. 145-60.
       [http://dx.doi.org/10.1016/B978-141604220-4.50016-X]

[4]   Bynoe T, Fleisher L. Anesthetic Emergencies in Emergencies of the Head and Neck Eisele D and McQuone S. St. Louis: Mosby 2000; pp. 97-109.

[5]   Myers E. Thyroidectomy in Operative Otolaryngology Head and Neck Surgery. Philadelphia: W.B. Saunders Company 1997; pp. 536-51.

[6]   Myers E. Tracheostomy in Operative Otolaryngology Head and Neck Surgery. Philadelphia: W.B. Saunders Company 1997; pp. 575-85.

[7]   Fang CH, Friedman R, White PE, Mady LJ, Kalyoussef E. Emergent Awake Tracheostomy- The Five-Year Experience at an Urban Tertiary Care Center. Laryngoscope 2015. E published ahead of print.

[8]   Meacham RK, Schindler J. Anesthesia care for the professional singer. Anesthesiol Clin 2015; 33(2): 347-56.
        [http://dx.doi.org/10.1016/j.anclin.2015.02.012] [PMID: 25999007]

[9]   Pacheco-Lopez PC, Berkow LC, Hillel AT, Akst LM. Complications of airway management. Respir Care 2014; 59(6): 1006-19.
        [http://dx.doi.org/10.4187/respcare.02884] [PMID: 24891204]

[10]   Johnson J. Parotid in Operative Otolaryngology Head and Neck Surgery. Philadelphia: W.B. Saunders Company 1997; pp. 504-18.

[11]   Koch W. Complications of Surgery of the Neck in Complications in Head and Neck Surgery. 2nd ed. Philadelphia: Mosby 2009; pp. 439-65.
        [http://dx.doi.org/10.1016/B978-141604220-4.50040-7]

[12]   Ragan B. Anesthesia for Otorhinolaryngologic (Ear, Nose, and Throat) Surgery in Anesthesiology. 2nd ed. New York: McGraw Hill 2012; pp. 1226-47.

[13]   Hoffman RA. Complications of Tympanomastoidectomy in Complications in Head and Neck Surgery. 2nd ed. Philadelphia: Mosby 2009; pp. 725-38.
        [http://dx.doi.org/10.1016/B978-141604220-4.50059-6]

[14]   Eibling DE. Epistaxis in Operative Otolaryngology Head and Neck Surgery. Philadelphia: W.B. Saunders Company 1997; pp. 2-20.

[15]   Jackman AH, Fried MP. Complications of nasal Surgery and Epistaxis management in Complications in Head and Neck Surgery. 2nd ed. Philadelphia: Mosby 2009; pp. 531-41.
        [http://dx.doi.org/10.1016/B978-141604220-4.50045-6]

[16]   Ow TJ, Parikh SR. Complications of Tonsillectomy and Adenoidectomy in Complications in Head and Neck Surgery. 2nd ed. Philadelphia: Mosby 2009; pp. 313-29.
        [http://dx.doi.org/10.1016/B978-141604220-4.50032-8]

[17]   Shah RK, Stocks C. Epiglottitis in the United States: national trends, variances, prognosis, and management. Laryngoscope 2010; 120(6): 1256-62.
        [PMID: 20513048]

[18]   Soder C. Airway Management of a Child with Epiglottitis in Management of the Difficult and Failed Airway. New York: McGraw Hill Medical 2008; pp. 389-93.

[19]   Fidkowski CW, Zheng H, Firth PG. The anesthetic considerations of tracheobronchial foreign bodies in children: a literature review of 12,979 cases. Anesth Analg 2010; 111(4): 1016-25.
        [PMID: 20802055]

[20]   Zur KB, Litman RS. Pediatric airway foreign body retrieval: surgical and anesthetic perspectives. Paediatr Anaesth 2009; 19 (Suppl. 1): 109-17.
        [http://dx.doi.org/10.1111/j.1460-9592.2009.03006.x] [PMID: 19572850]

[21]   Huchton D, Marsh B. Foreign Bodies in the Upper Aerodigestive Tract in in Emergencies of the Head and Neck Eisele D and McQuone S. St. Louis: Mosby 2000; pp. 156-67.

[22]   Cullen MM, Leopold DA. Nasal Emergencies in Emergencies of the Head and Neck Eisele, D and McQuone, S. St. Louis: Mosby 2000; pp. 239-62.

[23]   Baijal RG, Bidani SA, Minard CG, Watcha MF. Perioperative complications following awake and

deep extubation in children undergoing adenotonsillectomy. Pediatric Anesthesia 2015; 25: 392-9.
[http://dx.doi.org/10.1111/pan.12561]

[24]   Sun GH, Harmych BM, Dickson JM, Gonzalez del Rey JA, Myer CM III, Greinwald JH Jr.
        Characteristics of children diagnosed as having coagulopathies following posttonsillectomy bleeding.
        Arch Otolaryngol Head Neck Surg 2011; 137(1): 65-8.
        [http://dx.doi.org/10.1001/archoto.2010.227] [PMID: 21242549]

[25]   MacQuarrie K, Kirkpatrick D. Airway Management in a Patient with a Retropharyngeal Abscess in
        Management of the Difficult and Failed Airway. New York: McGraw Hill Medical 2008.

[26]   McQuone S. Neck Emergencies in Complications in Head and Neck Surgery. 2nd ed. Philadelphia:
        Mosby 2000; pp. 279-99.

CHAPTER 2

Thoracic Anesthesia

Chandrika R. Garner, Adair Q. Locke and **Thomas F. Slaughter**[*]

Wake Forest School of Medicine, Winston Salem, North Carolina, USA

Abstract: Given a higher prevalence of smoking, pulmonary and cardiovascular disease, and in many cases carcinoma, thoracic surgical patients experience a higher risk for perioperative morbidity and mortality than that of broader surgical populations. Careful preoperative assessment of functional status and a focus on optimizing preexisting conditions prove critical to successful surgical outcomes. As open thoracotomies decline in number, minimally invasive surgeries – including video assisted thoracoscopy (VAT) and robotic surgical approaches pose new challenges for intraoperative anesthetic management. Although double lumen endotracheal tubes remain the most common approach to lung isolation, an array of newer endobronchial blockers provide opportunities to facilitate surgery in patients with difficult airways as well as those requiring lobar isolation to tolerate surgical resection. Surgery of the esophagus and trachea continue to pose enormous challenges to both our intraoperative management and postoperative care. In thoracic surgery, perhaps more so than any other field, there is no doubt that anesthetic interventions in the preoperative, intraoperative, and postoperative settings directly impact patient survival and recovery. Evolving surgical techniques – particularly the move toward less invasive surgery – will challenge our current dogma pertaining to anesthetic management of the thoracic surgical patient – necessitating outcomes based research to further reduce adverse perioperative outcomes and enhance surgical recovery.

Keywords: Bronchial Blocker, Bronchoscopy, Double Lumen Tube, Esophagectomy, Hypoxemia, Lung Cancer, Mediastinoscopy, Non-small Cell Lung Cancer, One Lung Ventilation, Paravertebral Block, Small Cell Lung Cancer, Spirometry, Thoracotomy, Thoracic Anesthesia, Thoracic Epidural, Tracheal Resection, Tracheal Stenosis, Univent, VAT's.

INTRODUCTION

As a population, thoracic surgical patients experience at least moderate risk for perioperative morbidity and mortality. In many cases, these patients undergo pulmonary resections for cancer with underlying lung disease due to smoking and

---

[*] **Corresponding author Thomas F. Slaughter:** Wake Forest School of Medicine, Winston Salem, North Carolina, USA; Tel: (336) 758-5000; E-mail: tslaught@wakehealth.edu

Amballur D. John (Ed.)

other comorbidities. Patients undergoing thoracic surgery experience post-operative pulmonary and cardiac complications at rates exceeding that of the general surgical population. In addition to benefits afforded by any preoperative evaluation, this assessment serves 2 major purposes before thoracic surgery. **First**, a directed history and physical examination with targeted laboratory testing afford an opportunity to identify patients at increased risk for postoperative morbidity and mortality such that resources may be directed to mitigate risk. A **secondary goal** would be to identify patients most likely to require mechanical ventilatory support in the postoperative period – at least short term [1, 2]. In the case of most forms of lung cancer, mortality rates in the absence of surgery prove so dismal as to encourage fairly liberal criteria when assessing suitability for pulmonary resection. Increasing use of minimally invasive surgical procedures, lung sparing surgery, and postoperative pain management (including thoracic epidural analgesia) have extended the population eligible for surgery [3]. However, both patient and surgical team should be aware of the risks as well as potential for impaired quality of life after surgery. Not infrequently, surgical plans change on entry to the chest. A minimally invasive wedge resection may progress to pneumonectomy to offer the best chance for a cure. An understanding of the patient's underlying medical conditions – and ventilatory reserve in particular–proves crucial to team decisions about the course of action offering the greatest chance for recovery and a meaningful quality of life [4].

PREOPERATIVE CONSIDERATIONS IN THE PATIENT WITH LUNG CANCER

Given that a majority of patients undergoing thoracic surgical procedures will do so for lung cancer consideration of these diseases and underlying anesthetic concerns merit discussion. **In the U.S., lung cancer remains the leading cause of cancer related deaths exceeding that of breast, prostate, and colorectal cancers combined.** Cigarette smoking has been implicated in 90% of lung cancers with additional contributions by a number of genetic and environmental factors including exposure to asbestos, radon, and industrial carcinogens [5 - 10]. Although primary lung cancer may be categorized into more than 5 histologic categories, **for purposes of staging and treatment bronchogenic carcinoma is categorized as either: 1) small cell lung cancer (SCLC) or 2) non-small cell lung cancer (NSCLC)** [11 - 14] (Table **1**).

In most cases, micrometastatic disease is present at the time of diagnosis of SCLC, meaning that most often this disease process does not prove amenable to surgical resection. In contrast, survival in NSCLC proves unlikely without surgical resection of the primary tumor [15 - 17]. So, the **focus of the surgical preoperative assessment is 1)** to determine whether the primary tumor is resectable; and **2)** to determine whether the patient is likely to tolerate the planned procedure with acceptable perioperative morbidity and mortality.

Histologic Categories of Lung Cancer

Table 1. Histologic Categories of Lung Cancer.

Histologic Category	Incidence	Source	Characteristics
Squamous cell carcinoma	20%	Bronchial epithelium	Centrally located Local spread
Adenocarcinoma	35-40%	Mucus glands	Peripheral location Early metastasis
Large cell carcinoma	3-5%	Heterogeneous	Peripheral location Early metastasis
Carcinoma unspecified	20-25%	Undifferentiated	Aggressive course
Small cell carcinoma	10-15%	Bronchial	Centrally located Early metastasis

Anesthetic considerations specific to any lung cancer include: 1) direct localized effects from the primary tumor (*i.e.* tracheal deviation, mediastinal or pleural extension, abscess formation, pleural effusion); **2)** potential for mestastases (*i.e.* brain, liver, bone); **3)** toxicity resulting from prior chemotherapy (*i.e.* doxorubicin [cardiac], cisplatin [renal], bleomycin [pulmonary]; and **4)** paraneoplastic syndromes (*i.e.* hypercalcemia, Cushing's syndrome, syndrome of inappropriate antidiuretic hormone [SIADH], Lambert-Eaton syndrome [1, 2, 18].

Pulmonary Function Testing

Pulmonary Function Testing Suggestive of Increased Postoperative Morbidity

All thoracic surgical patients with underlying lung disease require preoperative assessment by spirometry. Numerous measures derived from spirometry – including forced vital capacity (**FVC**), forced expiratory volume in 1 sec (**FEV1**), maximal voluntary ventilation (**MVV**), and residual volume/total lung capacity (**RV/TLC**) – have been associated with adverse outcomes after surgery and pulmonary resection specifically [19 - 22] (Table **2**). A vital capacity (VC) 3-fold greater than tidal volume is considered necessary to generate an effective cough. Moreover, **MVV** less than 50% predicted has been associated with poor postoperative outcomes. Patients in otherwise good health with an FEV1 exceeding 2L are considered at low risk for either lobectomy or pneumonectomy. The most predictive spirometric test for postoperative respiratory complications may be the estimated postoperative FEV1%. Estimated postoperative FEV1% may be derived from the preoperative FEV1 after adjustment for the amount of lung to be resected – as depicted below.

Table 2. Pulmonary Function Testing Suggestive of Increased Postoperative Morbidity.

• Estimated postoperative FEV1% < 40%
• Estimated postoperative DLCO < 40%
• Maximal oxygen consumption (VO2max) < 10 ml/kg/min
• Forced vital capacity (FVC) < 50% predicted
• Forced expiratory volume in 1 sec (FEV1) < 2L
• FEV1/ FVC < 50%
• Maximum voluntary ventilation (MVV) < 50% predicted
• Residual volume/ total lung capacity > 50%
• Carbon monoxide diffusing capacity (DLCO) < 50% predicted
• Arterial carbon dioxide (PaCO2) > 45 mm Hg

Estimated Postoperative FEV1% = Preoperative FEV1 x (1 – fraction lung tissue resected/100)

An estimated postoperative FEV1% exceeding 40% suggests minimal risk for postoperative complications. In contrast, potential for respiratory complications increases with declining postoperative estimates for FEV1%. Patients with an estimated FEV1% < 30% after pulmonary resection are considered at high risk for morbidity and mortality and likely to require postoperative mechanical ventilation immediately after surgery [19 - 22]. Although no single test provides an all-encompassing risk assessment before thoracic surgery, the estimated postoperative FEV1% has been validated as a reasonable measure to assess potential for pulmonary morbidity and the need for postoperative mechanical ventilatory support. Similarly, diffusing capacity of carbon monoxide **(DLCO)** provides a measure of overall pulmonary gas exchange across the vascular bed, and the estimated postoperative DLCO proves a useful secondary assessment for morbidity and mortality after thoracic surgery [19]. The estimated DLCO proves relatively independent of estimated postoperative FEV1% and values less than 40% have been associated with both pulmonary and cardiac complications [23]. In patients with borderline risk as estimated by spirometry, ventilation/ perfusion scanning (V/Q scintigraphy) may provide a more refined estimate of postoperative residual lung function. Cardiopulmonary testing may prove useful in this setting as well [24]. Patients with a maximal oxygen uptake (VO2) <10 ml/kg/min experience high mortality rates after pulmonary resection. Similar non-invasive assessments of exercise capacity include the ability to walk greater than

300 meters in 6 minutes or the ability to climb 3 flights of stairs continuously [22]. Surprisingly, arterial blood gas values prove to be less reliable measures for assessing perioperative risk. Arterial oxygenation may be affected by exacerbation of the patient's underlying pulmonary disease before surgery; and, resection of the affected lung segments may lead to improved oxygenation postoperatively. Although hypercarbia proves a useful marker for increased perioperative risk, elevations in pCO_2 occur late in the disease process. Patients with impaired exercise capacity or suspicion of right or left ventricular dysfunction may benefit from echocardiographic evaluation to assess right and left ventricular function and to ensure medical optimization before surgery [25].

Preoperative Steps to Mitigate Perioperative Risks

Preoperative Optimization

Perioperative morbidity and mortality (respiratory and cardiac specifically) remain high in association with thoracic surgery and thoracotomy in particular. Efforts to mitigate preoperative risk factors will reduce adverse outcomes [26 - 29] (Table **3**). Smoking proves prevalent in the population of patients undergoing thoracic surgery and directly impacts both respiratory and cardiac morbidity. **Smoking** reduces mucociliary transport leading to increased secretions as well as inflammation and irritability of airways. Reductions in sputum production and improved spirometry measures occur within 2-3 months of discontinuing tobacco exposure. There are short term benefits to discontinuation of smoking as well with reductions in carboxyhemoglobin noted within 48 hrs [30, 31]. Acute respiratory infection – or exacerbation of chronic infections – should be treated with antibiotics before surgery [31]. In contrast, prophylactic antibiotics to suppress respiratory pathogens has not proved beneficial. Reactive airways disease (as reflected by wheezing before surgery) should be addressed as well. Mainstay **therapies for chronic obstructive pulmonary disease (COPD)** remain inhaled sympathomimetics and phosphodiesterase inhibitors. Beta 2-adrenergic agonists (*i.e.* albuterol, bitolterol, pirbuterol, levalbuterol, terbutaline) promote relaxation of airway smooth muscle and may be administered by multi-dose inhaler or nebulizer. Beta 2 agonists produce fewer cardiovascular effects than mixed adrenergic agents. Administration may occur *via* aerosolized nebulization *via* face mask or multi-dose inhalers. Administration by nebulizer eliminates variability in dosing associated with self-administered multi-dose inhalers. Anticholinergic agents, such as ipratropium bromide, reduce mucus secretions and inhibit vagally mediated bronchospasm. Most often, anticholinergic agents are administered in concert with beta 2-adrenergic agents. Potential for toxicity and a narrow therapeutic window have diminished the role for phosphodiesterase inhibitors (*i.e.* theophylline) in treatment of COPD.

Theophylline continues to be used in patients with sleep related breathing disorders and benefits patients by inducing bronchodilation and improving diaphragmatic function. Theophylline may possess anti-inflammatory effects as well. Empiric antibiotic therapy has no role in treatment of patients with chronic respiratory disease; however, acute exacerbations characterized by increased (or purulent sputum) may benefit from a short course of broad spectrum antibiotic therapy. A small subset of patients with COPD benefit from inhaled corticosteroid therapy; and, corticosteroids may prove beneficial for acute exacerbations as well. Supplemental oxygen may be indicated for arterial oxygen saturations less than 90%. Steroid therapy may prove beneficial in a subset of patients – most often those having benefitted from steroid therapy in the past. Steroids may be administered in inhaled form, parenterally, or orally. Steroids reduce mucosal inflammation and edema but prove of limited value for acute exacerbations of bronchospasm. A beneficial response to steroids accrues over a period of days to weeks. Many patients benefit from efforts to mobilize and eliminate respiratory secretions [32, 33]. Hydration *via* humidification of oxygen in combination with expectorants and mucolytic drugs (*i.e.* acetylcysteine) facilitate clearance of viscous secretions. Patient instruction in use of incentive spirometry, deep breathing, coughing, and postural drainage prove beneficial for both pre- and postoperative management [26]. Finally, every effort should be made to ensure that the patient's cardiovascular status has been optimized preoperatively [24]. Patients with pulmonary hypertension and/ or right heart failure may benefit from additional medical therapy, revascularization, or oxygen supplementation.

Table 3. Preoperative Steps to Mitigate Perioperative Risks.

• Smoking cessation
• Medical therapy to alleviate acute bronchospasm
• Antibiotic treatment of acute respiratory infections
• Steroid therapy
• Incentive spirometry
• Exercise therapy and improved nutrition
• Ensure optimization of cardiac status

INTRAOPERATIVE MONITORING

In addition to American Society of Anesthesiologists (ASA) recommended standard monitoring for patients undergoing general anesthesia, additional invasive monitoring may be indicated for thoracic and/or mediastinal surgical procedures. The patient's underlying medical condition and planned extent of the surgical procedure will dictate specific monitoring needs. In most planned intrathoracic or mediastinal procedures, arterial catheterization for continuous measurement of arterial blood pressure proves advisable [1, 22]. Potential for pneumothorax as well as vascular injury or obstruction to venous return poses risks for sudden hypotension. In addition, arterial cannulation provides an opportunity for assessment of arterial oxygenation and hematocrit during and after one-lung ventilation. Hypoxemia during one-lung ventilation remains common, and the ability to assess arterial oxygenation offers greater precision in management than simply following SpO_2 using pulse oximetry. Most often the arterial catheter may be placed after anesthetic induction to minimize patient discomfort. A common site for cannulation would be the radial artery given relatively low risk for ischemic injury. The dependent arm offers greater stability during patient positioning; however, many providers preferentially select the non-dominant hand in the unlikely event of a vascular or neurologic injury. In the case of mediastinoscopy, cannulation of the right radial artery provides a means to monitor for innominate artery compression by the mediastinoscope [34 - 36]. The pulse oximeter may be used in a similar manner with preferential cannulation of the left radial artery to ensure continuous access to accurate measures of systemic arterial pressure.

With the exception of pneumonectomy or reoperative thoracic surgery, central venous or pulmonary artery catheterization rarely will prove necessary in settings of thoracic or mediastinal surgery. The lateral decubitus position, one-lung ventilation, and PEEP may impose unpredictable changes to both central venous and pulmonary artery pressures – making these forms of monitoring unreliable. Central venous lines would more commonly be placed to provide venous access for fluid or blood administration in the event of excessive bleeding – as might occur with vascular injury in a minimally invasive or robotic thoracic pulmonary resection [37]. In addition, anticipated need for infusion of inotropic or vasoactive drugs intraoperatively favors placement of a central line as well [38]. Historically, pulmonary artery catheterization was used in cases of planned pneumonectomy as well as for monitoring of patients with pulmonary hypertension. Given advances in the medical management of pulmonary hypertension, and the previously discussed potential for one-lung ventilation to impair measures of central venous and pulmonary artery pressures, the potential for pulmonary artery catheterization to inform perioperative management for pulmonary resection proves limited. In most cases, the risks of pulmonary artery catheterization may exceed potential benefits. Should central venous or pulmonary artery catheterization be desired, placement of the line on the non-dependent (*i.e.* surgical) side will reduce potential for bilateral pneumothoraces. In patients with severe pulmonary hypertension or right heart failure, the more useful intraoperative monitor may be **transesophageal echocardiography (TEE)** [39]. TEE provides real-time assessment of right and left ventricular function as well as ventricular filling volumes. Changes in wall motion may indicate acute ischemia. Fairly accurate estimates of right ventricular and pulmonary artery pressures may be ascertained by hemodynamic calculations. The TEE probe should be placed after anesthetic induction but preceding positioning in the lateral decubitus position. Manipulation of the probe poses risk for movement of an endobronchial tube or blocker with potential for loss of lung isolation in the lateral position. However, fiberoptic bronchoscopy may be used to reposition the tube or blocker should this occur. Limiting manipulation of the TEE probe after positioning for one-lung ventilation generally proves advisable.

METHODS OF SECURING ONE LUNG VENTILATION

Indications for One Lung Ventilation (OLV)

There are multiple indications for one lung ventilation; both surgical and non-surgical indications for lung isolation exist. **Non-surgical indications** include hemoptysis, infection with concern for contamination of non-infected lung, differential compliance between lungs, bronchopleural fistula, and tracheal or bronchial injuries. **Surgical indications** for one lung ventilation include lung transplantation, minimally invasive (robotic or video-assisted) thoracic surgeries, thoracic procedures *via* thoracotomy, esophageal surgery, surgery on the thoracic aorta, anterior approaches to the thoracic spine, anterior mediastinal procedures, and minimally invasive cardiac procedures (Table **4**).

Indications for Lung Isolation (One Lung Ventilation)

Table 4. Indications for Lung Isolation (One Lung Ventilation).

• Unilateral lung isolation to prevent cross-contamination
o Massive bleeding
o Infection (*i.e.* pus)
• Minimally invasive thoracic surgery
o Video assisted thoracoscopy (VATS)
o Robotic thoracoscopy
• Air leak compromising ventilation
o Bronchopleural fistula
o Traumatic disruption of tracheobronchial tree
o Unilateral bulla
• Lung transplantation
• Unilateral bronchopulmonary lavage

(Table 4) cont.....

• Hypoxemia due to unilateral lung disease
• Surgical exposure (relative)
o Pulmonary resections
o Esophagectomy
o Thoracic aortic aneurysm repair
o Anterior thoracic spine procedures
o Minimally invasive cardiac surgery

Endobronchial Double Lumen Tubes

Endobronchial double lumen tubes (DLTs) remain the most common method for implementing one lung ventilation. There are many advantages of DLTs, including the ability to isolate collapse or ventilation of each lung, the ability to suction each lung, and relative ease of placement. DLTs are commercially available with the bronchial lumen extending into either the right or left mainstem bronchus. **Left sided double lumen tubes** prove appropriate for most procedures that require lung isolation. Bilateral sequential orthotopic lung transplantation may be performed with a left sided double lumen tube. As long as the surgeon is aware of the presence of the bronchial lumen in the left bronchus, left pneumonectomy is not an absolute contraindication to a left sided DLT. Left bronchial sleeve resections and resections of exophytic lesions involving the left bronchus are contraindications for placement of a left sided DLT. **Right sided DLTs** can prove more challenging to properly position due to variable take off of the right upper lobe. The bronchial lumen of the right sided double lumen tube has an additional opening to ensure ventilation of the right upper lobe necessitating careful positioning by fiberoptic bronchoscopy (Fig. **1**).

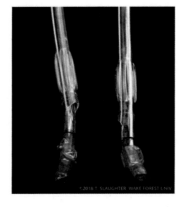

Fig. (1). Right and left endobronchial (double lumen endotracheal) tubes. Image provided by Thomas F. Slaughter, M.D., Wake Forest University.

Sizing of double lumen tubes may be based on CT imaging to ensure adequate tracheal and bronchial diameters. However, a general guideline would be to select a 39Fr DLT for an average sized male, 41Fr for a larger male, 37Fr for an average sized female, and 35 Fr for a small female (Tables **5** and **6**).

Table 5. Simplified Approach to Endobronchial Tube Size Selection.

Patient Demographic	Endobronchial Tube Size (Fr)
Average Female	35
Tall Female	37
Average Male	39
Tall Male	41

Table 6. Comparative external diameters of endotracheal tubes used for one lung ventilation.

SLT ID/ OD (mm)	Univent ID/ OD (mm)	EBT OD (Fr/mm)
10 / 13.5	8.0 / 13.5	41 / 13.7
		39 / 13.0
9.0 / 12.1		37 / 12.3
8.5 / 11.4		35 / 11.7

Placement of DLTs is facilitated by intubation with a Macintosh laryngoscope blade as it provides a larger oropharyngeal aperture for placement of the DLT. The size of even smaller adult DLTs far exceeds that of commonly employed single lumen endotracheal tubes. Once the blue bronchial cuff is placed through the vocal cords, the DLT is rotated to direct the bronchial cuff to the appropriate side. The DLT is advanced until the clear tracheal cuff is below the vocal cords and resistance is encountered. Removing the stylet prior to advancing the DLT is recommended by some to decrease risk for airway injury. The advantage of keeping the stylet in place during placement of the DLT is that rigidity of the tube with stylet in place may increase likelihood of proper positioning. Should resistance occur during insertion, repositioning or resizing of the DLT may be necessary. Once the stylet is removed, the DLT is advanced until encountering resistance. The tracheal cuff is then inflated and the adapter attached to begin ventilation. **Fiberoptic bronchoscopy must be performed to ensure optimal placement of the DLT**. The technique of sequential clamping, manual ventilation, and auscultation to confirm placement has not proved as accurate as fiberoptic bronchosopy. A simple algorithm for evaluating DLT placement by fiberoptic bronchoscopy is to begin by placing the fiberoptic bronchscope down the tracheal lumen (Fig. **2**). If carina is visualized, the bronchoscope is advanced to the bronchus not occupied by the bronchial cuff. The right bronchus will have a variable length and then will split into the right upper lobe (RUL) takeoff and the bronchus intermedius. The right upper lobe has a characteristic trifurcation which assists with confirmation of proper placement. The left mainstem bronchus is longer than the right mainstream bronchus with distal bifurcation to upper and lower lobes.

Additional landmarks useful in confirming placement of the DLT include the anterior tracheal rings and the posterior appearance of muscular striae. This proves particularly helpful when orientation of the bronchoscope has been altered or when pathological changes alter the normal anatomy.

Once the bronchial lumen is confirmed to be in the appropriate position, the next step is to insert the bronchoscope down the bronchial lumen to ensure that distal bronchial branches remain unobstructed. With a right sided DLT, one must ensure that the right upper lobe takeoff is ventilated through the opening in the bronchial lumen.

Standard Fiberoptic Bronchoscopy Images

If the carina cannot be visualized with the bronchoscope in the tracheal lumen, the DLT is either: **1)** too deep on the correct side, or **2)** in the incorrect bronchus. With the bronchoscope in the tracheal lumen, the DLT should be withdrawn slowly. If the DLT was in the correct bronchus – but too deep – the carina will appear. Subsequent visualization of the bronchial lumen allows for confirmation of appropriate bronchial tube positioning. If withdrawal of the DLT with the bronchoscope in the tracheal lumen does not bring the carina into view, the bronchial lumen likely was placed down the unintended bronchus. In this case, the carina will be viewed by placing the bronchoscope down the bronchial lumen of the DLT. In order to avoid damage to the bronchoscope, it should be withdrawn slightly before inserting the DLT further to avoid distortion and damage to the fiberoptic bronchoscope. With a right sided DLT, often no additional manipulation is needed to get the bronchial lumen into the right mainstem bronchus. With a left sided DLT, turning the patient's head to the right may facilitate placement. With the bronchoscope in the tracheal lumen, the bronchial cuff is inflated with 2-3 ml of air. A thin rim of blue cuff will be visualized (Fig. **2A**). The appropriate side of the adapter may then be clamped and the suction port opened to allow for one lung ventilation. Application of continuous suction to the open non-dependent lung may facilitate collapse of the operative lung. After positioning of the patient, bronchoscopy should be repeated to ensure that the DLT has not been displaced rostrally.

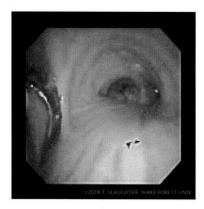

Fig. (2A). Left sided endobronchial (double lumen) tube viewed by fiberoptic bronchoscopy through the tracheal lumen just above the carina. Image provided by Thomas F. Slaughter, M.D., Wake Forest University.

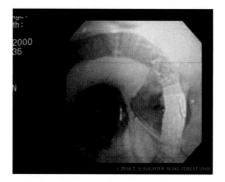

Fig. (2B). Left sided endobronchial tube viewed by fiberoptic bronchoscopy from the endobronchial lumen just above the carina. Image provided by Thomas F. Slaughter, M.D., Wake Forest University.

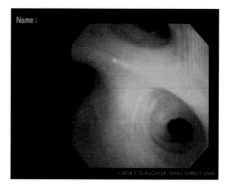

Fig. (2C). Left endobronchial double lumen tube view of right upper lobe by fiberoptic bronchoscopy through the tracheal lumen. Image provided by Thomas F. Slaughter, M.D., Wake Forest University

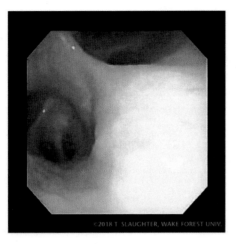

Fig. (2D). Left endobronchial double lumen tube view of left distal bronchus through the bronchial lumen. Image provided by Thomas F. Slaughter, M.D., Wake Forest University.

A single dose of dexamethasone 8-10 mg IV at anesthetic induction may prove beneficial by reducing risk for postoperative nausea and vomiting as well as airway edema. **At the conclusion of surgery**, extubation may be facilitated by elevating the head of the bed. If the patient is to remain intubated at the conclusion of surgery, exchanging the DLT for a single lumen endotracheal tube will decrease airway resistance, improve patient comfort, and facilitate airway suctioning and bronchoscopy if needed.

Univent Tube

The **Univent tube** (Fuji Systems; Tokyo, Japan) is a large single lumen endotracheal tube with a side channel containing a bronchial blocker. The blocker extends 8-10 cm beyond the tip of the tube to allow for passage into the appropriate bronchus (Fig. **3**). The bronchial blocker has a bifurcated proximal end with a pilot cuff to allow for inflation of the blocker balloon and a shaft to allow steering of the blocker's distal tip into the appropriate bronchus. Univent tubes may provide a smaller outer diameter than some DLTs, but remain larger than single lumen tubes with comparable internal diameters. The Univent tube is sized by internal diameter. Prior to placing the Univent tube, the operator must remove two wire stylets present with the shipping package. As with any device, it is prudent to test the cuffs and lubricate the exterior of the endotracheal tube. The blocker must then be withdrawn into the tube before intubation. The Univent blocker balloon is oval shaped as the channel containing the blocker causes increased bulk in the anterior/posterior axis. The <u>Univent tube is placed similarly to other single lumen endotracheal tubes except that the channel should be facing anteriorly to align with the glottic opening</u>. Once past the vocal cords, the tube may be rotated such that the blocker is directed towards the bronchus to be occluded. A bronchoscope will be used to confirm blocker placement in the appropriate bronchus. Under direct visualization, the blocker is inflated with 5-8 ml of air to occlude the bronchus for lung isolation. There should be enough room between the end of the blocker cuff and carina to prevent herniation of the blocker balloon into the trachea. Should the blocker herniate into the trachea peak airway pressures may increase with impaired ability to ventilate the patient. Simply removing air from the blocker cuff should resolve this issue until the blocker can repositioned with fiberoptic bronchoscopy. If needed, the blocker may be used to isolate the bronchus intermedius or one of the left side lobes. In these settings, less air will be needed in the blocker balloon to achieve a seal. Blocking the right mainstem bronchus with a Univent tube may prove challenging given potential for anatomical variations in the right upper lobe orifice. In some cases, the right upper lobe may be excluded partially despite blockade of the remainder of the right lung.

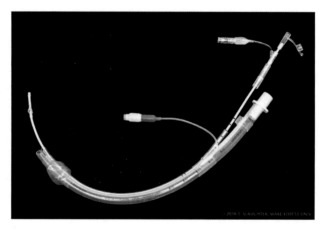

Fig. (3). Univent Tube (Fuji Systems; Tokyo, Japan). Image provided by Thomas F. Slaughter, M.D., Wake Forest University.

In some cases, (*i.e.* difficult airway, airway edema) the Univent tube may be retained to facilitate mechanical ventilation postoperatively. Prior to departure from the OR, the blocker should be withdrawn fully into the starting position. A flange on the exterior of the tube allows for "locking" the blocker into place. Efforts to label the blocker prove important to prevent staff from misidentifying as a feeding tube. Additional tape may be applied to decrease potential for the blocker to be inadvertently inserted during patient positioning in the intensive care unit. Some providers report cutting the pilot cuff to the blocker balloon to eliminate potential for accidental inflation of the blocker within the, Univent tube postoperatively.

Bronchial Blockers

A single lumen endotracheal tube with a bronchial blocker provides another option for achieving one lung ventilation. Bronchial blockers prove particularly useful in patients with difficult airways as well as those expected to remain intubated postoperatively. Several bronchial blockers are available, but basic principles of placement apply to all. Intubation with a standard single lumen endotracheal tube first must be accomplished. Prior to insertion blockers must be inspected, cuffs tested for patency, and the blocker lubricated. Placement is guided by fiberoptic bronchscopy. Blockers have varying steering methods for placement. If placement of the blocker on the left side proves challenging two tips may help. The **first** is to turn the patient's head to the left. The **second** is to use the FOB to place the ETT in the left mainstream bronchus and then to position the blocker through the ETT into the left bronchus before withdrawing the endotracheal tube to an appropriate position above the carina. Bronchial blockers have a balloon and lumen that may be used to apply CPAP or suction; however, given the length of the blockers and small internal diameter both options prove limited as compared to that achievable with a DLT. Once the blocker is positioned, the balloon should be inflated with the recommended amount of air under direct visualization with fiberoptic bronchoscopy. Once positioning is confirmed, the port around the blocker in the trifurcated adapter can be tightened to limit movement of the blocker and to decrease air leak within the anesthesia circuit. An alternative to placing the bronchial blocker through the trifurcated adapter and through the ETT is to place it beside the ETT *via* direct laryngoscopy. As with any blocker, the final positioning is confirmed under direct visualization using fiberoptic bronchoscopy.

The **Arndt endobronchial blocker** (Cook Medical) is one commonly used device (Fig. **4**). The Arndt bronchial blocker is available in 3 sizes with 7Fr and 9Fr sizes most commonly used in adults (Table **7**). The Arndt blocker is a wired blocker that requires fiberoptic bronchoscopy for guidance and proper placement. It is packaged with a trifurcated adapter to accommodate the blocker, a fiberoptic bronchoscope, and the Y-attachment piece of a breathing circuit to allow for continued ventilation during deployment of the blocker. The distal end of the blocker has a wire loop that serves as a snare to keep the blocker adjacent to the bronchoscope during placement. We find that attaching the blocker to the fiberoptic bronchoscope with the snare is most easily accomplished after placing each component in the trifurcated adapter – prior to attaching the trifurcated adaptor to the endotracheal tube. The bronchoscope and Arndt blocker should be lubricated to facilitate manipulation, and the cuff on the blocker should be completely deflated. The bronchoscope is then advanced, with the Arndt blocker attached *via* the wire loop, into the appropriate bronchus. Tension on the wire snare is then released, and the bronchoscope is withdrawn to visualize the tip of the Arndt blocker properly positioned. The tip of the blocker may be a centimeter or more proximal to the tip of the bronchoscope so care should be taken not to withdraw the blocker as the bronchoscope is removed. The guide wire and loop should be removed from the blocker after placement to increase the patent internal diameter of the blocker and to facilitate deflation of the lung. Once the wire is removed from the blocker it cannot be replaced. When using a 3.4 mm bronchoscope, the manufacturer recommends an endotracheal tube size no smaller than 7.5 for the 9Fr blocker and no smaller than 6.5 for the 7Fr blocker. With a larger 3.7 mm bronchoscope a larger endotracheal tube should be employed.

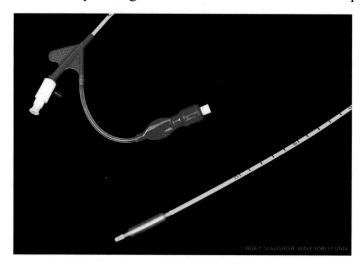

Fig. (4). Arndt endobronchial blocker (Cook Critical Care). Image provided by Thomas F. Slaughter, M.D., Wake Forest University.

Table 7. Arndt endobronchial blocker sizes.

Blocker Size (Fr)	Blocker Length (cm)	Balloon Volume (ml)	Smallest ETT Recommended (ID mm)
9	78	4-8	7.5
7	65	2-6	6.5

ETT = endotracheal tube; Fr = French; ID = internal diameter.

The Fuji Uniblocker (Fuji Systems Corp) comes in 2 sizes; the 9Fr is more relevant for adult use (Table **8**). It also has a trifurcated adapter that allows for bronchoscope guidance while the patient is being ventilated. The Fuji blocker is a "torque control" bronchial blocker (similar to the Univent) with the balloon tip having a slight angle to facilitate guidance from the external/proximal tip. The bronchoscope remains proximal to the blocker and is used to confirm rather than to guide placement of the blocker.

Table 8. Fuji Uniblockers (Fuji Systems; Tokyo, Japan).

Blocker Size (Fr)	Blocker Length (cm)	Balloon Volume (ml)
9	51	8
5	30	3

Fr = French

The Cohen blocker (Cook Medical) is available in a 9Fr size only. At 65 cm in length, it may be used in a 7.5 endotracheal tube with a 3.4 mm bronchoscope for guidance. With a larger bronchoscope, a larger endotracheal tube will be required. The bronchoscope is placed proximal to the tip of the blocker and under direct visualization the Cohen blocker tip is deflected by movement of a thumb wheel at the proximal end of the device (Fig. **5**).

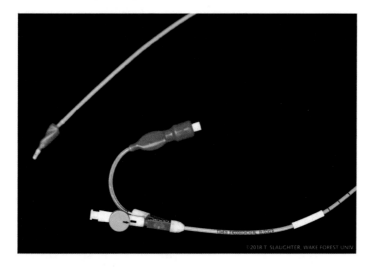

Fig. (5). Cohen Blocker (Cook Critical Care). Image provided by Thomas F. Slaughter, M.D., Wake Forest University.

The EZ-blocker (Teleflex Incorporated) is commercially available in a 7Fr size only. At 75 cm in length, it may be used with a 7.0 or larger endotracheal tube. The EZ-blocker is unique in that it has a bifurcated distal tip that may be used to block either the right or left mainstream bronchus without repositioning (Fig. **6**). Before the adapter and EZ-blocker can be placed, fiberoptic bronchoscopy is used to adjust the endotracheal tube depth such that there is approximately 4 cm between the endotracheal tube's distal end and the carina. This positioning facilitates mobility and placement of the blocker. The EZ-blocker is inserted into the single lumen endotracheal tube *via* a valved ring to eliminate air leak around the blocker after placement. The bronchoscope is used to position the EZ-blocker such that the bifurcated distal ends lie in each mainstem bronchus. To achieve lung isolation, the balloon lying in the appropriate bronchus is inflated. Once the appropriate blocker balloon is inflated ventilation by the endotracheal tube may be resumed. The distal ports on the EZ-blocker can be used to deliver oxygen by luer lock adapter (or capped when not in use).

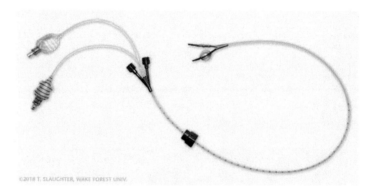

Fig. (6). EZ Blocker Endobronchial Blocker (Courtesy Teleflex Incorporated). Image provided by Thomas F. Slaughter, M.D., Wake Forest University.

Endobronchial intubation with ETT/MLT

An alternative to placement of a DLT or a bronchial blocker is endobronchial intubation with either a single lumen endotracheal tube or a microlaryngoscopy tube (MLT) (Covidien). MLTs are available in 4.0, 5.0, and 6.0 sizes. Unlike standard endotracheal tubes of this size, MLTs are long enough to place in an adult and have slightly larger cuffs to provide an adequate seal in an adult trachea. The advantage of a MLT over a standard endotracheal tube is that the smaller outer diameter lessens potential for trauma to the bronchus. In taller adults with a longer distance to the carina, standard single lumen endotracheal tubes might not prove long enough to provide bronchial isolation. Another disadvantage to using a single lumen endotracheal tube or MLT for endobronchial intubation is that there is no port access to the operative lung eliminating the ability to apply suction, to administer oxygen, or to apply PEEP to the non-dependent operative lung.

One Lung Ventilation and the Difficult Airway

There are many approaches to achieving one lung ventilation in the patient with a difficult airway. Various factors make patients difficult to ventilate or intubate;

some prove patient-specific and some disease specific. Patient related factors include obesity, large neck circumference, presence of facial hair, tongue size, thyromental distance, and limited mouth opening. Disease specific processes include distortion of upper airway anatomy due to cancer or prior radiation therapy. In some patients, placement of a single lumen endotracheal tube may prove possible but placement of a DLT proves extremely difficult. In any situation where DLT placement is the goal, an appropriately sized single lumen endotracheal tube should be available as an alternative.

The initial decision to be made when facing a patient with a difficult airway who requires lung isolation is whether anesthesia can be safely induced prior to securing the airway. If not intubation should be accomplished awake. Published case reports describe placement of a DLT in awake patients using video laryngoscopy [40]. In experienced hands, bronchoscopy can be used to place a DLT in awake patients. Due to the large external diameter of DLTs and the length of the DLT relative to a single lumen endotracheal tube, awake placement of a DLT will prove challenging. If awake intubation is required for safe airway management, a single lumen endotracheal tube may be placed by whatever technique proves most effective in the hands of the provider.

Once a single lumen endotracheal tube is in position, the provider can place a bronchial blocker regardless of whether intubation occurred orally or nasally [41]. If the single lumen endotracheal tube is placed orally, it can be exchanged for a DLT. Specialty airway exchange catheters with flexible tips may be used for this purpose (*i.e.* Cook® Airway Exchange Catheter – Extra Firm with Soft Tip). These airway exchange catheters are commercially available in 11 and 14Fr sizes with a length of 100cm – appropriate for the longer more rigid DLT.

Video laryngoscopy may be used to facilitate the tube exchange. Anterior displacement provided by the video laryngoscope facilitates passage of the DLT. Direct visualization also ensures that the providers can manipulate the DLT as needed to minimize injury to the glottis that might accompany blind passage of the DLT during exchange over the catheter. **Tube exchange with a video laryngoscope requires 2 providers**. One provider obtains and maintains a view of the glottis with the video laryngoscope. The second provider lubricates the airway exchange catheter and passes the catheter to a few centimeters beyond the end of the endotracheal tube. The second provider then deflates the cuff and slowly withdraws the endotracheal tube without displacing the exchange catheter. The first provider, still maintaining the view, establishes control of the exchanged catheter at the mouth as the endotracheal tube is removed from the exchange catheter. The second provider removes the stylet within the DLT and places the distal bronchial opening over the tip of the exchange catheter. The second provider advances the DLT over the exchange catheter and maintains control of the distal end of the exchange catheter. The first provider then gently passes the bronchial and then tracheal openings through the vocal cords. The exchange catheter is removed, and DLT placement confirmed by fiberoptic bronchoscopy. This process may be reversed for exchange of a DLT for a single lumen endotracheal tube if necessary at the conclusion of surgery.

The Univent tube may be used for awake fiberoptic intubation, but due to its larger outer diameter relative to a standard endotracheal tube, it proves less desirable for nasal intubation.

In patients with a difficult airway not requiring awake intubation, video laryngoscopy may be used to place a DLT. If a video laryngoscope is to be used, the curvature of the DLT must match the curvature of the video laryngoscope stylet. Specialty stylets for the video laryngoscopes that are long enough for use with DLTs are commercially available. In the absence of these stylets, the stylet that is packaged with the DLT can be molded to match the video laryngoscope. Compared with the C-mac for patients without difficult airways, the Glidescope has been shown to be associated with greater time to intubation when used for placement of DLTs [42].

The patient with a tracheostomy presents a unique challenge. There are multiple alternatives for lung isolation in this patient population. A cuffed tracheostomy tube may be placed and a bronchial blocker inserted through it or in patients with a larynx placed orally. Case reports describe placing a MLT as well as an EZ blocker beside a tracheostomy tube [43, 44]. If a cuffed tracheostomy tube is not available, a reinforced endotracheal tube can be used with a bronchial blocker as described above. If the stoma proves large, it may be possible to employ the distal portion of a DLT guided into position with fiberoptic bronchoscopy. Again, if a laryngectomy has not been performed intubation *via* the orotracheal route remains a possibility.

PHYSIOLOGY OF ONE LUNG VENTILATION

Proper lung isolation is critical for most intrathoracic procedures, particularly for video assisted thoracoscopy and minimally invasive robotic thoracic procedures. The anesthesiologist is challenged with maintaining adequate ventilation and oxygenation with a single lung, often times in patients with underlying pulmonary disease. Induction of anesthesia, one lung ventilation, and the lateral position disrupt normal ventilation and perfusion matching and increase intrapulmonary shunt, but the overall incidence of hypoxemia has declined sharply with improvements in lung isolation techniques and with the use of modern inhaled anesthetic agents.

The **lateral decubitus position** results in alterations in lung compliance and pulmonary perfusion patterns. In the spontaneously ventilating patient, a greater proportion of ventilation shifts to the dependent lung in the lateral position as its alveoli sit on a steeper portion of the compliance curve. The induction of anesthesia and muscle paralysis, however, results in a decreased FRC of the dependent lung. Compliance is reduced to a greater extent in the dependent lung than the nondependent lung due to cephalad displacement of the lower hemidiaphragm, and the flexed (jackknife) position. An open contralateral hemithorax will contribute to reduced compliance as loss of negative intrapleural pressure shifts mediastinal contents toward the dependent lung. A greater proportion of ventilation therefore shifts to the upper lung during two lung ventilation. Blood flow patterns are altered when a patient is lateral. Pulmonary blood flow is greater in the dependent lung due to the influence of gravity (Fig. **7**). Ventilation favoring the upper lung and perfusion favoring the lower lung results in uncoupling of ventilation-perfusion matching and a widened $P(A\text{-}a)O_2$ gradient.

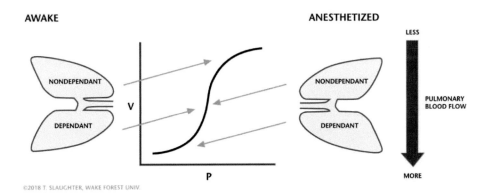

©2018 T. SLAUGHTER, WAKE FOREST UNIV.

Fig. (7). Lung compliance and blood flow in the awake and anesthetized patient. In the awake patient, the nondependent lung is less compliant and receives a lower proportion of ventilation. In the anesthetized patient, lung volumes are decreased in both lungs, and the nondependent lung moves toward the compliant portion of the pressure-volume curve, while the dependent lung moves downward to the less complaint portion of the curve. Under anesthesia, during two lung ventilation there is ventilation-perfusion mismatch as the nondependent lung receives more ventilation while the dependent lung receives more blood flow.

When one lung ventilation is initiated, shunt fraction increases due to continued blood flow to the collapsed lung (Fig. **8**). The degree to which blood is shunted to the nonventilated lung will contribute directly to hypoxemia. Since the right lung receives a greater proportion of blood flow, shunt fraction is higher for right sided surgery [45]. Several factors may reduce shunt flow to the nonventilated lung including gravity's influence on pulmonary perfusion, retraction of the surgical lung, and hypoxic pulmonary vasoconstriction. Typical shunt flow during one lung ventilation is 20-30%.

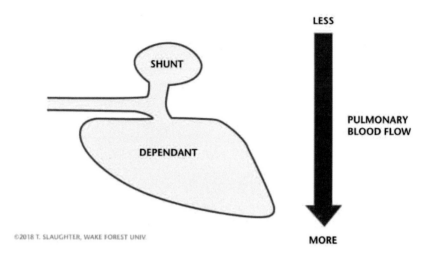

Fig. (8). Once one lung ventilation is initiated, the dependent lung receives a greater proportion of blood flow. Blood that is still directed toward the non-dependent, non-ventilated lung becomes shunt flow.

Hypoxic pulmonary vasoconstriction (HPV) is thought to reduce shunt flow through the nonventilated lung by 40-50% [46, 47]. HPV has a biphasic response to hypoxia beginning within seconds and plateauing by 15 minutes. With sustained moderate hypoxia, a second phase of increasing pulmonary vascular resistance occurs and peaks after 2 hours [48]. Certain physiologic conditions and pharmacologic agents inhibit HPV potentially exacerbating hypoxemia. COPD, cirrhosis, sepsis, and hypothermia all negatively impact HPV. The halogenated volatile anesthetics inhibit HPV in a dose dependent manner while propofol does not [49]. Older agents, including enflurane and halothane, more profoundly impacted HPV; however, modern inhalational anesthetic agents prove weaker inhibitors. Studies comparing the inhalational anesthetics isoflurane, sevoflurane, and desflurane failed to demonstrate consistent and clinically significant differences in arterial oxygenation and shunt fraction as compared to intravenous anesthetics [50, 51]. One explanation is that the cardiac output-lowering effects of volatile anesthetics decreases mixed venous P02 (PvO_2). Decreased PvO_2 stimulates HPV, which may counteract direct effects of the volatile agents. Vasodilators including hydralazine, nitroprusside, nitroglycerin, and lisinopril also inhibit HPV. Examples of various pharmacologic and physiologic variables and their effects on HPV are listed below (Table **9**).

Table 9. Modifiers of Hypoxic Pulmonary Vasoconstriction [47, 110, 111].

Promote HPV	Inhibit HPV	Little/ No effect
Acidosis	Alkalosis	Inhaled nitric oxide (-/ 0)
Hypercapnia	Hypocapnia	Isoflurane (-/0)
Hyperthermia	Hypothermia	Desflurane (-/0)
Systemic hypertension	COPD	Sevoflurane (-/0)
Decreased pulmonary oxygen partial pressure (PvO2)	Increased pulmonary oxygen partial pressure (PvO2)	Ketamine
Decreased alveolar oxygen partial pressure (PAO2)	Cirrhosis	Opioids
Lung retraction	Pregnancy	Diltiazem
Epidural anesthesia (+/0)	Sepsis	Clonidine
Almitrine	Hemodilution	---
Propofol (+/0)	Increased left atrial pressure	---
Propranolol	Nitrous oxide	---
Norepinephrine	Halothane	---
Phenylephrine	Calcium channel blockers	---
Lidocaine	Hydralazine	---
Ipratroprium	Nitroglycerin	---
---	Nitroprusside	---
---	Dopamine (-/0, dose dependent)	---
---	Dobutamine	---
---	Losartan	---
---	Lisinopril	---
---	Sildenafil	---

VENTILATORY STRATEGIES DURING ONE LUNG VENTILATION

Goals of management during one lung ventilation include: **1)** optimizing surgical visualization and operative conditions, **2)** maintaining adequate ventilation and oxygenation, **3)** and mitigating postoperative acute lung injury (ALI). While mechanisms underlying **ALI** prove complex and multifactorial, one lung ventilation increasingly has been implicated in this injury process. Intraoperative risk factors for post-thorocotomy ALI include peak inspiratory pressures exceeding 35-40 cm H_2O, plateau pressures greater than 25 cm H_2O, excessive perioperative fluid administration, blood transfusion, pneumonectomy, lung transplantation, and prolonged one lung ventilation. Preexisting patient factors include a history of alcohol abuse, poor postoperative predicted lung function, and preexisting lung injury (such as trauma, infection or chemotherapy) [47].

While controversy remains, low tidal volume ventilation increasingly is recommended to reduce potential for ALI. Protective ventilation strategies may reduce the incidence of postoperative ALI as well as atelectasis in thoracic surgical patients (Licker). The use of low tidal volumes (4-6 ml/kg of ideal body weight), routine use of PEEP, recruitment maneuvers, and permissive hypercapnia have been advocated for lung protection. Permissive hypercapnia to $PaCO_2$ values of 70 mm Hg is generally well-tolerated but should be used with caution in patient with cardiac impairment or arrhythmias – and avoided in patients with increased intracranial pressure [47]. Volume control or pressure control ventilation may be employed during one lung ventilation. Some advocate for pressure control ventilation during one lung ventilation given lower peak airway pressures (due to decelerating flow waveform), potential for alveolar recruitment, and improved distribution of inspired gas. The use of volume control *versus* pressure control ventilation during one lung ventilation has not consistently been demonstrated to offer improved oxygenation [52, 53]. Peak airway pressures are lower on pressure control ventilation, but much of the reduction of peak pressures occurs in the respiratory circuit rather than the bronchus of the dependent lung [54]. At this time, there is insufficient evidence to recommend one mode of ventilation over another during one lung ventilation. **Peak pressure goals** should be less than 35 cm H_2O with a plateau pressure less than 25 cm H_2O. The combination of low tidal volumes and higher ventilatory rates may predispose to auto-PEEP. For this reason, the application of PEEP must be considered on a case by case basis. Specific care should be taken to avoid alveolar over-distension in patients with COPD. Excessive PEEP may worsen oxygenation during one lung ventilation by increasing pulmonary vascular resistance with diversion of blood to the operative lung. In patients with normal or restrictive lung disease, a PEEP of 5-10 cm H_2O generally be will be well tolerated. An FIO_2 of 1.0 is administered during induction of anesthesia and prior to initiation of one lung ventilation to promote resorption atelectasis. During one lung ventilation, FIO_2 is generally maintained at 1.0; although some authors advocate lower FIO_2 concentrations to lessen potential for oxygen toxicity [45].

Managing Hypoxemia

Despite advancements in one lung ventilation techniques, **hypoxemia occurs in 5-10% of procedures requiring one lung ventilation**. A PaO_2 less than 60 mm Hg (or hemoglobin saturation less than 90%) generally suggest the need for intervention to improve oxygenation. Several factors may predict likelihood for desaturation during one lung ventilation. Having a right-sided operation increases likelihood for hypoxemia since the right lung is larger than the left. An abnormally low oxygen tension (PaO_2) on preoperative blood gas analysis or during two lung ventilation has been correlated with lower PaO_2 on one lung ventilation. If a preoperative ventilation-perfusion scan is available, it may help predict intraoperative arterial oxygenation. The degree of preoperative perfusion to the operative lung inversely correlates to PaO_2 levels achieved during one lung ventilation. Patient position can play a role also. The lateral decubitus position offers improved oxygenation over the semi-lateral and supine positions by preferentially distributing blood to the dependent, ventilated lung [55].

Approach to Hypoxemia During One Lung Ventilation (Table 10)

Table 10. Approach to hypoxemia during one lung ventilation.

• Reinflate operative lung if rapid, severe desaturation
• Ensure adequate systemic blood pressure
• Reassess double lumen tube/ bronchial blocker position with fiberoptic bronchoscopy
• Consider bronchospasm as potential etiology
• Consider adding PEEP to dependent lung
• Apply a recruitment maneuver to dependent lung
• Apply CPAP 2-5 cm to nondependent lung
• Periodic reinflation of nondependent lung
• Consider selective lobar insufflation with bronchial blocker
• Consider selective lobar collapse of operative lobe with bronchial blocker
• In pneumonectomy or transplant paitents, consider pulmonary artery clamp on operative lung

The **most common treatable causes of hypoxemia** include displacement of the double lumen endotracheal tube or bronchial blocker, occlusion of a major bronchus by a bronchial balloon, occlusion of bronchi by secretions or blood, or an inadequate ventilation strategy leading to atelectasis. If desaturation proves rapid and severe, the operative lung should be reinflated and FiO_2 increased to 1.0 until the cause of desaturation is determined and remedied. The position of the endobronchial blocker should be reassessed with a flexible bronchoscope (Fig. **2**). The endobronchial cuff may be excluding a lobe from ventilation. Flexible bronchoscopy may also reveal thick secretions or blood impairing adequate ventilation. Bronchospasm should be ruled out as a potential contributor. A recruitment maneuver followed by application of extrinsic PEEP may improve oxygenation in some patients, although it may be deleterious in others if intrinsic PEEP already exists – particularly in elderly patients or those with emphysematous lungs. Hypoxemia may transiently worsen during the recruitment maneuver as intrapulmonary pressures rise shunting blood to the non-ventilated lung. If these maneuvers prove unsuccessful, application of CPAP to the nondependent lung often improves oxygenation by decreasing shunt fraction. The nondependent lung is first inflated with a tidal volume breath through the double lumen tube or the bronchial blocker suction channel. Anywhere from 2-10 cm of CPAP is applied using a system with an oxygen source and pressure relief valve that may be dialed to various levels of CPAP [56]. Such systems may be constructed from available anesthesia equipment or several systems are available commercially (Fig. **9**). The disadvantage of CPAP is that even partial reinflation of the operative lung may not prove acceptable to the surgical team – especially during thoracoscopic or minimally invasive robotic procedures. If CPAP is applied, it should be maintained at the lowest possible level to maintain adequate oxygenation. Pressures of 2-5 cm H_2O typically prove sufficient. Periodic reinflation of the nondependent lung provides another strategy to mitigate hypoxemia but may impede surgical progress. **More advanced techniques** include insufflation of selected lobar segments of the nondependent lung using a fiberoptic bronchoscope and selective lobar collapse of only the operative lobe. If other methods fail during pneumonectomy or lung transplant and severe hypoxemia continues, a pulmonary artery clamp may be applied to reduce transpulmonary shunt. Administration of inhaled nitric oxide (iNO) to the ventilated lung generally has not improved arterial oxygenation. Combinations of iNO and almitrine have demonstrated benefit, but almitrine's potential for toxicity resulted in its removal from many markets. Combinations of inhaled nitric oxide or an inhaled prostacyclin along with pulmonary vasoconstrictors like phenylephrine may improve oxygenation but warrant further study [57, 58].

THORACIC SURGICAL DIAGNOSTIC PROCEDURES

(Fiberoptic Bronchoscopy, Rigid Bronchoscopy, and Mediastinoscopy)

Although the majority of **flexible fiberoptic bronchoscopies** are performed under topical anesthetic with minimal sedation, expanding applications including tumor laser ablation, balloon dilatation and stent placement, and bronchial thermoplasty have led to longer procedures with increasing necessity for either deep sedation or general anesthesia. In contrast, **rigid bronchoscopy and mediastinoscopy** most often are performed under general anesthesia – and more commonly in an operative setting [34, 59, 60]. Regardless of procedure planned, preoperative assessment may identify airway concerns or other comorbidities suggesting the need to relocate from an off-site location to an operative site. In the case of flexible fiberoptic bronchoscopy, topical anesthesia with adjunctive sedation proves a popular approach to optimize procedural conditions and maximize patient satisfaction. Topical anesthetics must be administered judiciously as local anesthetic toxicity has been reported in these settings. In adults, lidocaine 4% (4-6 ml) may be nebulized to produce reasonable anesthesia of the pharynx and tracheobronchial tree [35, 61, 62]. Commercial sprays containing benzocaine prove popular in this role, although excess administration may lead to methemoglobinemia. Transtracheal injection of local anesthetic (lidocaine 4% 2-3ml) and blockade of glossopharyngeal nerves will enhance suppression of the gag reflex. Total intravenous anesthesia (TIVA) approaches include continuous infusions of propofol (25-100 mcg/kg/min) or dexmedetomidine. Low dose narcotic administration will suppress the cough reflex but increase potential for respiratory depression. The antisialogogue effects of glycopyrrolate (0.1-0.2 mg/80 kg) administered preoperatively often prove beneficial.

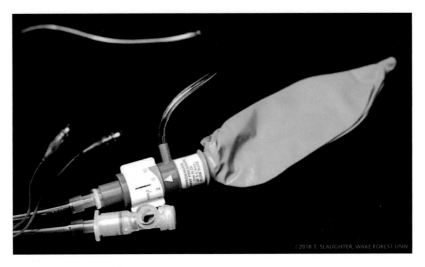

Fig. (9). CPAP (Continuous Positive Airway Pressure) Device. Image provided by Thomas F. Slaughter, M.D., Wake Forest University.

In contrast, **rigid bronchoscopy** most often is performed under general anesthesia with neuromuscular blockade. Rigid bronchoscopy offers greater ability to suction the airway in the case of hemorrhage and may be used preferentially to remove foreign objects or to bypass strictures – or obstructions due to tumor. The most common anesthetic challenge associated with any bronchoscopy is that of ensuring adequate ventilation and oxygenation during the procedure. In the case of flexible fiberoptic bronchoscopy, the procedure is performed commonly with sedation and spontaneous ventilation – unless a preexisting endotracheal tube is in place. Rigid bronchoscopy is more commonly performed with positive pressure ventilation provided *via* a sideport on the bronchoscope [34, 35, 60]. High frequency jet ventilation (HFJV) has been reported in this setting as well.

Inhalation agents may be used in this setting although leakage into the environment and provider exposure may favor TIVA techniques. **Major complications** prove rare in bronchoscopy; however, biopsies or laser treatments may precipitate massive hemorrhage – and laryngospasm or bronchospasm may prove life threatening. Given the combination of topical anesthesia and sedation, aspiration proves a concern. Patients considered at high risk for aspiration preoperatively may require endotracheal intubation as a precaution. Tension pneumothorax may lead to sudden cardiovascular collapse.

In patients without airway obstruction/ compression, general anesthesia with endotracheal intubation proves the most common anesthetic approach for mediastinoscopy [36, 63]. Compression of the innominate artery may occur during these procedures and may be monitored with either a right radial arterial line or pulse oximetry of the right hand. Measurement of non-invasive blood pressure in the left upper extremity provides a means to attain actual blood pressure in this setting. Given proximity to pulmonary and innominate vasculature, mediastinoscopy poses a risk for massive bleeding [36]. For this reason, a common approach would be to place an arterial line with 2 large peripheral IVs after anesthetic induction. Ensuring that compatible blood is available by type and cross may prove prudent as well. Other less common complications associated with mediastinoscopy include pneumothorax, air embolism, and injury to phrenic or recurrent laryngeal nerves.

ESOPHAGEAL SURGERY

Although **esophageal surgery** may be indicated for a number of "benign" conditions – including achalasia or esophageal perforation, in most cases esophagectomy is undertaken for esophageal carcinoma. Squamous cell carcinoma (associated with alcohol and tobacco exposure) remains the most common histologic diagnosis for esophageal cancer worldwide; however, adenocarcinoma is now the most rapidly increasing cancer in the U.S. Several risk factors have been associated with adenocarcinoma including tobacco smoke, gastroesophageal reflux disease (GERD), Barrett's esophagus, and obesity. In most cases, esophageal cancer proves non-resectable at the time of diagnosis. However, any potential for cure will necessitate surgical resection with concurrent chemotherapy and/or radiation treatment. Multiple surgical approaches to esophagectomy have been reported – most recently incorporating minimally invasive strategies. Regardless, perioperative morbidity and mortality remain high with mortality rates of 5-8% reported [64, 65]. Factors contributing to both morbidity and mortality include the patient's underlying medical condition and coexisting disease, patient age, tobacco use, tumor stage, extent of surgery, and experience of the surgical team.

Specific anesthetic needs will be dictated by the surgical approach. Common surgical methods for esophageal resection include: **1)** transhiatal and **2)** transthoracic approaches. Increasingly endoscopic techniques are being incorporated to eliminate the need for laparotomy and/or thoracotomy. Although minimally invasive approaches appear to reduce postoperative ICU length of stay, it remains unclear whether overall morbidity and mortality are reduced [64].

As with any thoracic surgery, efforts to optimize the patient's underlying medical condition and overall health before surgery is indicated. Patients with esophageal cancer frequently experience malnutrition relating to reduced oral intake and catabolic activity of the disease process. In general, these patients are considered at increased risk for aspiration and anesthetic induction techniques incorporating a rapid sequence induction (with elevation of the back and application of cricoid pressure) – or awake intubation – may prove prudent. In addition to standard ASA recommended monitors, the potential for compression of the heart or great vessels – or vascular injury – justifies invasive arterial blood pressure monitoring. In addition, the surgical team may desire central venous catheterization to facilitate postoperative assessment of fluid balance. In most cases, lung isolation will be required necessitating placement of an endobronchial tube or blocker after anesthetic induction [66]. Other concerns specific to esophageal resection include: **1)** a desire to restrict fluid administration and **2)** incorporation of protective ventilatory strategies. There is some concern that excess fluid administration may lead to postoperative morbidity in the form of tissue edema, impaired wound healing, increased risk for anastomotic leak, and increased pulmonary and cardiac morbidity. Complicating volume restrictive strategies is the concern for a tenuous blood supply at the site of surgical anastomosis and common occurrence of vasodilation and hypotension associated with thoracic epidural analgesia [65, 66]. Recent evidence suggests that administration of low-dose vasopressors or inotropes proves preferable to either hypotension or excess volume administration in these settings.

Pulmonary related complications account for the majority of both morbidity and mortality after esophageal surgery. **Common complications** include aspiration, atelectasis, pneumonia, pulmonary edema, and acute respiratory distress syndrome (ARDS) [64, 66]. Perioperative volume restriction accompanied by protective intraoperative ventilatory strategies are thought to mitigate risk. Protective ventilatory strategies include employing pressure-controlled ventilation with low tidal volumes (*i.e.* 5-6 ml/kg), judicious application of PEEP, permissive hypercapnia, control of peak ventilatory pressures (*i.e.* <35 cm H_2O), and early postoperative extubation. Adequate postoperative analgesia – most often provided by thoracic epidural analgesia – proves critical to facilitate clearance of respiratory secretions with coughing and early mobilization [67]. As with any type of thoracic surgery, cardiac dysrhythmias remain common after esophageal surgery. Atrial fibrillation and other supraventricular tachycardias occur most often during the initial 2-3 days after surgery and should elicit investigation for cardiac ischemia as well as anastomotic leaks. Leak at the anastomotic site may occur in as many as 14% of cases and will be associated with significant collateral injury secondary to inflammation and necrosis of adjacent tissue [65, 66]. Small leaks may be managed with drainage and antibiotics; however, larger leaks require surgical intervention. Failure to identify anastomotic leaks early may result in empyema, mediastinitis, sepsis, and death.

VIDEO ASSISTED THORACOSCOPY AND MINIMALLY INVASIVE ROBOTIC THORACIC SURGERY

As technology and experience with minimally invasive thoracic surgery continues to evolve, indications for these techniques continues to expand. **Video assisted thoracoscopy (VATS)** is employed for pulmonary resection and cancer staging, resection of mediastinal masses, pericardial windows, drainage of empyemas, and management of pleural effusion – to name a few. Although **anesthetic** concerns for minimally invasive thoracic surgery prove, in large part, similar to that for thoracotomy; there are considerations specifically relevant to VATS as well as robotic thoracic surgery [68 - 70]. Both VATS and robotic thoracic surgery are performed in the lateral decubitus position and require lung isolation (*i.e.* one lung ventilation). Placement of an endobronchial double lumen tube (as opposed to blocker) is most often preferred to minimize potential for displacement of the endobronchial cuff after repositioning the patient. In contrast to open thoracotomy, lung isolation proves critical for surgical visualization during minimally invasive procedures. For this reason, application of CPAP to the non-dependent lung will interfere with visualization and likely prove unacceptable to the surgical team. A major advantage of minimally invasive surgical approaches proves to be less postoperative pain and more rapid postoperative recovery [69 - 71]. However, the potential for conversion to open thoracotomy always persists and for this reason some surgical teams prefer preoperative placement of a thoracic epidural catheter for all patients [70, 72]. A major consideration for minimally invasive thoracic surgical procedures is the use of carbon dioxide (CO_2) insufflation into the pleural cavity to enhance visualization of the surgical field [73, 74]. Excessive insufflation pressures may produce mediastinal shift (or impair venous return) resulting in sudden hypotension and/or bradycardia. Insufflation of CO_2 should elicit **heightened awareness** for signs of venous gas embolism as well as hypercarbia. Tension pneumothorax of the non-operative lung and subcutaneous emphysema may occur as well. Given potential for hemodynamic compromise related to insufflation – as well as the possibility of vascular injury – adequate venous access and arterial blood pressure monitoring are indicated [73, 74]. In patients for whom adequate peripheral venous access proves impossible, placement of a central venous line may be indicated. In the case of **robotic surgery**, docking of the surgical robot with intrathoracic placement of surgical trocars limits the ability to reposition the patient rapidly. In some cases, access to the patient's airway will be constrained once the robot is docked [75]. Therefore, placement of venous and arterial access – as well as assurance of optimal lung isolation – must occur in the supine position before turning the patient lateral. Given the time required to disengage the robotic arms and the potential for vascular injury, availability of adequate venous access and blood prove particularly critical in the case of robotic assisted thoracic surgical procedures [75].

TRACHEAL RESECTION AND RECONSTRUCTION

The most common indications underlying tracheal resection and reconstruction include tracheal stenosis and cancer. **Tracheal stenosis** may occur in response to prior endotracheal intubation or tracheostomy, and cancer – although relatively uncommon – most often proves attributable to squamous cell or adenoid cystic carcinoma. Less common etiologies for tracheal injury include inflammatory responses to trauma (or burns) and compression from nearby tumors, thyroid goiter, or vascular abnormalities [76]. Patients with tracheal pathology frequently present clinically with dyspnea on exertion and cough progressing to orthopnea and hemoptysis. Hoarseness may occur with involvement of the larynx or recurrent laryngeal nerve. Any patient with tracheal stenosis (or obstruction) undergoing a diagnostic or therapeutic procedure must be **approached with extreme caution given potential for acute airway obstruction** [77]. Symptoms of orthopnea and/ or stridor prove particularly concerning. Neither a standard airway examination nor chest x-ray prove of great value in assessing risk for airway obstruction. High resolution computed tomography of the trachea proves valuable in these patients. In cases of high grade tracheal obstruction, bronchoscopy may be delayed until immediately before surgical intervention to allow for emergent surgical intervention should acute airway obstruction occur at the time of the diagnostic examination [78, 79]. Pulmonary function testing – and flow-volume loops in particular – have assumed a less important role with advances in high resolution imaging. Ventilator or steroid dependency – or a history of prior radiation therapy – serve as relative contraindications to surgery given increased risk for wound dehiscence at anastomotic sites. However, recent efforts directed toward tracheal transplantation and tissue engineering likely will expand the population eligible for tracheal surgery in the future.

Anesthetic planning for tracheal resection and reconstruction must be carefully informed by consultation with the surgical team and review of findings on computed tomography and diagnostic bronchoscopy. These surgeries are not typically associated with major bleeding; however, the upper extremities are tucked so placement of at least 2 peripheral IVs and a radial arterial catheter proves advisable. If total intravenous anesthesia (TIVA) is planned during the period of tracheal reanastomosis, some form of monitoring for depth of anesthesia may be helpful. The **great concern** for these patients remains acute airway obstruction with anesthetic induction or airway instrumentation. In patients experiencing orthopnea, planning should incorporate securing the airway in a sitting position. Whether the airway is best secured with the patient breathing spontaneously – or after anesthetic induction – must be determined in concert with the surgical team and the patient's preference. Should an induction with spontaneous ventilation be desired, this may be accomplished by either mask ventilation or with an LMA. Regardless, preparations by the team must include alternatives for rescue in the event of acute airway obstruction [78, 79]. A variety of endotracheal tubes ranging in size from 4.0 to 7.0 (with and without steel reinforcement) and a pediatric fiberoptic bronchoscope suitable for placement in the smaller endotracheal tubes should be present. Rigid bronchoscopy may prove life-saving given its ability to transverse an obstruction and to facilitate suctioning and jet ventilation. Should acute airway obstruction occur after anesthetic induction – and not prove amenable to placement of an LMA or endotracheal tube, **potential methods to rescue** may include: **1)** rigid bronchoscopy, **2)** jet ventilation (supraglottic or transtracheal), **3)** tracheotomy, or **4)** institution of cardiopulmonary bypass (CPB) or extracorporeal membrane **oxygenation (ECMO). For cases at particularly high risk for airway obstruction, arterial and/or venous cannulas may be placed preoperatively under local anesthesia to facilitate initiation of ECMO or CPB** should airway obstruction occur. In most cases, the surgical team will place a sterile reinforced endotracheal tube distal to the tracheal stenosis or obstruction during surgical dissection. However, in the case of pathology affecting the distal trachea or carina, there are reports of jet ventilation *via* catheters traversing the surgical site as well as independent ventilation of each lung distal to the site of surgical resection [78, 80 - 82]. In most cases, the surgical team will replace the endotracheal tube across the site of the surgical anastomosis on closure of the trachea. There is a strong desire to extubate these patients at completion of surgery to eliminate any potential for the endotracheal tube to abrade the surgical anastomotic site. Prolonged postoperative mechanical ventilation may contribute to dehiscence of the surgical anastomosis. Needless to say, these patients prove at high risk for airway obstruction postoperatively. The anesthetic should be planned to minimize potential for excessive administration of narcotics or neuromuscular blockers at conclusion of the procedure. The surgical repair will necessitate cervical flexion to reduce strain on the anastomotic site. In many cases, the surgical team may place a retention suture between the chin and chest to facilitate flexion of the neck. Emergent reintubation poses extreme risk for disruption of the tracheal suture line and should be avoided if at all possible. Regardless, should the need to reintubate the patient occur blood in the airway and cervical flexion will complicate the process and may necessitate emergent surgical tracheotomy. **Again, careful planning and coordination by the entire surgical team is necessary to mitigate risks throughout the perioperative period for these patients.**

POSTOPERATIVE CONSIDERATIONS

The vast majority of thoracic surgical patients will be extubated at the conclusion of their procedure; and, criteria for extubation prove similar to that for other general anesthetic procedures. In fact, concerns for mechanical ventilation to "stress" suture lines and promote acute lung injury and/ or bronchopulmonary fistula formation creates pressure to extubate patients after thoracic surgery even under less than ideal conditions. **Common conditions underlying failure to extubate** in this setting include inadequate reversal of neuromuscular relaxation or excess sedation relating to the intraoperative administration of narcotics and/or inhalational agents (Table **11**). Should the anticipated time to extubation prove short, the endobronchial tube may be retained into the PACU setting; however, longer expectations for mechanical ventilatory support – as might be associated with inadequate oxygenation postoperatively – would favor exchange to a single lumen endotracheal tube. Given the size and relatively specific positioning of endobronchial tubes, exchange to a single lumen endotracheal tube will reduce pressure on glottic structures, improve patient comfort, allow for easier suctioning of the airway, and reduce the potential for malpositioning of the endotracheal tube with patient emergence in the PACU or ICU setting. A leak test may be performed by assessing ability of the patient to ventilate around the endobronchial tube (with deflated tracheal cuff) should there be concerns about airway edema. Obviously, in the case of difficult initial intubation – or concerns for airway edema – the endobronchial tube may be retained – or exchanged using an airway exchange catheter with appropriate ancillary airway devices present.

Conditions Associated with Need for Mechanical Ventilation After Thoracic Surgery

Table 11. Conditions Associated with Need for Mechanical Ventilation After Thoracic Surgery. (Modified from Ramsay JG and Murphy M *"Postoperative Respiratory Failure and Treatment"* **in** Thoracic Anesthesia, 3rd Edition. **Kaplan JA, Slinger PD (Eds). Elsevier Science: Philadelphia p. 406, 2003)**

Residual neuromuscular blockade	Massive blood/ fluid replacement
Residual anesthetic (*i.e.* lack of responsiveness)	Ongoing bleeding

(Table 11) cont.....

FiO2 requirement > 50%	Surgical complication
Respiratory distress	Perioperative MI or congestive heart failure
Preop mechanical ventilation	Need to isolate contaminant (*i.e.* drainage)
Predicted postop FEV1 < 30%	Massive air leak
Prolonged intraoperative course	Excessive airway secretions and/or blood
Hypothermia	Morbid obesity

(Modified from Ramsay JG and Murphy M "*Postoperative Respiratory Failure and Treatment*" in Thoracic Anesthesia, 3ʳᵈ Edition. Kaplan JA, Slinger PD (Eds). Elsevier Science: Philadelphia p. 406, 2003).

PAIN MANAGEMENT

Pain associated with a thoracotomy incision proves extreme with multiple components including incision of skin and underlying muscles, intercostal nerve injury, dislocation of costophrenic joints, possibly rib fractures or resections, chest tube drains, and pleural inflammation resulting from stripping and surgical manipulation within the thoracic cavity [83, 84]. Failure to achieve adequate postoperative analgesia contributes to impaired cough, inability to clear secretions, atelectasis, and impaired mobility (Table **12**). Although **thoracic epidural analgesia** remains the gold-standard therapy for managing pain after thoracic surgery, a multimodal approach to postoperative analgesia best meets patient needs to facilitate recovery and reduce length of stay. Selection of an analgesic strategy requires a considered patient specific approach and should be determined at the time of preoperative evaluation. Postoperative pain management strategies will be determined in part by the planned surgical procedure, the patient's underlying medical condition and preferences, need for perioperative anti-platelet/ anticoagulant therapy, and in the case of continuous regional anesthetic infusions, the provider's ability to provide postoperative support and supervision of the analgesic plan [85]. Thoracic epidural analgesia (TEA) remains the "gold standard" for pain management after thoracic surgical procedures (Table **13**). TEA improves the ability to cough and mobilize secretions and facilitates postoperative mobility while simultaneously reducing the need for postoperative narcotics and their associated adverse effects [67, 85 - 88]. Risks associated with epidural analgesia including hypotension, potential for epidural hematoma, and relatively high failure rates have more recently increased interest in thoracic paravertebral analgesia as an alternative regional analgesic approach. Paravertebral catheters may be placed under ultrasound guidance – or directly by the surgeon at conclusion of the intraoperative procedure. Paravertebral analgesia appears associated with reduced risks as compared to TEA and offers potential for similar analgesia [85, 87 - 89]. With either TEA or paravertebral analgesia, there is little evidence to suggest that addition of adjunctive drugs to local anesthetic infusions proves beneficial. In patients for whom TEA or paravertebral analgesia prove contraindicated, alternatives may include single-shot intrathecal narcotic administration or intercostal analgesia provided by injection or continuous infusion by catheter. The use of intrathecal narcotics will necessitate close postoperative monitoring for respiratory depression. Interpleural infusions and cryoanalgesia have proved of decreasing interest given concerns for local anesthetic toxicity and long-term paresthesias, respectively. Multimodal approaches to management of postoperative pain prove superior to local anesthetics alone and may incorporate systemic narcotics, acetaminophen, and non-steroidal anti-inflammatory drugs – with appropriate precautions for patients at risk of hepatic or renal insufficiency [85, 87, 90]. Non-steroidal anti-inflammatory drugs prove a powerful adjuvant to reduce inflammation as well as referred shoulder pain associated with chest tubes. Additional adjunctive drugs used for postoperative pain include the corticosteroids (*i.e.* dexamethasone), gabapentoids (*i.e.* gabapentin and pregabalin), and ketamine; however, optimal dosing regimens and risks for adverse effects remain unclear [83, 85, 87, 91 - 93]. In most cases a multimodal analgesic plan with a thoracic epidural catheter employing a low dose of local anesthetic remains the preferred approach after thoracic surgical procedures. Prolonged pain after thoracotomy proves common – occurring in as many as 50% of patients. A subset of these patients transition to experience a chronic pain syndrome [84, 87, 92, 94]. In many patients, this pain proves mild; however, in 3-5% the pain may prove disabling. Referral of these patients to Pain Medicine specialists is indicated. Local anesthetic injection of trigger points and cryotherapy of intercostal nerves may alleviate symptoms.

Implications for Lack of Adequate Analgesia After Thoracic Surgery

Table 12. Implications for Lack of Adequate Analgesia after Thoracic Surgery.

• Impaired coughing and mobility
• Increased respiratory complications
• Increased potential for reintubation
• Prolonged length of stay
• Patient dissatisfaction
• Increased potential for post-thoracotomy pain syndrome

Approaches to Postoperative Analgesia

Table 13. Approaches to Postoperative Analgesia.

Regional Analgesia
• Thoracic epidural analgesia
• Paravertebral analgesia

(Table 13) cont.....

• Intrathecal narcotics
• Intercostal nerve blocks
• Percutaneous wound infiltration
• Intrapleural infusions
Systemic Analgesics
• Non-steroidal anti-inflammatory drugs (NSAIDs)
• Acetaminophen
• Systemic narcotics
Adjuvant Drugs
• Corticosteroids (*i.e.* dexamethasone)
• Ketamine
• Gabapentanoids (*i.e.* gabapentin, pregabalin)

COMPLICATIONS OF THORACIC SURGERY

Given the age and comorbidities commonly associated with adult patients requiring thoracic surgery, the fact that they experience elevated risks for postoperative morbidity and mortality should prove no surprise. Needless to say, the patient's preexisting condition and the extent of surgery contribute significantly to adverse perioperative outcomes; however, some risks prove specific to the surgical approach as well.

Airway Concerns

Given the size and rigidity of endobronchial tubes, placement may lead to traumatic or compressive injuries [95]. Laryngeal edema has been associated with prolonged intubation but most often proves limited in course resolving after extubation with simple elevation of the bed. In more severe cases with stridor, administration of steroids and aerosolized racemic epinephrine may expedite recovery. Dislocation of arytenoids and vocal cord injury have been reported with endobronchial intubation. The recurrent laryngeal nerve may be injured during surgical resection – in some cases leading to permanent paralysis of the vocal cord in adducted position [96 - 98].

Pulmonary Complications

Atelectasis proves nearly ubiquitous after thoracic surgery. Numerous factors contribute including patient obesity, underlying respiratory dysfunction, surgical trauma, and postoperative pain contributing to splinting with inadequate cough and retained secretions [99 - 101]. As FRC declines postoperatively, ventilation/

perfusion mismatching leads to an increase in alveolar-arterial gradient and resulting hypoxemia. In patients with marginal ventilatory reserve, acute respiratory failure may ensure requiring reintubation and mechanical ventilatory support [100]. Treatment of atelectasis focuses around control of postoperative pain to facilitate coughing, clearance of secretions, and early postoperative mobilization [85, 102]. Incentive spirometry proves particularly helpful to increase FRC.

Small air leaks prove common after thoracic surgery. In most cases, reexpansion of the lung facilitated by chest tubes leads to closure of the leak(s) over a period of days. A persistent air leak may lead to bronchopleural fistula which is associated with significantly increased patient morbidity and mortality. In addition to posing threat of infection, bronchopleural fistulae result in air loss to the pleural space necessitating increased minute ventilation. Patients with limited ventilatory reserve may be tipped into respiratory failure [99 - 101, 103]. Should mechanical ventilation be required in the presence of a bronchopleural fistula, low tidal volumes with increased ventilatory rate, limited peak inspiratory pressure, and permissive hypercapnia proves prudent. High frequency ventilation and differential mechanical ventilation using an endobrochial tube and synchronized ventilators have proved alternative approaches. Resolution of a bronchopleural fistula proves challenging – often requiring multiple surgeries possibly including myoplasty. Long-term mortality in these patients may approach 20%.

Less common complications associated with thoracic surgery include tension pneumothorax and torsion of a residual lobe. Placement of a chest tube should prevent tension pneumothorax. However, sudden hemodynamic collapse at the conclusion of a thoracic surgical procedure should elicit an immediate question as to whether the chest tubes are connected to suction. Obstruction or disconnection of chest tube suction may underlie development of a tension pneumothorax despite presence of chest tubes. Physical signs of tension pneumothorax include decreased breath sounds in the affected lung field, unilateral wheezing, and a "hollow" sound elicited by percussion of the affected chest. Should there be a delay in replacing a chest tube, emergent decompression may be performed using an IV catheter placed in the mid-clavicular line. A rare complication associated with upper lobectomy is that of torsion of the right middle lobe or lingual, respectively. Without the upper lobe to restrict movement, the remaining middle lobe may twist on itself. Initially, a large intrapulmonary shunt results which may lead to respiratory decompensation. If left untreated, the torsion may progress to pulmonary infarction [67, 101, 103 - 105]. A diagnosis proves evident during fiberoptic bronchoscopy as the bronchus proves compressed.

Cardiac Complications

Perioperative myocardial infarction remains a major cause of perioperative morbidity and mortality in this population. Thorough preoperative evaluation to identify patients at greatest risk and to allow for preoperative efforts to mitigate risk remains essential [29, 99, 101, 106]. Given the propensity for thoracic epidural anesthesia to cause vasodilation – as well as the sympathetic stimulation resulting from the surgery, vigilance to limit hypotension and tachycardia during the perioperative period appears prudent as well. Supraventricular dysrhythmias (*i.e.* multifocal atrial tachycardia, atrial flutter, and atrial fibrillation) prove common after thoracic surgery. Patient age and the extent of surgical resection appear associated [24, 30, 107]. Other contributing factors may include preexisting cardiac disease, surgical manipulation, and abnormalities of acid/base balance). In most cases, these conditions will be treated medically; however, hemodynamic instability may necessitate emergent cardioversion. An uncommon, but potentially **lethal complication** specific to thoracic surgery is that of cardiac herniation. Most often, this complication would occur after pneumonectomy in the presence of a pericardial defect. Entrapment of the heart within the defect leads to sudden cardiovascular collapse due to obstruction to venous return. Other signs that may be associated with cardiac herniation include jugular venous distention and an axis change in the ECG. Rapid identification and immediate reoperation prove critical to recovery.

Hemorrhage

Bleeding after thoracotomy proves uncommon; however, associated mortality may be significant. Massive blood loss may occur into the pleural space with loss of suture or staple from pulmonary venous or arterial vessels. Bronchial and intercostal vessels offer additional sources for significant bleeding. Signs may include bleeding from chest tube(s) or simply unexplained hypotension postoperatively. Pending return to surgery these cases are handled as with any other case of traumatic blood loss – with administration of crystalloid replacement – and blood products if necessary. In the case of massive hemoptysis, asphyxia remains the most immediate threat [37]. Immediate placement of an endobronchial tube may be lifesaving. An alternative approach reported includes rigid bronchoscopy with tamponade of the bleeding using an endobronchial blocker and/ or cotton pledgets soaked in a vasoconstrictor.

Neurologic Injuries

Thoracic surgery poses multiple risks for neurologic injury related to both positioning as well as the surgical dissection. The lateral decubitus position may lead to pressure and ischemic injury of the eye, ear, nose, and dependent skin –

particularly areas with a bony prominence such as the pelvis and sacrum. Excessive elevation of the non-dependent arm – or pressure on the dependent arm – may result in brachial plexus injury. Given their anatomic location, the radial, ulnar, sciatic, and peroneal nerves prove particularly vulnerable to pressure injury in the lateral position [108] (Table **14**). Generous use of soft padding and an axillary roll may mitigate risk for peripheral nerve injury. From the standpoint of the surgical procedure itself, intercostal nerve injury due to surgical dissection or pressure injury (*i.e.* retractors) remain common. Patients may experience postoperative numbness or pain in affected dermatomes [97, 103, 109]. Intercostal nerve injury may precede debilitating chronic pain syndrome in 2-3% of patients [84, 92, 94]. Both the recurrent laryngeal and phrenic nerves may be injured during surgical dissection [95 - 97]. Injury to the recurrent laryngeal may be associated with unilateral vocal cord paralysis and hoarseness. Phrenic nerve injury is characterized by elevation of the affected hemidiaphragm on CXR. In patients with marginal respiratory reserve, this may prove a serious complication leading to prolonged mechanical ventilation and increased risk for pneumonia.

Positioning Injuries Associated with Thoracic Surgery

Table 14. Positioning Injuries Associated with Thoracic Surgery (Modified from Gallagher C, Sladen R, Lubarsky D. "Thoracotomy Postoperative Complications" in Problems in Anesthesia "Thoracic Anesthesia" (Brodsky JB, ed) p. 400 4(2): 1990).

Structure	Injury
Eye	Corneal abrasion; ischemic injury (i.e. loss of vision)
Ear	Pressure necrosis
Nose	Pressure necrosis
Skin	Pressure ulcers
Brachial plexus	Palsy due to stretching or pressure
Radial nerve	Pressure induced carpal tunnel syndrome
Ulnar nerve	Palsy due to pressure on ulnar groove
Sciatic nerve	Palsy due to compression on dependent pelvis
Common peroneal nerve	Foot drop due to pressure on dependent fibula

(Modified from Gallagher C, Sladen R, Lubarsky D. "Thoracotomy Postoperative Complications" in Problems in Anesthesia "Thoracic Anesthesia" (Brodsky JB, ed) p. 400 4(2): 1990.)

CONCLUSION

Thoracic anesthesia remains a complex and challenging subspecialty of anesthesiology. Surgical advances including minimally invasive video assisted thoracoscopy (VATs) and robotic surgery offer life-saving (or life-prolonging) surgery for increasing numbers of patients. As age and comorbidities of this patient population grow, careful preoperative assessment and a thorough understanding of pulmonary and cardiovascular physiology prove critical to mitigating patient risk in the perioperative setting. A thorough preoperative evaluation with evaluation of respiratory and optimization of overall functional status remains the foundation for successful outcomes. Intraoperatively, technical facility with laryngoscopy, video laryngoscopy, and fiber-optic bronchoscopy prove essential to achieving lung isolation with both double lumen endotracheal tubes as well as endobronchial blockers. As video assisted (VAT) and robotic thoracoscopy increasingly displace open thoracotomy as preferred surgical approaches, evolution in our approaches to anesthetic care of these patients must occur. Mediastinoscopy, esophageal resection and tracheal surgery pose unique challenges as well. Increasingly, the importance of intraoperative fluid replacement, ventilatory management, and postoperative analgesia to patient morbidity and mortality has become apparent – with many questions yet to be answered by rigorous clinical research trials. Strong communication and cooperation between all perioperative staff remains key to safe and successful outcomes in thoracic surgery.

CONSENT FOR PUBLICATION

Not applicable.

CONFLICT OF INTEREST

The author (editor) declares no conflict of interest, financial or otherwise.

ACKNOWLEDGEMENT

Declared none.

REFERENCES

[1] Choi H, Mazzone P. Preoperative evaluation of the patient with lung cancer being considered for lung resection. Curr Opin Anaesthesiol 2015; 28: 18-25.
[http://dx.doi.org/10.1097/ACO.0000000000000149]

[2] Cottrell JJ, Ferson PF. Preoperative assessment of the thoracic surgical patient. Clin Chest Med 1992; 14: 47-53.

[3] Deng B, Cassivi SD, de Andrade M, *et al.* Clinical outcomes and changes in lung function after segmentectomy *versus* lobectomy for lung cancer cases. J Thorac Cardiovasc Surg 2014; 148: 1186-92 e3.

[4] Ediebah DE, Coens C, Zikos E, *et al.* Does change in health-related quality of life score predict survival? Analysis of EORTC 08975 lung cancer trial. Br J Cancer 2014; 110: 2427-33.
[http://dx.doi.org/10.1038/bjc.2014.208]

[5] Burris JL, Studts JL, DeRosa AP, Ostroff JS. Systematic review of tobacco use after lung or head/neck cancer diagnosis: Results and recommendations for future research. Cancer Epidemiol Biomarkers Prev 2015; 24(10): 1450-61.

[http://dx.doi.org/10.1158/1055-9965.EPI-15-0257]

[6]   Al-Zoughool M, Pintos J, Richardson L, *et al.* Exposure to environmental tobacco smoke (ETS) and risk of lung cancer in Montreal: a case-control study. Environ Health 2013; 12: 112.
        [http://dx.doi.org/10.1186/1476-069X-12-112]

[7]   Dresler C. The changing epidemic of lung cancer and occupational and environmental risk factors. Thorac Surg Clin 2013; 23: 113-22.
        [http://dx.doi.org/10.1016/j.thorsurg.2013.01.015]

[8]   Field RW, Withers BL. Occupational and environmental causes of lung cancer. Clin Chest Med 2012; 33: 681-703.
        [http://dx.doi.org/10.1016/j.ccm.2012.07.001]

[9]   Gamble J. Lung cancer and diesel exhaust: a critical review of the occupational epidemiology literature. Crit Rev Toxicol 2010; 40: 189-244.
        [http://dx.doi.org/10.3109/10408440903352818]

[10]   Ngamwong Y, Tangamornsuksan W, Lohitnavy O, *et al.* Additive Synergism between Asbestos and Smoking in Lung Cancer Risk: A Systematic Review and Meta-Analysis. PLoS One 2015; 10: e0135798.
        [http://dx.doi.org/10.1371/journal.pone.0135798]

[11]   Field RW, Smith BJ, Platz CE, *et al.* Lung cancer histologic type in the surveillance, epidemiology, and end results registry *versus* independent review. J Natl Cancer Inst 2004; 96: 1105-7.
        [http://dx.doi.org/10.1093/jnci/djh189]

[12]   Melloni BB. Lung cancer in never-smokers: radon exposure and environmental tobacco smoke. Eur Respir J 2014; 44: 850-2.
        [http://dx.doi.org/10.1183/09031936.00121314]

[13]   Puggina A, Broumas A, Ricciardi W, Boccia S. Cost-effectiveness of screening for lung cancerwith low-dose computed tomography: a systematic literature review. Eur J Public Health 2015.
        [http://dx.doi.org/10.1093/eurpub/ckv170.069]

[14]   Sharp L, Brewster D. The epidemiology of lung cancer in Scotland: a review of trends in incidence, survival and mortality and prospects for prevention. Health Bull (Edinb) 1999; 57: 318-31.

[15]   Kanou T, Okami J, Tokunaga T, *et al.* Prognosis associated with surgery for non-small cell lung cancer and synchronous brain metastasis. Surg Today 2014; 44: 1321-7.
        [http://dx.doi.org/10.1007/s00595-014-0895-3]

[16]   Zhang J, Gold KA, Lin HY, *et al.* Relationship between tumor size and survival in non-small-cell lung cancer (NSCLC): an analysis of the surveillance, epidemiology, and end results (SEER) registry. J Thorac Oncol 2015; 10: 682-90.
        [http://dx.doi.org/10.1097/JTO.0000000000000456]

[17]   Zhou F, Jiang T, Ma W, Gao G, Chen X, Zhou C. The impact of clinical characteristics on outcomes from maintenance therapy in non-small cell lung cancer: A systematic review with meta-analysis. Lung Cancer 2015; 89: 203-11.
        [http://dx.doi.org/10.1016/j.lungcan.2015.06.005]

[18]   Wood DE. Preoperative assessment of the thoracic surgery patient: introduction. Semin Thorac Cardiovasc Surg 2001; 13: 90-1.
        [http://dx.doi.org/10.1053/stcs.2001.26634]

[19]   Dales RE, Dionne G, Leech JA, Lunau M, Schweitzer I. Preoperative prediction of pulmonary complications following thoracic surgery. Chest 1993; 104: 155-9.
        [http://dx.doi.org/10.1378/chest.104.1.155]

[20]   Kretzschmar MA, Hachenberg T. Thoracic anesthesia. Curr Opin Anaesthesiol 2015; 28: 1.
        [http://dx.doi.org/10.1097/ACO.0000000000000158]

[21]   Phunmanee A, Tuntisirin C, Zaeoue U. Preoperative spirometry to predict postoperative complications in thoracic surgery patients. J Med Assoc Thai 2000; 83: 1253-9.

[22]   Trzaska-Sobczak M, Skoczynski S, Pierzchala W. Pulmonary function tests in the preoperative evaluation of lung cancer surgery candidates. A review of guidelines. Kardiochir Torakochirurgia Pol 2014; 11: 278-82.
[http://dx.doi.org/10.5114/kitp.2014.45677]

[23]   Culver BH. Preoperative assessment of the thoracic surgery patient: pulmonary function testing. Semin Thorac Cardiovasc Surg 2001; 13: 92-104.
[http://dx.doi.org/10.1053/stcs.2001.25041]

[24]   Teplick R. Preoperative cardiac assessment of the thoracic surgical patient. Chest Surg Clin N Am 1997; 7: 655-96.

[25]   Ueda S, Isogami K, Kobayashi S, Osawa N, Konnai T. Preoperative assessment of myocardial ischemia in thoracic surgery for lung cancer. Kyobu Geka 2007; 60: 1129-33.

[26]   Agostini P, Cieslik H, Rathinam S, *et al.* Postoperative pulmonary complications following thoracic surgery: are there any modifiable risk factors? Thorax 2010; 65: 815-8.
[http://dx.doi.org/10.1136/thx.2009.123083]

[27]   Aldrich JM, Gropper MA. Can we predict pulmonary complications after thoracic surgery? Anesth Analg 2010; 110: 1261-3.
[http://dx.doi.org/10.1213/ANE.0b013e3181d785c0]

[28]   Amar D, Munoz D, Shi W, Zhang H, Thaler HT. A clinical prediction rule for pulmonary complications after thoracic surgery for primary lung cancer. Anesth Analg 2010; 110: 1343-8.
[http://dx.doi.org/10.1213/ANE.0b013e3181bf5c99]

[29]   Yang M, Ahn HJ, Kim JA, Yu JM. Risk score for postoperative complications in thoracic surgery. Korean J Anesthesiol 2012; 63: 527-32.
[http://dx.doi.org/10.4097/kjae.2012.63.6.527]

[30]   Jaklitsch M, Billmeier S. Preoperative evaluation and risk assessment for elderly thoracic surgery patients. Thorac Surg Clin 2009; 19: 301-12.
[http://dx.doi.org/10.1016/j.thorsurg.2009.07.004]

[31]   Quraishi SA, Orkin FK, Roizen MF. The anesthesia preoperative assessment: an opportunity for smoking cessation intervention. J Clin Anesth 2006; 18: 635-40.
[http://dx.doi.org/10.1016/j.jclinane.2006.05.014]

[32]   Nomori H, Kobayashi R, Fuyuno G, Morinaga S, Yashima H. Preoperative respiratory muscle training. Assessment in thoracic surgery patients with special reference to postoperative pulmonary complications. Chest 1994; 105: 1782-8.
[http://dx.doi.org/10.1378/chest.105.6.1782]

[33]   Kozian A, Kretzschmar MA, Schilling T. Thoracic anesthesia in the elderly. Curr Opin Anaesthesiol 2015; 28: 2-9.
[http://dx.doi.org/10.1097/ACO.0000000000000152]

[34]   Dincq AS, Gourdin M, Collard E, *et al.* Anesthesia for adult rigid bronchoscopy. Acta Anaesthesiol Belg 2014; 65: 95-103.

[35]   Jose RJ, Shaefi S, Navani N. Anesthesia for bronchoscopy. Curr Opin Anaesthesiol 2014; 27: 453-7.
[http://dx.doi.org/10.1097/ACO.0000000000000087]

[36]   Thomsen RW. Mediastinoscopy and video-assisted thoracoscopic surgery: anesthetic pitfalls and complications. Semin Cardiothorac Vasc Anesth 2008; 12: 128-32.
[http://dx.doi.org/10.1177/1089253208319873]

[37]   Lohser J, Donington JS, Mitchell JD, Brodsky JB, Raman J, Slinger P. Case 5-2005: anesthetic management of major hemorrhage during mediastinoscopy. J Cardiothorac Vasc Anesth 2005; 19:

678-83. [clin conf].
[http://dx.doi.org/10.1053/j.jvca.2005.07.016]

[38]   El-Tahan MR. Anesthetic management of thoracoscopic lobectomy in a patient with severe
        biventricular dysfunction: thoracic anesthesia perspectives. J Cardiothorac Vasc Anesth 2015; 29: e48-
        9.
        [http://dx.doi.org/10.1053/j.jvca.2014.12.003]

[39]   Ashes C, Roscoe A. Transesophageal echocardiography in thoracic anesthesia: pulmonary
        hypertension and right ventricular function. Curr Opin Anaesthesiol 2015; 28: 38-44.
        [http://dx.doi.org/10.1097/ACO.0000000000000138]

[40]   Seo H, Lee G, Ha S, Song JG. An awake double lumen endotracheal tube intubation using the Clarus
        Video System in a patient with an epiglottic cyst: a case report. Korean J Anesthesiol 2014; 66: 157-9.
        [http://dx.doi.org/10.4097/kjae.2014.66.2.157]

[41]   Arndt GA, Buchika S, Kranner PW, DeLessio ST. Wire-guided endobronchial blockade in a patient
        with a limited mouth opening. Can J Anaesth 1999; 46: 87-9.
        [http://dx.doi.org/10.1007/BF03012521]

[42]   Russell T, Slinger P, Roscoe A, McRae K, Van Rensburg A. A randomised controlled trial comparing
        the GlideScope(®) and the Macintosh laryngoscope for double-lumen endobronchial intubation.
        Anaesthesia 2013; 68: 1253-8.
        [http://dx.doi.org/10.1111/anae.12322]

[43]   Howell S, Ata M, Ellison M, Wilson C. One-lung ventilation *via* tracheostomy and left endobronchial
        microlaryngeal tube. J Cardiothorac Vasc Anesth 2014; 28: 1052-4.
        [http://dx.doi.org/10.1053/j.jvca.2013.12.022]

[44]   Matei A, Tommaso Bizzarri F, Preveggenti V, Mancini M, Vicchio M, Agnoletti V. EZ-Blocker and
        One-Lung Ventilation *via* Tracheostomy. J Cardiothorac Vasc Anesth 2015; 29: e32-3.
        [http://dx.doi.org/10.1053/j.jvca.2015.02.005]

[45]   Brassard CL, Lohser J, Donati F, Bussieres JS. Step-by-step clinical management of one-lung
        ventilation: continuing professional development. Can J Anaesth 2014; 61: 1103-21.
        [http://dx.doi.org/10.1007/s12630-014-0246-2]

[46]   Eisenkraft JB. Effects of anaesthetics on the pulmonary circulation. Br J Anaesth 1990; 65: 63-78.
        [http://dx.doi.org/10.1093/bja/65.1.63]

[47]   Lohser J. Evidence-based management of one-lung ventilation. Anesthesiol Clin 2008; 26: 241-72.
        [http://dx.doi.org/10.1016/j.anclin.2008.01.011]

[48]   Bindslev L, Jolin A, Hedenstierna G, Baehrendtz S, Santesson J. Hypoxic pulmonary vasoconstriction
        in the human lung: effect of repeated hypoxic challenges during anesthesia. Anesthesiology 1985; 62:
        621-5.
        [http://dx.doi.org/10.1097/00000542-198505000-00014]

[49]   Van Keer L, Van Aken H, Vandermeersch E, Vermaut G, Lerut T. Propofol does not inhibit hypoxic
        pulmonary vasoconstriction in humans. J Clin Anesth 1989; 1: 284-8.
        [http://dx.doi.org/10.1016/0952-8180(89)90028-7]

[50]   Lumb AB, Slinger P. Hypoxic pulmonary vasoconstriction: physiology and anesthetic implications.
        Anesthesiology 2015; 122: 932-46.
        [http://dx.doi.org/10.1097/ALN.0000000000000569]

[51]   Pruszkowski O, Dalibon N, Moutafis M, *et al*. Effects of propofol *vs*. sevoflurane on arterial
        oxygenation during one-lung ventilation. Br J Anaesth 2007; 98: 539-44.
        [http://dx.doi.org/10.1093/bja/aem039]

[52]   Pardos PC, Garutti I, Pineiro P, Olmedilla L, de la Gala F. Effects of ventilatory mode during one-lung
        ventilation on intraoperative and postoperative arterial oxygenation in thoracic surgery. J Cardiothorac
        Vasc Anesth 2009; 23: 770-4.

[http://dx.doi.org/10.1053/j.jvca.2009.06.002]

[53]   Unzueta MC, Casas JI, Moral MV. Pressure-controlled *versus* volume-controlled ventilation during one-lung ventilation for thoracic surgery. Anesth Analg 2007; 104: 1029-33.
[http://dx.doi.org/10.1213/01.ane.0000260313.63893.2f]

[54]   Roze H, Lafargue M, Batoz H, *et al.* Pressure-controlled ventilation and intrabronchial pressure during one-lung ventilation. Br J Anaesth 2010; 105: 377-81.

[55]   Karzai W, Schwarzkopf K. Hypoxemia during one-lung ventilation: prediction, prevention, and treatment. Anesthesiology 2009; 110: 1402-11.
[http://dx.doi.org/10.1097/ALN.0b013e31819fb15d]

[56]   Hogue CW Jr. Effectiveness of low levels of nonventilated lung continuous positive airway pressure in improving arterial oxygenation during one-lung ventilation. Anesth Analg 1994; 79: 364-7.
[http://dx.doi.org/10.1213/00000539-199408000-00029]

[57]   Doering EB, Hanson CW III, Reily DJ, Marshall C, Marshall BE. Improvement in oxygenation by phenylephrine and nitric oxide in patients with adult respiratory distress syndrome. Anesthesiology 1997; 87: 18-25.
[http://dx.doi.org/10.1097/00000542-199707000-00004]

[58]   Raghunathan K, Connelly NR, Robbins LD, Ganim R, Hochheiser G, DiCampli R. Inhaled epoprostenol during one-lung ventilation. Ann Thorac Surg 2010; 89: 981-3.
[http://dx.doi.org/10.1016/j.athoracsur.2009.07.059]

[59]   Murcia Sanchez E, German MJ, Ibanez V, Perez-Cerda F. Anesthetic management for mediastinoscopy in a patient with severe pulmonary hypertension. Rev Esp Anestesiol Reanim 2007; 54: 55-6.

[60]   Pathak V, Welsby I, Mahmood K, Wahidi M, MacIntyre N, Shofer S. Ventilation and anesthetic approaches for rigid bronchoscopy. Ann Am Thorac Soc 2014; 11: 628-34.
[http://dx.doi.org/10.1513/AnnalsATS.201309-302FR]

[61]   Kaur H, Dhooria S, Aggarwal AN, Gupta D, Behera D, Agarwal R. A Randomized Trial of 1% *vs.* 2% Lignocaine by the Spray-as-You-Go Technique for Topical Anesthesia During Flexible Bronchoscopy. Chest 2015; 148: 739-45.
[http://dx.doi.org/10.1378/chest.15-0022]

[62]   Wahidi MM, Jain P, Jantz M, *et al.* American College of Chest Physicians consensus statement on the use of topical anesthesia, analgesia, and sedation during flexible bronchoscopy in adult patients. Chest 2011; 140: 1342-50.
[http://dx.doi.org/10.1378/chest.10-3361]

[63]   Swanson NJ. Mediastinoscopy: its anesthetic considerations. AANA J 1977; 45: 290-5.

[64]   Buise M, Van Bommel J, Mehra M, Tilanus HW, Van Zundert A, Gommers D. Pulmonary morbidity following esophagectomy is decreased after introduction of a multimodal anesthetic regimen. Acta Anaesthesiol Belg 2008; 59: 257-61.

[65]   Ng JM. Perioperative anesthetic management for esophagectomy. Anesthesiol Clin 2008; 26: 293-304.
[http://dx.doi.org/10.1016/j.anclin.2008.01.004]

[66]   Ng JM. Update on anesthetic management for esophagectomy. Curr Opin Anaesthesiol 2011; 24: 37-43.
[http://dx.doi.org/10.1097/ACO.0b013e32834141f7]

[67]   Gu CY, Zhang J, Qian YN, Tang QF. Effects of epidural anesthesia and postoperative epidural analgesia on immune function in esophageal carcinoma patients undergoing thoracic surgery. Mol Clin Oncol 2015; 3: 190-6.
[http://dx.doi.org/10.3892/mco.2014.405]

[68]   Hsin MK, Yim AP. Management of complications of minimally invasive thoracic surgery.

Respirology 2010; 15: 6-18.
[http://dx.doi.org/10.1111/j.1440-1843.2009.01653.x]

[69]   Lochowski MP, Kozak J. Video-assisted thoracic surgery complications. Wideochir Inne Tech Malo Inwazyjne 2014; 9: 495-500.
[http://dx.doi.org/10.5114/wiitm.2014.44250]

[70]   McKenna RJ Jr. Complications and learning curves for video-assisted thoracic surgery lobectomy. Thorac Surg Clin 2008; 18: 275-80.
[http://dx.doi.org/10.1016/j.thorsurg.2008.04.004]

[71]   Kuritzky AM, Ng T. Video-assisted thoracic surgery *vs.* Muscle-sparing thoracotomy: Prioritizing randomized trial to assess complications and long-term survival over cost comparisons: In reply to spartalis and colleagues. J Am Coll Surg 2015; 221: 890-1.
[http://dx.doi.org/10.1016/j.jamcollsurg.2015.07.001]

[72]   Solaini L, Prusciano F, Bagioni P, di Francesco F, Solaini L, Poddie DB. Video-assisted thoracic surgery (VATS) of the lung: analysis of intraoperative and postoperative complications over 15 years and review of the literature. Surg Endosc 2008; 22: 298-310.
[http://dx.doi.org/10.1007/s00464-007-9586-0]

[73]   Campos JH. An update on robotic thoracic surgery and anesthesia. Curr Opin Anaesthesiol 2010; 23: 1-6.
[http://dx.doi.org/10.1097/ACO.0b013e3283336547]

[74]   Zhang Y, Wang S, Sun Y. Anesthesia of robotic thoracic surgery. Ann Transl Med 2015; 3: 71.

[75]   Campos J, Ueda K. Update on anesthetic complications of robotic thoracic surgery. Minerva Anestesiol 2014; 80: 83-8.

[76]   Sandberg W. Anesthesia and airway management for tracheal resection and reconstruction. Int Anesthesiol Clin 2000; 38: 55-75.
[http://dx.doi.org/10.1097/00004311-200001000-00005]

[77]   Mentzelopoulos SD, Romana CN, Hatzimichalis AG, Tzoufi MJ, Karamichali EA. Anesthesia for tracheal resection: a new technique of airway management in a patient with severe stenosis of the midtrachea. Anesth Analg 1999; 89: 1156-60.
[http://dx.doi.org/10.1213/00000539-199911000-00013]

[78]   Hobai IA, Chhangani SV, Alfille PH. Anesthesia for tracheal resection and reconstruction. Anesthesiol Clin 2012; 30: 709-30.
[http://dx.doi.org/10.1016/j.anclin.2012.08.012]

[79]   Young-Beyer P, Wilson RS. Anesthetic management for tracheal resection and reconstruction. J Cardiothorac Anesth 1988; 2: 821-35.
[http://dx.doi.org/10.1016/0888-6296(88)90109-3]

[80]   Loizzi D, Sollitto F, De Palma A, Pagliarulo V, Di Giglio I, Loizzi M. Tracheal resection with patient under local anesthesia and conscious sedation. Ann Thorac Surg 2013; 95: e63-5.
[http://dx.doi.org/10.1016/j.athoracsur.2012.08.068]

[81]   Vachhani S, Tsai JY, Moon T. Tracheal resection with regional anesthesia. J Clin Anesth 2014; 26: 697-8.
[http://dx.doi.org/10.1016/j.jclinane.2014.10.001]

[82]   Zhu B, Ma LL, Ye TH, Huang YG. Anesthesia management of tracheal resection. Chin Med J (Engl) 2010; 123: 3725-7.

[83]   Baki ED, Oz G, Kokulu S, *et al.* Comparison of transcutaneous electrical nerve stimulation and paravertebral block for postthoracotomy pain relief. Thorac Cardiovasc Surg 2015; 63: 514-8.
[http://dx.doi.org/10.1055/s-0035-1544212]

[84]   Kinney MA, Hooten WM, Cassivi SD, *et al.* Chronic postthoracotomy pain and health-related quality

of life. Ann Thorac Surg 2012; 93: 1242-7.
[http://dx.doi.org/10.1016/j.athoracsur.2012.01.031]

[85]   De Cosmo G, Aceto P, Gualtieri E, Congedo E. Analgesia in thoracic surgery. Minerva Anestesiol 2009; 75: 393-400. [review].

[86]   Nielsen DV, Bhavsar R, Greisen J, Ryhammer PK, Sloth E, Jakobsen CJ. High thoracic epidural analgesia in cardiac surgery. Part 2--high thoracic epidural analgesia does not reduce time in or improve quality of recovery in the intensive care unit. J Cardiothorac Vasc Anesth 2012; 26: 1048-54.
[http://dx.doi.org/10.1053/j.jvca.2012.05.008]

[87]   Romero A, Garcia JE, Joshi GP. The state of the art in preventing postthoracotomy pain. Semin Thorac Cardiovasc Surg 2013; 25: 116-24.
[http://dx.doi.org/10.1053/j.semtcvs.2013.04.002]

[88]   Steinthorsdottir KJ, Wildgaard L, Hansen HJ, Petersen RH, Wildgaard K. Regional analgesia for video-assisted thoracic surgery: a systematic review. Eur J Cardiothorac Surg 2014; 45: 959-66.
[http://dx.doi.org/10.1093/ejcts/ezt525]

[89]   Cioffi U, Raveglia F, Rizzi A, Di Mauro P, De Simone M, Baisi A. Paravertebral analgesia in video-assisted thoracic surgery: A new hybrid technique of catheter placement for continuous anesthetic infusionf. Thorac Cardiovasc Surg 2015; 63: 533-4.
[http://dx.doi.org/10.1055/s-0034-1396426]

[90]   Nosotti M, Rosso L, Tosi D, et al. Preventive analgesia in thoracic surgery: controlled, randomized, double-blinded studydagger. Eur J Cardiothorac Surg 2015; 48: 428-34.
[http://dx.doi.org/10.1093/ejcts/ezu467]

[91]   Brulotte V, Ruel MM, Lafontaine E, Chouinard P, Girard F. Impact of pregabalin on the occurrence of postthoracotomy pain syndrome: a randomized trial. Reg Anesth Pain Med 2015; 40: 262-9.
[http://dx.doi.org/10.1097/AAP.0000000000000241]

[92]   Hu J, Liao Q, Zhang F, Tong J, Ouyang W. Chronic postthoracotomy pain and perioperative ketamine infusion. J Pain Palliat Care Pharmacother 2014; 28: 117-21.
[http://dx.doi.org/10.3109/15360288.2014.908992]

[93]   Ryu HG, Lee CJ, Kim YT, Bahk JH. Preemptive low-dose epidural ketamine for preventing chronic postthoracotomy pain: a prospective, double-blinded, randomized, clinical trial. Clin J Pain 2011; 27: 304-8.
[http://dx.doi.org/10.1097/AJP.0b013e3181fd5187]

[94]   Wildgaard K, Ringsted TK, Aasvang EK, Ravn J, Werner MU, Kehlet H. Neurophysiological characterization of persistent postthoracotomy pain. Clin J Pain 2012; 28: 136-42.
[http://dx.doi.org/10.1097/AJP.0b013e3182261650]

[95]   Thangathurai D, Roffey P, Mogos M, Raid M, Mikhail M. Anesthetic implications of recurrent laryngeal nerve palsy after esophagectomy. J Cardiothorac Vasc Anesth 2004; 18: 822.
[http://dx.doi.org/10.1053/j.jvca.2004.08.032]

[96]   Benouaich V, Porterie J, Bouali O, Moscovici J, Lopez R. Anatomical basis of the risk of injury to the right laryngeal recurrent nerve during thoracic surgery. Surg Radiol Anat 2012; 34: 509-12.
[http://dx.doi.org/10.1007/s00276-012-0946-7]

[97]   Krasna MJ, Forti G. Nerve injury: injury to the recurrent laryngeal, phrenic, vagus, long thoracic, and sympathetic nerves during thoracic surgery. Thorac Surg Clin 2006; 16: 267-75. [vi.].
[http://dx.doi.org/10.1016/j.thorsurg.2006.05.003]

[98]   Welter S, Cheufou D, Darwiche K, Stamatis G. Tracheal injuries, fistulae from bronchial stump and bronchial anastomoses and recurrent laryngeal nerve paralysis: management of complications in thoracic surgery. Chirurg 2015; 86: 410-8.
[http://dx.doi.org/10.1007/s00104-014-2862-3]

[99]   Suemitsu R, Sakoguchi T, Morikawa K, Yamaguchi M, Tanaka H, Takeo S. Effect of body mass index

on perioperative complications in thoracic surgery. Asian Cardiovasc Thorac Ann 2008; 16: 463-7.
[http://dx.doi.org/10.1177/021849230801600607]

[100] Fernandes EO, Teixeira C, Silva LC. Thoracic surgery: risk factors for postoperative complications of lung resection. Rev Assoc Med Bras 2011; 57: 292-8.
[http://dx.doi.org/10.1590/S0104-42302011000300011]

[101] Rotman JA, Plodkowski AJ, Hayes SA, *et al.* Postoperative complications after thoracic surgery for lung cancer. Clin Imaging 2015; 39: 735-49.
[http://dx.doi.org/10.1016/j.clinimag.2015.05.013]

[102] Popping DM, Elia N, Marret E, Remy C, Tramer MR. Protective effects of epidural analgesia on pulmonary complications after abdominal and thoracic surgery: a meta-analysis. Arch Surg 2008; 143: 990-9.
[http://dx.doi.org/10.1001/archsurg.143.10.990]

[103] Cooper L. Postoperative complications after thoracic surgery in the morbidly obese patient. Anesthesiol Res Pract 2011; 2011: 865634.
[http://dx.doi.org/10.1155/2011/865634]

[104] Christensen JD, Seaman DM, Washington L. Imaging of complications of thoracic and cardiovascular surgery. Radiol Clin North Am 2014; 52: 929-59.
[http://dx.doi.org/10.1016/j.rcl.2014.05.003]

[105] Yano M, Yokoi K, Numanami H, *et al.* Complications of bronchial stapling in thoracic surgery. World J Surg 2014; 38: 341-6.
[http://dx.doi.org/10.1007/s00268-013-2292-2]

[106] De Decker K, Jorens PG, Van Schil P. Cardiac complications after noncardiac thoracic surgery: an evidence-based current review. Ann Thorac Surg 2003; 75: 1340-8.
[http://dx.doi.org/10.1016/S0003-4975(02)04824-5]

[107] Komori C, Hanaoka K. Anesthesia for thoracic surgery in elderly patients. Kyobu Geka 2005; 58: 607-12.

[108] Cheney FW, Domino KB, Caplan RA, Posner KL. Nerve injury associated with anesthesia: a closed claims analysis. Anesthesiology 1999; 90: 1062-9.
[http://dx.doi.org/10.1097/00000542-199904000-00020]

[109] Hogan QH. Pathophysiology of peripheral nerve injury during regional anesthesia. Reg Anesth Pain Med 2008; 33: 435-41.
[http://dx.doi.org/10.1097/00115550-200809000-00006]

[110] Ishibe Y, Shiokawa Y, Umeda T, Uno H, Nakamura M, Izumi T. The effect of thoracic epidural anesthesia on hypoxic pulmonary vasoconstriction in dogs: an analysis of the pressure-flow curve. Anesth Analg 1996; 82: 1049-55.

[111] Pearl RG, Finn JC. Hemodynamic effects of diltiazem during vasoconstrictor pulmonary hypertension in sheep. Anesth Analg 1990; 71: 493-7.
[http://dx.doi.org/10.1213/00000539-199011000-00007]

CHAPTER 3

Cardiac Anesthesia

Jeffrey Dodd-o[*]

Johns Hopkins Medical Institutions, Baltimore, Maryland, USA

Abstract: Cardiac anesthesia encompasses the care of patients with cardiac disease; it is not limited to the care of patients undergoing cardiac surgery. In order to provide a successful cardiac anesthetic, it is imperative to understand fundamental aspects of cardiovascular physiology. These concepts include preload, afterload, and contractility; and how they relate to pressure-work *versus* volume-work for the heart. These concepts guide the management of specific disease conditions such as aortic stenosis, aortic insufficiency, mitral stenosis, mitral insufficiency, hypertrophic cardiomyopathy, as well as systolic heart failure and diastolic heart failure. A brief introduction to ventricular assist devices is included as well.

Keywords: Afterload, Aortic Insufficiency, Aortic Stenosis, Contractility, Diastolic Heart Failure, Hypertrophic Cardiomyopathy, Mitral Insufficiency, Mitral Stenosis, Preload, Pressure Work, Systolic Heart Failure, Ventricular Assist Devices (VADS), Volume Work.

INTRODUCTION

Cardiac anesthesia encompasses the care of patients with cardiac disease; it is not limited to the care of patients undergoing cardiac surgery. In order to provide a successful cardiac anesthetic, it is imperative to understand the fundamental aspects of cardiovascular physiology (Figs. **1 - 4**). These concepts include preload, afterload, and contractility; and how they relate to pressure-work *versus* volume-work for the heart. These concepts guide the management of specific disease conditions such as aortic stenosis, aortic insufficiency, mitral stenosis, mitral insufficiency, hypertrophic cardiomyopathy, as well as systolic heart failure and diastolic heart failure. A brief introduction to ventricular assist devices is included as well.

[*] **Corresponding author Jeffrey Dodd-o:** Johns Hopkins Medical Institutions, Baltimore, Maryland, USA; Tel: (410) 955-5000; E-mail: jdoddo@jhmi.edu

Amballur D. John (Ed.)

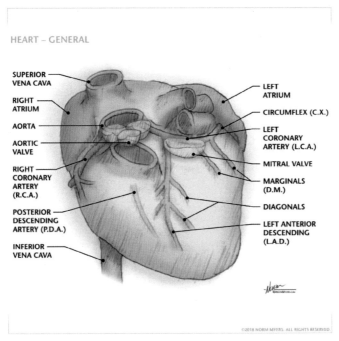

Fig. (1). Heart General. Image provided by Norm Myers.

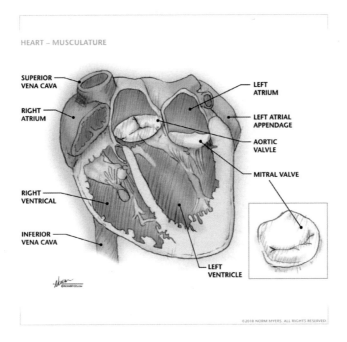

Fig. (2). Heart Musculature. Image provided by Norm Myers.

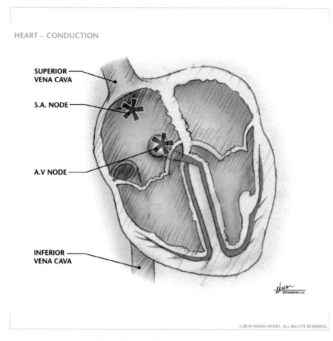

Fig. (3). Heart Conduction. Image provided by Norm Myers.

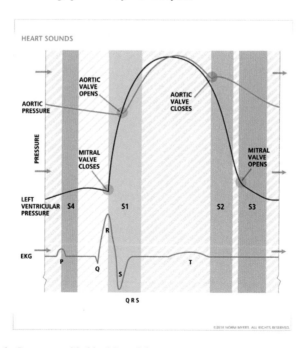

Fig. (4). Heart Sounds. Image provided by Norm Myers.

PRELOAD, AFTERLOAD AND CONTRACTILITY

PRELOAD

Preload, on a cellular level, is the amount of linear distending force on a myocyte. This determines the position of the myocyte's intracellular contractile elements relative to one another. The relative position of these intracellular contractile elements changes their sensitivity to calcium [1]. Since calcium allows the contractile myofilaments to interact with one another, any change in sensitivity to calcium alters the efficiency and effectiveness of the myocyte's contraction efforts. On a ventricular level, preload refers to the amount of blood contained within the ventricle at end diastole (*i.e.* – immediately prior to contraction initiation). It is not difficult to imagine how this volume could influence the linear distending force on each myocyte comprising the ventricle. Thus, preload determines the contractile efficiency and effectiveness of the individual myocytes comprising the chamber, and of the chamber as a whole. However, preload also refers to the amount of blood available to be ejected by the ventricle. In this regard, preload determines the maximal stroke volume possible by the ventricle in that preload is the amount of blood available to be ejected in any given beat.

AFTERLOAD

Afterload is the **amount of force preventing contraction of a myocyte or a chamber**. From a myocardial chamber point of view, it is determined principally by the point of greatest impediment to flow between that chamber and the capillary system. It can therefore be generated by a stenotic cardiac valve, by constricted resistance vessels, or by any point in between. Afterload to atrial contraction could also be generated by a regurgitant aortic (for left atrium) or pulmonary (for right atrium) valve. For example, aortic regurgitation raises the pressure in the left ventricle during ventricle diastole, when the atrium is trying to contract. Similarly, a drop in ventricular compliance from any cause (concentric ventricular hypertrophy, ischemia compromising ventricular relaxation, infiltrative myocardial process) will make ventricular distension more difficult and raise afterload to atrial contraction.

CONTRACTILITY

Contractility is the force with which a myocyte can shorten or a chamber can become smaller. It is influenced by the construct of the myocytes' intracellular contractile apparatus, the relative position of the component contractile elements when contraction is initiated (*i.e.* preload), the availability of ions (calcium) and mediators (cAMP) which promote the interaction of contractile elements, the sensitivity of the myofilaments to these factors promoting myofilament interaction, and the availability of energy (to allow the aligned contractile elements to move relative to one another). <u>Intracellular cAMP</u> levels can be raised by beta-receptor stimulation and by phosphodiesterase III inhibitors. Because these two approaches share neither the same mechanism nor receptor (β-agonist increases cAMP production through β-receptor stimulation, phosphodiesterase III inhibitors prevent cAMP breakdown through inhibition of its metabolizing enzyme), these two agents can be used simultaneously with syngeneic effects.

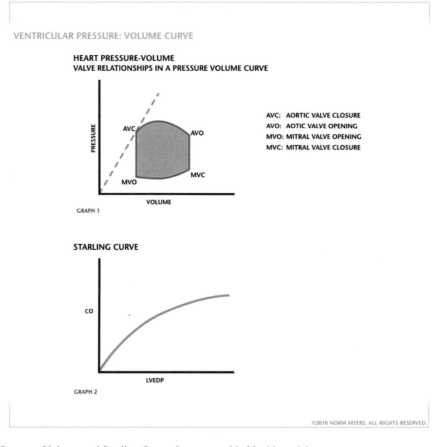

Fig. (5). Pressure Volume and Starling Curve. Image provided by Norm Myers.

Interaction Between Preload, Afterload and Contractility

The influence of preload and contractility on cardiac output is classically represented by the **Frank-Starling Curve** (Fig. **5**, Graph 2). A look at the **left ventricular pressure volume relationship** (Fig. **5**, Graph 1, Fig. **6**) may better depict the interaction between preload, afterload, contractility, compliance and cardiac output. When viewing the ventricular pressure-volume relationship, there are separate relationships for diastole and systole. In Fig. (**6**) **Points A and D** represent the End Systolic Volume. **Point D** is the onset of isovolumetric relaxation, while **Point A** is the opening of the mitral valve and the onset of passive (followed by active) ventricular filling. **Points B and C** represent End Diastolic Volume, and ventricular preload especially. **Point B** is the point at which isovolumetric ventricular contraction begins, and intraventricular pressure rises. **Point C** is the point at which ventricular pressure has risen high enough to open the aortic valve, and the ventricle begins to eject. **Point D** is the point at which the pressure in the ventricle no longer exceeds that of the aorta. The aortic valve closes, ventricular ejection stops, and isovolumetric ventricular relaxation begins.

Note that:

1. Volume is on the X axis and Pressure in on the Y axis
2. The height along the Y axis at which point "B" occurs is the maximum pressure that the atrium can generate. When the ventricular pressure rises above this point, ventricular filling ceases. During ventricular filling (early filling and atrial contraction), the ventricular volume therefore, increases (*i.e.* you move to the right along the X axis of the diastolic PV curve) until the height of this curve on the Y axis surpasses the pressure that can be generated by the atrium.
3. The horizontal distance between **point C** and **point D** is the **stroke volume**. As adaptations allow preload to be further increased, points "B" and "C" move farther to the right along the "volume axis" of the Diastolic PV relationship curve. The horizontal distance between EDV (point "C") and ESV (point "D") increases. Stroke volume therefore increases. As afterload increases (*i.e.* points "C" and "D" occur higher on the Y axis), point "D" intersects the systolic PV curve at a point farther right along the X axis. Thus, stroke volume is decreased.
4. As **diastolic compliance** decreases, the diastolic PV curve gets more vertical. Atrial contraction fills the LV until the ventricular pressure exceeds the limit of pressure that the atrium can generate. If the diastolic PV curve gets more vertical, the atrial pressure limit is reached without traveling as far along the X-axis (point B). Thus, the volume within the ventricle at EDV is less and stroke volume decreases.
5. As inotropy increases (*i.e.* the systolic PV relationship gets more steep), **point "D"** on the curve **will move more to the left**. This means the ESV will be smaller, and the stroke volume will be larger.
6. The relationship between preload and cardiac output depicted by the Frank-Starling Curve is not shown by the Left Ventricular PV curve. The change in cardiac output as a function of preload depicted by the **Frank-Starling Curve** reflects as change in the contractile function of the ventricle as its preload is

increased. The systolic contractility curve of the <u>Left Ventricular PV curve</u> assumes a constant preload. Any effect on stroke volume of a preload-dependent change in contractile function, which is the real relationship displayed in the Frank-Starling Curve, is not captured by the Left Ventricular PV curve.

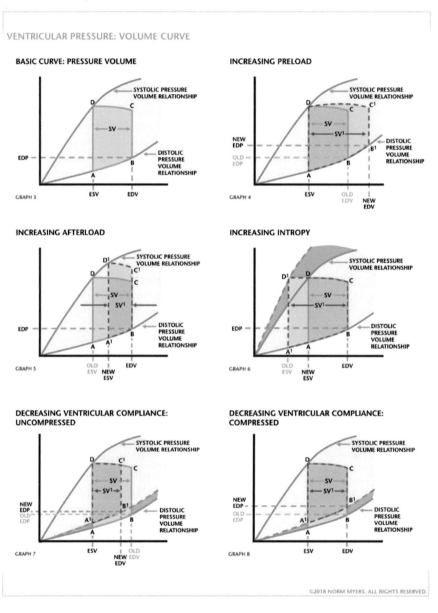

Fig. (6). Pressure Volume Curves Effect of Preload and Afterload. Image provided by Norm Myers.

7. On the systolic pressure:volume curve, a more vertical slope represents greater contractility independent of preload, while a more horizontal slope represents a lesser contractility. When examining the diastolic pressure:volume relationship, a more vertical slope depicts decreased compliance and a more horizontal slope depicts increased compliance.

PRESSURE WORK, VOLUME WORK AND THEIR ROLE IN CARDIAC VALVULAR DISEASE

Physiologic Response to Pressure Loading

Hearts adapted to chronic pressure load (*e.g.* Aortic stenosis, severe hypertension) do so by increasing wall thickness without increasing the chamber size (*i.e.* concentric hypertrophy). This reduces the energy demands on individual myocytes, as dictated by the Physics Law of LaPlace (Tension = [pressure*radius]/[2*wall thickness]). The **Law of LaPlace** states that the tension placed on any segment of the wall of a sphere is directly related to the pressure contained within the sphere and to the radius of a sphere. It is indirectly related to the thickness of the wall of the sphere. Limiting the radius of a ventricular chamber and increasing the thickness of the chamber wall therefore, limit the tension which must be generated by any myocyte in order to contract that chamber. Thus, individual myocytes are not at the limit of their capacity to generate tension, and could generate more (if needed) to overcome a sudden increase in the afterload. **Concentric hypertrophy** is therefore an effective mode of adaptation to a pressure load. Unfortunately, the burden of generating pressure still increases the energy requirements of the wall as a whole. Because the neovascularization to the pressure-loaded, hypertrophic heart is inadequate, oxygen supply:demand may be further compromised.

As with any adaptive process, concentric hypertrophy does have potentially **deleterious sequelae**. The process is associated with an increase in collagen and fibrous deposition. This limits the ease and extent of myocyte elastic recoil following contraction. This translates into decreased chamber compliance, and the need for a greater distending force within the chamber to allow a comparable volume of blood entry. Finally, endocardial ischemia can develop. Because myocardial perfusion is provided by vessels traveling from the epicardium to the endocardium, elevating the pressure within the chamber decreases the transmyocardial perfusion pressure gradient and impairs perfusion to the endocardium. That is to say, the blood perfusing left ventricular wall myocytes travels from the epicardium to the endocardium. The perfusing pressure in the epicardial coronary vasculature is the aortic pressure during diastole, because the left ventricle gets perfused only during diastole. In the absence of coronary occlusive disease, the downstream pressure in the endocardial vessels is equal to the pressure in the LV chamber (*i.e.* LVEDP). Decreasing LV compliance therefore risks compromising LV myocardial perfusion by increasing LVEDP and decreasing the perfusing gradient across the LV wall.

It is easy to envision how a process which causes ventricular pressure work can increase intraventricular end diastolic pressure at a rapidly escalating rate. In the case of aortic stenosis, for example, an increasingly stenotic valve raises the ventricular wall stress to promote concentric hypertrophy. This brings with it a decrease in ventricular compliance and a rise in LVEDP. Along with this, a progression of aortic stenosis impedes ventricular emptying. More blood therefore remains in the ventricle at end ejection, compounding the rise in intraventricular pressure. This results in more wall stress, and promotes further concentric hypertrophy.

Pressure-loaded ventricles whose impediment to ejection is suddenly removed (*e.g.* correction of aortic stenosis or a sudden "normalization" of systolic pressure in a chronically hypertensive patient) should demonstrate contractile function which is similar or better than it was when the pressure load was present. The potential risk is one of inadequate chamber filling. **Ventricular compliance** takes considerable time to recover following relief of a pressure load. Thus, elevated intraventricular pressures continue to be necessary to adequately fill the ventricle. With ventricular emptying facilitated by resolution of aortic stenosis or hypertension, more time is required to completely fill the ventricle. Adequate ventricular filling can sometimes be improved with rate controlling agents.

Physiologic Response to Volume Loading Conditions

Volume loaded cardiac states (*i.e.* cardiomegaly) suggest systolic contractile function is becoming insufficient to maintain adequate end organ perfusion.Insufficient end organ perfusion may represent either a low- or a high-cardiac output state. In **low cardiac output** cardiomegaly, increased ventricular volume is an adaptation that allows the heart to approximate a normal stroke volume and cardiac output in spite of having a reduced ejection fraction. That is to say, a ventricle which is trying to achieve a stroke volume of 60 ml with an ejection fraction of 30% will require twice the starting volume as a heart which is trying to achieve that same stroke volume with an ejection fraction of 60% (*i.e.* starting volume 200 ml *vs.* 100 ml). Cardiomegaly can therefore occur as an adaptation to decreased cardiac output from myocardium weakened by ischemia, infarction or inflammation (infectious or autoimmune).

In **high output** cardiomegaly, alternatively, increased ventricular volume is an adaptation to allow the heart to achieve abnormally high cardiac outputs which have become necessary because ejected blood is not efficiently directed towards end organ perfusion. In this setting, intracardiac shunts (*e.g.* mitral/tricuspid regurgitation, or a defect in the atrial or ventricular septum) or systemic shunts (*e.g.* arterio-venous shunts from dialysis fistulae, hepatic failure, *etc.*) may direct large portions of the arterial flow to the venous system without ever perfusing the microvasculature. In conditions of high output failure, the strength of contraction suggested by a normal or elevated ejected volume on imaging studies may be deceptive. That is to say, conditions in which microvascular perfusion is bypassed decrease the resistance against which the heart must contract and may therefore give a false impression as to the contractile strength of the heart. *In this regard, a patient with an LVEF of 40% in hepatic failure likely has a weaker heart than an otherwise healthy patient with an LVEF of 40%. Resolving the hepatic failure will, therefore, unmask this poor function.*

The list of conditions which can depress contractile function and precipitate hypervolemia is long. Many of these conditions share activation of the rennin-angiotensin-aldosterone and adrenergic systems as an associated feature. They also share a **histologic pattern** of collagen loss, fibrosis which is only patchy in distribution, and intracellular loss of cytoskeleton and myofibril proteins. Never-the-less, progression of the functional and histologic deterioration cannot be prevented by pharmacologic blockade of the rennin-angiotensin-aldosterone or adrenergic systems. There is some hope that functional deterioration may be reduced by blocking an injury cascade whereby increased release of macrophage chimases leads to free radical production and dephosphorylation of focal adhesion kinases [2].

As explained above, dilated cardiac conditions often represent a state of compromised contractility. This may be the case in spite of normal values of ventricular ejection fraction values as determined by surface imaging. In these patients it is therefore important to avoid intra-operative conditions which increase resistance to antegrade flow out of the aortic valve. It is also prudent to have available inotropes which can augment ventricular contractile function. This is particularly important to keep in mind when the dilated cardiac condition is associated with a high output cardiac state whose etiology will be corrected by the surgical procedure (*e.g.* mitral regurgitation). Since such procedures acutely close shunts which bypass microvascular perfusion, the entire cardiac output suddenly becomes subjected to the increased afterload of the systemic microvasculature. This can unmask pre-existing compromised contractile function and result in systolic heart failure.

Ramifications of Pressure Load *vs.* Volume Load For Anesthesiologist

The body employs distinct adaptive mechanisms to deal with pressure and volume loading. These different mechanisms have contrasting effects on energy supply:demand ratios. A ventricle which is chronically exposed to high afterload will concentrically hypertrophy. This reduces wall stress by LaPlace's Law. The cost for this concentric hypertrophy is a higher energy requirement to sustain the increased tissue mass. By contrast, a heart in whose cardiac output is inadequate due to limited energy supply (*i.e.* ischemia) or peripheral dilation which shunts blood away from vital organs (*i.e.* low afterload) avoids concentric hypertrophy. In these settings, the heart increases systemic perfusion through volume loading and production of supra-normal cardiac output.

The **supply:demand balance** should also guide the anesthesiologist's cardiovascular intervention when supporting a patient whose heart is tasked with pressure or volume work. When **pressure work** is required, as in the setting of valvular stenosis, the energy requirement for ventricular contraction is high. To limit this energy need, it is ideal to minimize the heart rate as much as possible. Since ventricular perfusion is highest during ventricular diastole, a slower heart rate also allows for improved ventricular perfusion. **Thus, the general rule is to keep the heart rate <u>S</u>low in the setting of valvular <u>S</u>tenosis**.

By contrast, energy demands are less limiting when cardiomegaly has developed to compensate for **volume work** (Frank-Starling Effect). Particularly when cardiomegaly has developed as an adaptation to valvular insufficiency, and most notably when it is aortic valve insufficiency, a prolonged diastolic phase can be detrimental to systemic perfusion. With valvular insufficiency, forward flow occurs only when chamber pressures are elevated to a level above that of the distal chamber. That is to say, the left ventricle can eject antegrade only when its pressure exceeds that of the aorta. When the ventricle relaxes, its pressure drops below that of the aorta and antegrade flow ceases. If there is aortic valvular insufficiency, there is nothing to prevent aortic blood flowing back into the left ventricle when left ventricular pressure drops below that of the aorta. In this situation, when energy requirements of the thin LV are relatively low and the negative consequences of prolonged diastole are high, a more rapid heartrate is advantages. Thus, the general rule is to keep the heart rate **<u>R</u>**apid in the setting of valvular **<u>R</u>**egurgitation.

Acute overload (pressure or volume) tends to cause much more lability and unanticipated chamber failure. This is related to a **cascade** of a sudden rise in wall chamber pressure –> rapid rise in wall tension –> decrease in perfusion pressure (especially if there is new hypotension simultaneously) –> ischemia.

ANESTHETIC CONSIDERATIONS FOR SPECIFIC LESIONS

AORTIC STENOSIS (AoS)

PRE-OP INFO: Distinguish whether ventricle is dilated (systolic function beginning to fail) *vs.* concentric hypertrophy; Determine presence of associated Aortic Insufficiency (adds volume loading and drops diastolic pressure to lower coronary perfusion pressure); Distinguish sinus rhythm *vs.* atrial fibrillation (atrial sinus contribution up to 40%); Determine left ventricular function (Is current rhythm same as rhythm at time of evaluation?) and aortic valve area

INTRA-OP: defibrillation pads; monitor leads II, V_5, available beta-blocker and amiodarone; available pure α agonist; available volume resuscitation; pre-load reducer (TNG) rather than pure afterload reducing agent (nitroprusside); The most common risk in aortic stenosis is heart failure precipitated by ischemia, hypovolemia, or dysrhythmia; The concentrically hypertrophic left ventricle, if undilated, typically has retained systolic contractile function but has some degree of diastolic dysfunction. This poor ventricular compliance leads to elevated left ventricular end diastolic pressure (LVEDP). If diastolic hypotension occurs systemically, the combined effect of low perfusion pressure and high endocardial pressure compromises coronary perfusion pressure (coronary perfusion pressure = aortic diastolic pressure – LVEDP). Compounding the supply:demand imbalance is the fact that the time for coronary perfusion is shortened in diastolic dysfunction because the isovolumetric phase of relaxation makes up an increasing proportion of diastole.

In addition, the noncompliant left ventricle is very dependent on preload. **Hypovolemia** can dramatically reduce left ventricle (LV) filling, with stroke volume suffering. Alternatively, too much volume in a noncompliant ventricle raises LVEDP and can compromise left atrial emptying. The resultant atrial distension can precipitate a **dysrhythmia** and loss of atrial kick. As stated earlier, atrial kick can be responsible for up to 40% of LV filling. Finally, any increase in ischemia can further compromise LV compliance, precipitating any of the above events. A prudent approach would therefore include awareness of whether the LV has begun dilating. If dilation has begun, assume poor heart function. If not, prepare for a noncompliant, hypertrophic heart with the considerations stated above. High filling pressures are required to adequately fill the noncompliant ventricle. This often requires maintained atrial kick. Consider defibrillation pads and have an antidysrhythmic such as amiodarone available. When LVEDP is high perfusion of the ventricular requires a longer diastole and higher diastolic pressure. Attempt to avoid tachycardia, and keep afterload high. Unfortunately, the stenotic Aortic Valve limits stroke volume, so too slow a heart rate compromises cardiac output. Ideal heart rate is ~55-70. Too little volume risks inadequate LV filling. Too much volume risks elevating LVEDP, resulting in ischemia and/or dysrhythmia. Consider some monitor of heart function, particularly as it pertains to volume requirements (PA catheter *vs.* TEE). A low diastolic arterial pressure can compromise coronary perfusion pressure with rapid decompensation of hemodynamics. This often requires pure alpha-agonists and/or volume to reverse if the heart is concentrically hypertrophic. Consider continuous arterial pressure monitoring with arterial catheter, especially if aortic stenosis is severe.

MITRAL STENOSIS

PRE-OP: Understand right ventricle (RV) function, rhythm, assume poor LV function

INTRA-OP: Maximize RV perfusion (keep CVP low, systolic blood pressure high, heart rate low; avoid hypoxemia/hypercarbia); Available inhaled nitric oxide or inhaled epoprostenol; Defibrillator pads, beta-blocker and amiodarone; available intra-aortic balloon pump (IABP) to support RV perfusion

Mitral stenosis is critically sensitive to volume status. Chronic mitral stenosis creates a pressure work load which can result in pulmonary hypertension and increased resistance to RV output. This can lead to RV hypertrophy, diastolic RV dysfunction, and a volume sensitive RV analogous to the volume-sensitive LV of aortic stenosis. Also similar to the LV of aortic stenosis, the hypertrophied RV of MS develops an elevated right ventricle end diastolic pressure (RVEDP). This compromises RV perfusion, a process compounded by low arterial systolic and/or diastolic pressure (the RV is perfused during systole and diastole). Left atrial distension and/or RV ischemia can ultimately lead to **dysrhythmia**. Increased flow across MV from tachycardia or hypervolemia can increase the gradient across the MV. This can further dilate the left atrial, precipitate dysrhythmias and lead to RV failure. These patients can also develop LV failure. Often, the process leading to MS is Rheumatic heart disease. This typically also affects LV contractile function. LV contractile function can be further compromised by any process which raises RV pressure. If elevated RV pressure shifts the interventricular septum to the left, this can further compromise function of the already dysfunctional LV.

With these concerns in mind, a **reasonable approach** would be to attempt to support RV function by maintaining sinus rhythm, avoiding tachycardia, avoiding RV distention and avoiding arterial hypotension. Tachycardia will also shorten diastole, when left ventricular filling through the stenotic mitral valve is supposed to be occurring. This combination of tasks can be difficult to balance. Adequate *i.v.* access, the potential benefit of continuous arterial pressure monitoring, immediate access to antidysrhythmics and a defibrillator, as well as the availability of an IABP (in case RV hypoperfusion cannot otherwise be avoided) should each be considered. If CVP is not particularly elevated preoperatively, measuring CVP may be helpful as a rise in CVP could indicate pending RV failure. Inotropic support with an agent such as epinephrine that will not drop arterial pressure is often a good strategy. Another option may be dobutamine or milrinone, though these can each drop arterial tone and thereby decrease RV coronary perfusion pressure. In addition to tachycardia and arterial diastolic hypotension, hypercarbia and hypoxemia will worsen the RV cnergy supply:demand ratio (as well as raise RVEDP) by causing pulmonary arterial hypertension and increase RV afterload. This should be considered when contemplating sedating a spontaneously-ventilating patient.

AORTIC INSUFFICIENCY (AoI)

PRE-OP: Distinguish acute *vs.* chronic (acute often with less LV dilation)

INTRA-OP: keep high HR, low afterload

Aortic insufficiency creates a volume load, ultimately adapted to by ventricular dilation. Because excessive pressure generation is not necessary, increasing myocyte numbers (concentric hypertrophy) is not a part of the adaptive process. The ventricle is able to dilate to reduce myocyte stress while still compensating for the volume needs. The slow increase in volume load allows the ventricle to dilate before any significant increase in LVEDP can occur. A low wall tension is therefore maintained. Because pressure generated by the myocytes (*i.e.* LVEDP) and radius of the LV wall have opposite effects on myocyte tension, at some point the compensatory mechanism for volume overload becomes maladaptive. That is to say, the benefit of dilating (maintaining low ventricular chamber pressure) is outweighed by the effect the delirious impact of increasing diameter (increasing myocyte tension). As myocyte tension requirements exceed capabilities, LV ejection fraction begins to decline.

Aortic insufficiency can also develop suddenly. This is less well tolerated than gradually developing Aortic Insufficiency. With acute aortic insufficiency, the volume load rises to a high level before adaptation by the ventricle can occur. There is a sudden rise in LVEDP, and a sudden need for increased HR to compensate for the drop in blood pressure and decreased effective forward flow throughout the aorta. The combination of increased work load (increase HR) and decreased perfusion pressure (elevated LVEDP and decreased arterial diastolic pressure) deleteriously effects ventricular oxygen supply:demand.

Aortic insufficiency of <u>either chronic or acute onset can create increased pressure work for the left atrium (LA)</u>. The ventricular volume loading occurs during ventricular diastole. While this does not create a particular pressure load for the relaxing ventricle, the left atrium is trying to contract and eject into the ventricle at this time. The rapidly filling ventricle is therefore at a higher pressure during the atrial contraction phase of diastole than it would normally be. This increases LA afterload, leading to LA enlargement and risking atrial fibrillation.

<u>Regurgitation from aortic insufficiency occurs because the aortic pressure is higher than the LV pressure during ventricular diastole</u>. The general approach is therefore to lower the aortic pressure and to limit the time spent in ventricular diastole. This can be accomplished with pure afterload reducers (nitroprusside, nicardipine), combined preload and afterload reducers (nitroglycerine), or agents which purely increase intracellular cAMP (dobutamine, milrinone). The choice depends upon the need to increase the HR or to add inotropic support. Epinephrine is an alternative to give chronotropic and inotropic support in a patient who cannot tolerate a further drop in arterial pressure. Because the likelihood for a sudden ventricular <u>decompensation is more likely with acute or severe aortic insufficiency, continuous arterial pressure monitoring is more likely to be helpful in these situations</u>.

MITRAL REGURGITATION (MR)

PRE-OP: Acute *vs.* chronic (acute often with less LA dilation; acute with greater potential for unexpected RV failure; chronic with assumed LV dysfunction); determine etiology of MR (exclude ischemia as etiology of functional MR); if afib, exclude anticoagulation before neuraxial approach

INTRA-OP: <u>Mitral regurgitation, like aortic insufficiency, is a regurgitant lesion and therefore tends to lead to volume overload</u>. As a regurgitant lesion, MR can develop either acutely or gradually over time. The <u>acute</u> appearance again leaves no time for chamber adaptation, and is therefore more <u>poorly tolerated</u>. It leads to volume overload to the left atrium during ventricular systole, and volume overload to the left ventricle during ventricular diastole (excess filling from the high pressure LA). Of these, <u>the acutely rising left atrial pressure is the etiology of greatest symptomatology</u>. It results in pulmonary vascular congestion, leading to dyspnea. Furthermore, the left atrial and pulmonary vascular pressure rise occurs simultaneous with right ventricular systole. This increased afterload prohibiting right ventricular systole can lead to right ventricular failure. Additionally, the low antegrade flow during left ventricular systole leads to lower systemic arterial pressure. A lower systemic arterial pressure combined with elevated biventricular diastolic pressure (from biventricular diastolic volume overload) can compromise the energy supply:demand ratio to both ventricles. In most cases, however, <u>it is right ventricular failure which tends to be the greater problem</u>. This is likely due to the fact that the regurgitant mitral valve allows the ventricle to eject against a lower afterload, decreasing the pressure work requirement (and the deleterious effects of pressure work on energy supply:demand) of the left ventricle.

The goal, then, is to promote antegrade flow out of the ventricle (to decrease pulmonary edema and right heart pressure work) and decrease the duration of time spent in ventricular diastole (when LV filling from the high pressure LA leads to LV volume overload). <u>Avoidance of arterial hypertension or of bradycardia are therefore typically the objectives</u>. One **caveat to note** is the <u>importance of understanding the etiology of mitral regurgitation</u>. Ischemic coronary disease can lead to mitral regurgitation by either regional wall motion abnormalities or infarction. If this is the case, enthusiasm for avoiding bradycardia and pursuing arterial hypotension have to be tempered by the realization that tachycardia and diastolic hypertension could lead to myocardial ischemia that will worsen the MR. When the potential for myocardial ischemia is high, ischemia monitoring with lead II and V5 of the EKG, continuous arterial monitoring as an early indication of decompensation, and/or PA catheter to help exclude low cardiac output as the etiology of arterial hypotension may be more useful.

HYPERTROPHIC CARDIOMYOPATHY/HYPERTROPHIC OBSTRUC-TIVE CARDIOMYOPATHY (HCM/HOCM)

PRE-OP INFO: Presence or absence of left ventricular outflow tract obstruction; Presence or absence of MR; Rhythm.

INTRA-OP: defibrillation pads; monitor leads II, V_5, available beta-blocker and amiodarone; available pure α agonist; available volume resuscitation

HYPERTROPHIC CARDIOMYOPATHY, with or without obstruction, <u>refers to the development of a nondilated cardiomyopathy with ventricular wall hypertrophy that is asymmetric</u>. It results in a noncompliant, hypercontractile left ventricle that requires high LVEDP to adequately fill. <u>When present, the obstruction is typically due to the anterior leaflet being caught in the LV outflow tract during ventricular systole</u> (systolic anterior movement of the mitral valve leaflet, **SAM**). Though the reason for this anterior leaflet getting caught in the LVOT is debatable ("pushed" there by a drag effect or "sucked" there by a Venturi effect [1], the <u>end physiologic effect is combining the pathologies of aortic stenosis and intermittent mitral insufficiency</u>.

Patients with <u>HCM/HOCM are often completely asymptomatic or only intermittently symptomatic</u>. In the absence of obstruction, symptomatology is typically related to a high catecholamine state and resolves quickly with resolution of the catecholamine surge. The added component of obstruction, though, makes exacerbations harder to correct. The coexisting MR leads to pulmonary congestion, acute pulmonary hypertension, and (sometimes) RV failure. The factors making systolic anterior motion of the mitral valve (SAM) more likely to occur include an elongated, mobile anterior mitral leaflet or chordae to this leaflet a left ventricular outflow tract (LVOT) narrowed by asymmetric septal hypertrophy, ventricular hypovolemia, and/or ventricular hypercontractility. While many of these factors are inherent (anterior mitral leaflet/chordae hypermobility, asymmetric septal hypertrophy), some can be mitigated (ventricular hypovolemia and hypercontractility). The goal of therapy, then, is to limit the presence of these mitigating conditions.

The approach to **HCM/HOCM**, then, is similar to the approach to aortic stenosis – maintain SR, maintain ventricular filling, and avoid tachycardia. One difference between HCM/HOCM and aortic stenosis is that the impediment to LV ejection in HCM/HOCM is dynamic and not fixed. That is to say, the LVOT obstruction limits stroke volume in HCM/HOCM only when the LVOT is narrowed. Thus, slowing the HR and increasing preload can actually relieve LVOT obstruction, increase stroke volume and increase cardiac output. This allows for more aggressive HR control in HCM/HOCM than in Aortic stenosis if it results in avoidance of LVOT obstruction (HR 50-60 range).

Because acute development of SAM can lead to the sudden decompensations, beat to beat arterial pressure monitoring may be more beneficial even than in aortic stenosis. Because dysrhythmias, particularly tachydysrhythmias, that prevent adequate ventricular filling can be so devastating, antidysrhythmics such as beta-blockers, amiodarone and defibrillator pads should be considered. Ventricular hypovolemia, ventricular hypercontractility and low arterial vascular tone should be avoided as these all narrow the LVOT and set the stage for SAM in someone whose mitral apparatus makes them predisposed. Finally, inotropes which increase ventricular contractility and HR should be avoided in favor of pure (phenylephrine) or predominant (norepinephrine) α-adrenergic agents to treat hypotension unless LVOT obstruction and SAM have been ruled out.

HEART VALVES AND ANTICOAGULATION

When one considers anticoagulation for valve replacement patients, the primary considerations include: **1)** mechanical or biological; **2)** replace semilunar valve or not semilunar valve. **Mechanical Valves** increase the likelihood of thromboembolism and valve thrombosis. The risk of valve thrombosis is higher in the mitral or tricuspid position than in the aortic or pulmonary position due to the lower flow velocities across valves in the mitral or tricuspid positions. While many surgeons will prefer anticoagulation for the first 3 months following replacement of any valve (regardless of position or whether or not it is mechanical), the increased thromboembolic and valve thrombosis risks result in lifelong anticoagulation for mechanical valves. Without anticoagulation, the risk of mechanical mitral and aortic valve to cause embolism is 1.3% *vs.* 0.8%, respectively, while risk of valve thrombosis is 0.5% *vs.* 0.1%, respectively.

In an outpatient setting, only vitamin K antagonists (warfarin) are recommended as anticoagulation. None of the oral thrombin or factor Xa inhibitors have thus far proven efficacious

The 2012 American College of Chest Physicians (ACCP) guidelines recommend the following:

For a **tissue valve** that has been in place >3months in either the aortic or mitral position, aspirin (75-100 mg daily) is recommended unless the patient has additional risk factors (atrial fibrillation, LVEF <30%, prior thromboembolism or a hypercoagulable state). If the patient has one of these risk factors, concurrent warfarin (INR goal 2.0-3.0) is recommended. In a patient for whom Coumadin is recommended but who cannot take Coumadin, an aspirin dose of 75-325 mg/day is recommended.

For a mechanical aortic valve that is in the Aortic position in place ≥ 3 months and is either a bileaflet valve or a Medtronic hall valve, the **INR** goal should be 2.0-3.0 as long as the patient does not also have an additional risk factor (atrial fibrillation, LVEF <30%, prior thromboembolism or a hypercoagulable state). If the patient has one of these risk factors, a mechanical aortic valve that is neither bileaflet nor a Medtronic Hall valve*, or has a mechanical valve in a mitral or tricuspid position, goal INR should be 2.5-3.5.

Anticoagulation during the first 3 mos following valve replacement is a bit more aggressive. Patients in sinus rhythm and without other indication for anticoagulation should receive aspirin (75-100 mg) after having bioprosthetic valve placed in the aortic position. During the first 3 mos following bioprosthetic valve placement in the mitral position, vitamin K antagonism titrated to an INR of 2.0-3.0 is recommended. Following mechanical valve placement with bileaflet and Medtronic hall valves in the aortic position, an INR of 2.5-3.5 may be better than a goal of 2.0-3.0. For transcatheter aortic valve replacement, aspirin (50-100 mg/day) plus clopidogrel (75 mg/day) is recommended for the first 3 mos. If Coumadin is to be interrupted for surgery, the following guidelines would be in agreement with recommendations by the 2012 ACCP, 2008 SCA, 2008 STS and 2008 SCAI.

Following the first 3 mos after valve replacement (when thrombosis and thromboembolic risks are highest), most patients can tolerate short periods of Coumadin cessation with little risk. The **exceptions** are: **1)** those patients with specific risk factors (atrial fibrillation, prior thromboembolism, LVEF < 30%, surgery for malignancy or sepsis, hypercoagulable state), **2)** mechanical valves in the aortic position that are neither bileaflet nor Medtronic Hall valves (*e.g.* aortic ball valves and tilting disc valves such as Lillehei Kaster, Omniscience, and Starr Edwards valves), **3)** mechanical valves in the mitral or tricuspid position, **4)** two or more mechanical valves.

Discontinue warfarin 5 days prior to planned surgery, and admit patient when INR drops below the target range. Do not give large doses of vitamin K to reverse the warfarin, as this will prolong the time to re-establish a therapeutic INR following surgery. Therapeutically anticoagulate with *i.v.* unfractionated (aPTT goal 1.5-2) or SQ low molecular weight (1 mg/kg every 12 hrs) when INR drops below target range. While unfractionated or low molecular weight heparin may be used, unfractionated is often preferred. This is driven primarily by the ease of reversibility. Stop low molecular weight heparin 12 hrs prior to surgery. Resume low molecular weight or unfractionated heparin as soon as possible (considering bleeding risk) following surgery. Resume warfarin as soon as possible (considering bleeding risk) following surgery. Stop heparin once INR has become therapeutic.

For patients that are not high risk of thrombosis or thromboembolic event, stop Coumadin 5 days prior to surgery and test INR one day prior to surgery. If the INR is 1.5 to 1.9 on the day before surgery, consider low dose oral vitamin K (*e.g,* 1.0-2.5 mg). Such a dose is likely to reduce the INR to 1.4 or less within 24 hours [3].

*Examples of mechanical valves that are neither bileaflet nor Medtronic Hall valves include aortic ball valves and tilting disc valves such as Lillehei Kaster, Omniscience, and Starr Edwards valves.

PACEMAKERS

Pacemakers, a commonly-used tool to optimize rate and synchrony of chamber contraction, vary in the number of chambers paced, the combination of chambers paced, as well as the response to tachycardia. They can pace a single atrium, a single ventricle, or a combination of atria and ventricles. Because the indications for number and specific chambers paced are determined by the underlying cardiac disease, knowing the number and specific chambers paced has classically given information about underlying disease. Thus, **a single chamber ventricular pacer is placed for bradycardia in a patient with otherwise good heart function.** A **duel**

chamber, <u>atrial-ventricular pacemaker is placed for bradycardia in a patient whose compromised ventricular function requires the additional filling delivered</u> by appropriately-timed atrial contraction. **A biventricular pacemaker** is <u>placed when ventricular function is compromised</u> (LVEF $\leq$ 30%) due, at least in part, by asynchronously contracting ventricles as indicated by a prolonged QRS ($\geq$ 130 ms). Thus, patients with a single chamber pacemaker have historically had significantly better underlying ventricular function than those having biventricular pacing. It is important to note, however, <u>that this paradigm is evolving</u>. Thus, biventricular pacing has recently been shown to be superior to single lead right ventricular pacing in patients with LVEF up to 50%, heart block (1st, 2nd, 3rd degree or right or left bundle branch) and bradycardia requiring pacing.

It is important to realize that many of the interventions designed for chronic therapy of systolic heart dysfunction can either have their efficacy compromised by tools used commonly by surgeons in the operating room (*e.g.* Cautery can interfere with pacemakers) or can compromise the efficacy of tools anesthesiologists use in the operating room to maintain anesthesia, analgesia and hemodynamic stability (*i.e.* sympathetic antagonists prescribed for chronic use may block the efficacy of pharmacologic sympathetic agonists commonly used by anesthesiologists). This makes <u>it important to understand the patient's dependence on their pacemaker, and to anticipate the effect of the patient's particular pharmacologic heart failure cocktail on our ability to influence hemodynamics.</u>

In a patient with a pacemaker, it <u>is therefore ideal to understand whether the patient can maintain adequate systemic perfusion and blood pressure if the paceris stopped</u>. If not, consider reprogramming the pacemaker to an asynchronous backup rate to avoid hemodynamic deterioration due to electromagnetic (*e.g.* cautery) inhibition of the pacemaker. A perhaps more invasive alternative is a backup transcutaneous or transvenous pacemaker may be considered as an option. **Does the pacemaker have an antitachycardia response?** If so, it <u>is often best to have this inactivated and external defibrillator pads placed to avoid inadvertent stimulation of this response</u> (often involving electrical cardioversion) by electrocautery. Does adequate battery life remain? What is the response to a magnet? These questions can be defined by interrogating the pacemaker and/or defibrillator. Interrogation should be performed within 6 months (if defibrillator function) or 1 yr (if simple pacemaker) of anesthesia induction. While battery life can obviously be known only with interrogation, it is important to realize that even the response to magnet is not consistent. **With pacemakers, 60%** go to high rate asynchronous pacer, **25%** go to asynchronous pacer not high rate, **15%** go to short duration asynchronous pacer. With **pacer/AICDs**, <u>usually inactivate the anti-tachycardiac response but response of the pacemaker is variable</u>.

Finally, if bipolar electrocautery is used, care should be taken in location of grounding pad placed. By locating the pad so that the pacemaker and wires are not between the site of surgery and the grounding pad, electromagnetic activity from the cautery should be directed away from the pacing/defibrillator device and reduce the risk of interference.

INOTROPIC SUPPORT – PHARMACOLOGIC

Pharmacologic infusions are the therapeutic mainstay to regain and sustain cardiac output and end organ perfusion in patients with systolic heart failure. These agents can be chosen individually, based on the patient's blood pressure and the anticipated effects of specific agents on blood pressure. They can be used in combination, taking advantage of different mechanisms of action of various agents, to achieve additive effects.

EPINEPHRINE – beta agonist and alpha agonist. Beta-agonism stimulates beta receptors in the heart and vasculature (as well as the bronchial system of the lungs) to increase intracellular cAMP. The cardiac stimulation increases heart rate, strength of myocyte contraction, and myocyte irritability, while the vascular effects would cause peripheral (and bronchial) dilation. Alpha stimulation causes peripheral vascular constriction to maintain peripheral tone (no such effect on bronchial tree). The net effect is to increase heart rate and increase blood pressure, but increasing the risk of cardiac dysrhythmia. Bronchial dilation also occurs.

DOBUTAMINE – beta-agonist without alpha agonism. Due to the unopposed nature of beta-stimulation, similar hemodynamic consequences to epinephrine can be seen except that blood pressure often drops. A choice between dobutamine and ephinephrine is therefore often determined by whether the patient can tolerate a drop in arterial blood pressure. If both are used simultaneously, it is important to realize that they both function by stimulating the same beta-receptors. From an inotropic standpoint, then, one would not expect a bit "additive" effect.

Dobutamine can be useful in helping RV:PA coupling when LV diastolic dysfunction or RV systolic failure occur in the setting of pulmonary hypertension exists. **Levosimendan** may be even more effective than dobutamine in the setting of pulmonary hypertension, though, due to additional pulmonary vasodilatory effects.

MILINRIONE – like dobutamine, milrinone results in an in increased intracellular cAMP. Unlike dobutamine, milrinone accomplishes this by inhibiting enzymatic metabolism of intracellular cAMP rather than stimulating cAMP production through beta-receptor activation. Milrinone with epinephrine should therefore be more effective than dobutamine with epinephrine in synergistically increasing intracellular cAMP and augmenting increasing each other's inotropic effects. Another difference *versus* dobutamine is that milrinone has a more delayed onset of action and longer half-life. The "delayed onset" effects can be overcome by giving a "loading dose" of milrinone. One must be ready to treat the potential for hypotension.

DOPAMINE – Inotropic benefit along with some peripheral constriction. Though there may be some inotropic benefit through stimulation of dopamine receptors at very low doses ($\leq$ 2 mcg/kg/min), most of the inotropic benefit comes from stimulating beta1 receptors. At higher doses ($\geq$ 10 mcg/kg/min), stimulation of alpha receptors causes some peripheral constriction as well. From an inotropic standpoint, the benefit of combining dopamine with dobutamine or epinephrine would be expected to be small and the result mainly of stimulating dopamine receptors. There would, however, be an anticipated additive inotropic effect by combining dopamine with milrinone.

Two agents Under Development Include Levosimendan and Istaroxime.

LEVOSIMENDAN – increases calcium sensitivity in cardiac myocyte. It simultaneously opens ATP-sensitve potassium channels in vascular smooth muscle and mitochondria. The result is increased inotropy, peripheral dilation and cardioprotection. Though the hemodynamic effects resemble those of dobutamine, levosimendan has the advantage of reducing all-cause mortality in chronic heart failure patients taking beta-blockers who are hospitalized for acute exacerbation [4].

ISTAROXIME – Istaroxime inhibits NA:K ATPase and potentiates the Sarcoplasmic/Endoplasmic Reticulum Calcium ATPase (SERCA2a(11)). Na:K ATPase inhibition increases intracellular calcium by preventing calcium extrusion from the cell and triggering release of calcium from the sarcoplasmic reticulum. The result of increased intracellular calcium in is increased inotropy. SERCA2a potentiation facilitates calcium sequestration, aiding in relaxation. Istaroxime also has antidysrhythmic effects through a mechanism which is unclear.

VASOPRESSORS

PHENYLEPHRINE – alpha adrenergic receptor stimulator – causes peripheral constriction by stimulation of alpha adrenergic receptors

NOREPINEPHRINE – alpha adrenergic and beta receptor stimulator – more potent and more efficacious an alpha stimulator than phenylephrine. Thus, peripheral constriction begins at a lower dose and achieves a higher peak with norepinephrine than with phenylephrine. Additionally, norepinephrine contains a degree of beta-stimulation which is not present with phenylephrine. The relative alpha:beta effect of norepinephrine is the opposite of the relation in epinephrine. That is, norepinephrine has greater alpha effect than beta, while epinephrine has greater beta effect than alpha.

EPHEDRINE – causes release of norepinephrine from nerve terminals. As expected, it therefore has the same general effects as exogenous norepinephrine (increased peripheral tone, maintenance of heart rate), though to a much lower degree (due, in part, to the supra-physiologic doses of norepinephrine given exogenously). Because it is dependent on the release of stored norepinephrine in nerve terminals, ephedrine will be less efficacious in settings which can deplete these stores (shock).

VASOPRESSIN – vascular constriction based on stimulation of (vasopressin) receptors which are distinct from alpha adrenergic receptors. There are varying opinions as to the comparative effects of vasopressin *vs.* norepinephrine on the pulmonary vasculature and on the different systemic vascular beds. In short, there are times when norepinephrine is more effective at raising blood pressure. There are times when vasopressin is more effective at raising blood pressure. There are times when the combination of norepinephrine and vasopressin can raise the blood pressure when neither one individually is effective. Disagreement exists as to its effect on pulmonary vasculature, although there is some suggestion that vasopressin has relatively fewer pulmonary effects than norepinephrine.

INOTROPIC SUPPORT – MECHANICAL

One option for support in cases where pharmacologic agents are insufficient is intra-aortic balloon pump (IABP) (Fig. **7**). An **IABP** is a balloon placed high in the descending thoracic aorta. It inflates at the moment of aortic valve closure and deflates at the moment of aortic valve opening. By inflating at this moment, the IABP pushes additional blood into the ascending aorta during diastole, increasing the pressure with which the coronary arteries are perfused. Deflation immediately before aortic valve opening drops the pressure within the ascending aorta at the moment of ventricular systole. This facilitates blood expulsion from the left ventricle. Thus, coronary perfusion is improved and ventricular work is reduced.

Positioning and timing are critical to the effectiveness of the IABP. The closer it is placed to the aortic valve; the greater effect it has on pressure changes in this area. However, the curved shape of the aortic arch prevents placement of the balloon in this area, due to the trauma that could ensue from inflating a straight balloon within a curved vessel. Additionally, the pressure changes produced by inflating and deflating the IABP will be most influential if occurring suddenly at the moment of aortic valve closing and opening, respectively.

Although many relative contraindications for IABP exist, <u>Aortic Insufficiency is an absolute contraindication</u>. An incompetent aortic valve prohibits pressure buildup with IABP inflation and leads instead to exacerbation of the volume overload resultant from aortic insufficiency.

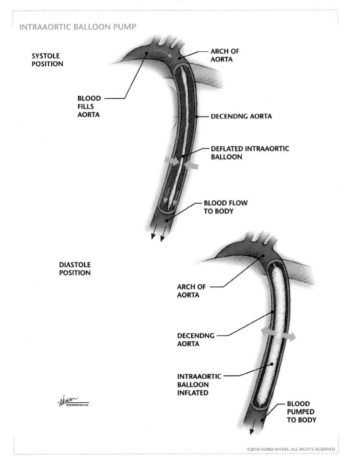

Fig. (7). Intraaortic Balloon Pump. Image provided by Norm Myers.

SYSTOLIC AND DIASTOLIC HEART FAILURE

Simply stated, systolic failure is inability of the heart to empty while diastolic failure is inability of the heart to fill.

SYSTOLIC HEART FAILURE

Systolic dysfunction is an <u>impairment of contractile function</u>. Etiologies can be ischemic and nonischemic in etiology. It can occur in association with, or independent of, diastolic dysfunction. The hypoperfusion resultant from systolic dysfunction ultimately triggers compensatory mechanisms which include changes in heart rate, chamber size and thickness, and stimulation of sympathetic, renin-angiotensin, as well as natriuretic systems. These <u>compensatory mechanisms, when progressing to an extreme, can themselves become cardiotoxic</u>. **Chronic therapy** to treat heart failure includes devices to re-establish optimal rate and synchrony of chamber contraction, as well as <u>pharmaceuticals</u> to reduce the toxicity of sympathetic, renin-angiotensin and natriuretic system stimulation. Interventions to provide short-term hemodynamic support for acute systolic decompensation include minimizing factors that can precipitate decompensation (*e.g.* Ischemia, tachycardia), increasing contractile function (inotropes) while minimizing afterload as much as possible. The acute and chronic therapies, then can sometimes conflict.

PRE-OP – presence/absence of pacemaker. If present, understand patient's pacer-dependence, associated defibrillator (turn off and have external defibrillator), response to magnet, remaining battery life. If present, may need to be interrogated after surgery. Understand which classes of heart failure medications patient taking chronically, and effect that may have on responsiveness to inotropes/vasopressors.

INTRA-OP – Appropriate pressors available, consider Pulmonary Artery catheter and central access/intra-arterial pressure monitoring catheter, amiodarone available (higher risk of, and less tolerance for, dysrhythmia)

Agents commonly used to support hemodynamics include inotropes (epinephrine, milrinone, dopamine), alpha-agonists (phenylephrine, ephedrine, norepinephrine) and vasopressin. The effectiveness of some of these agents can be attenuated by the chronic therapy often prescribed to patients with systolic heart dysfunction. Thus, beta-blockers can reduce the chronotropic effects of epinephrine and milrinone. In such a scenario, dopamine (with or without glycopyrolate or atropine) may be a more effective pharmacologic choice to reverse symptomatic bradycardia. Chronic carvedilol or labetolol therapy may render alpha-agonists ineffective in raising blood pressure. Here, vasopressin may be an effective alternative. ACE-inhibitors and ARBs can also reduce responsiveness to alpha-agonists, possibly by reducing alpha-adrenergic receptor density. This may be the reason for the relatively greater responsiveness to vasopressin in these cases.

DIASTOLIC HEART FAILURE

Diastolic dysfunction is an <u>abnormality of ventricular filling, relaxation, and/or compliance</u>. It can occur in the setting of normal or abnormal systolic function. The presence of diastolic dysfunction in patients with normal or near normal ventricular ejection fraction is termed <u>Heart Failure with Preserved Ejection</u>

Fraction (HFPEF). Morbidity and mortality are higher in HFPEF *versus* patients in preserved ejection fraction without diastolic dysfunction.

Risk factors for diastolic dysfunction included advanced age, female sex, DM, obesity, hypertension and coronary artery disease. With the exclusion of coronary artery disease, these are the same risk factors for HFPEF.

Diastole is the time between aortic valve closure and mitral valve closure. **It has 4 phases**: **1)** isovolumetric relaxation; **2)** early filling; **3)** diastasis; **4)** atrial contraction. **Isovolumetric relaxation** is the time between Aortic valve closure and mitral valve opening. During this phase, the mitral annulus moves away from the ventricular apex, ultimately dropping the ventricular pressure below that of the atrium and creating a suction that leads to phase 2. **Early filling** is from the point of mitral valve opening until the onset of diastasis. During early filling, the mitral annulus continues to move away from the ventricular apex. Because the intraventricular pressure drops below that of the atrium, blood passively enters the ventricle from the atrium until both chamber pressures become equal. In a normal ventricle, this accounts for 70-80% of ventricular filling. **Diastasis** begins when atrial and ventricular chamber pressures equalize, such that flow between the chambers stops. **Atrial contraction** then begins, pushing the final 20-30% of blood into the ventricle.

Diastole involves cardiac relaxation, filling and elastic recoil. Relaxation (a.k.a. **lusitropy**) is an active, energy-consuming process that is most apparent during the first 2 phases of diastole. Energy is utilized to dissociate calcium from tropomyosin C, lyse actin-myosin bridges, and remove calcium from the cytoplasm. **Filling** occurs during stage 2 and 4 of diastole, typically in a 70-80% *vs.* 20-30% ratio. It is dependent on ventricular (lusitropy, elastic recoil and end systolic volume) and atrial (volume, elastic recoil and contractile strength) factors. **Elastic recoil** is dependent on collagen deposition and fibrosis as well as cytoskeleton changes. Pericardial constriction can also limit ventricular expansion

Progression of the disease is graded into four levels (I-IV) based on echocardiographic findings that translate to clinical manifestations. **Grade I (mild)** disease shows slower mitral annular excursion away from the apex in early diastole. It corresponds to increased atrial and lower ventricular volume when the mitral valve closes at diastasis, is more dependent on atrial contraction to fill the ventricle, and manifests clinically as shortness of breath only with moderate or severe exercise. In **Grade II (moderate)** disease, the inability of passive filling to increase ventricular volume has been corrected by the body's retention of fluid to raise atrial pressure. This higher atrial pressure facilitates early ventricular filling. It also, however, increases pulmonary vascular congestion and leads to dyspnea with only mild exertion. In **Grade III (restrictive)** diastolic dysfunction, the LV pressure is so high as to prevent additional filling with atrial contraction. Ventricular filling is then limited to early diastole, and retrograde blood flow into the pulmonary vasculature can occur during atrial contraction. Patients experience dyspnea at rest. These symptoms can usually be relieved by the administration of nitroglycerin or maneuvers (Valsalva) which reduce atrial pressure. In **Grade IV** diastolic dysfunction, the process is so progressed that the symptoms and echocardiographic findings are not reversible by maneuvers designed to acutely lower atrial pressure.

With <u>Grades I and II</u> diastolic dysfunction, <u>impaired relaxation</u> is the overriding problem. This is worsened by tachycardia (which shortens relaxation time) and can be compensated for with increased pre-load and maintained atrial kick. In <u>Grades III and IV diastolic dysfunction</u>, impaired relaxation is compounded by elevated elastic recoil and restrictive physiology. While tachycardia can still worsen pulmonary congestion if ischemia is precipitated, bradycardia can also be problematic. Because diastolic dysfunction limits ventricular filling, stroke volume is effectively fixed and cardiac output is dependent on heart rate. Bradycardia therefore limits cardiac output. Furthermore, increased volume is unhelpful – atrial pressures are already high and the additional volume just adds to pulmonary congestion.

Clinical Approach

<u>Diastolic dysfunction is very common – 50% of new diagnoses of heart failure involve diastolic dysfunction</u>. Because it can occur in the absence of systolic dysfunction, respect for the possibility of diastolic dysfunction should be exercised in any patient with the previously-stated risk factors. An echocardiograph report, if present, can comment on the presence and grade of diastolic dysfunction. With this as a guide, <u>avoiding tachycardia</u> (which shortens diastolic relaxation time) <u>and maintaining sinus rhythm</u> (to help ventricular filling) <u>are good general approaches</u>. Their importance increases as one progresses from Grade I to Grade IV diastolic dysfunction. <u>Fluid management varies by Stage</u> of diastolic dysfunction. <u>Stage I and II</u> are fairly fluid tolerant, so fluid administration is often helpful overall. <u>Stage III and IV</u>, on the other hand, have pulmonary congestion at baseline. Additional fluid administration should therefore be done only judiciously. No agents are pure facilitators of muscle relaxation, though beta-agonists can be lusitropic at low doses if tachycardia can be avoided. By benefiting right ventricular contractile function, these beta-agonists may also help to compensate for the pulmonary congestion that can occur in diastolic dysfunction. Nitroglycerine can reduce preload to help with pulmonary vascular congestion as well. Finally, avoiding conditions such as

myocardial ischemia and tachycardia which worsen diastolic performance are important. In this regard, alpha agents (phenylephrine, norepinephrine) may be a useful adjunct to support the arterial diastolic blood pressure while minimizing tachycardia. Because of the high left ventricular diastolic pressure common in diastolic dysfunction, a high diastolic blood pressure is necessary to assure transmyocardial perfusion pressure as coronary perfusion is occurring.

VENTRICULAR ASSIST DEVICES

A **ventricular assist device (VAD)** (Fig. **8**) assumes some of the work of the ventricle. In the case of a left ventricular assist device (LVAD), it takes blood from the left atrium or left ventricle and pumps it into the aorta. The typical source of blood for an LVAD is the left ventricular apex, and the typical destination is the descending thoracic aorta. Because native left ventricular ejected volume is only a fraction of the volume as is provided by the LVAD, LVAD output into the descending thoracic aorta often flows retrograde up the aorta to assure adequate perfusion to the coronaries, head vessels, left subclavian and intercostal vessels.

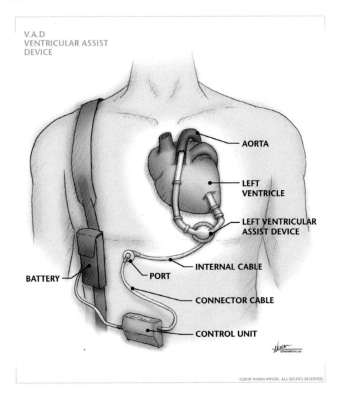

Fig. (8). V.A.D. – Ventricular Assist Device. Image provided by Norm Myers.

There are **2 general types of VADs** – **pulsatile flow VADs** and **laminar flow VADs**. The **pulsatile flow VADs** are first generation VADs and are conceptually more similar to the native ventricle in their function than are laminar flow VADs. The pulsatile VADs consist of a chamber which fills with blood and then ejects. Tissue valves on the inflow and outflow cannulae of the VAD assure unidirectional flow of the ejected blood. The VAD can be set to eject either at a certain rate or when if fills to a preset volume. The device is connected to an external controller which allows manual adjustment of the pump frequency and ejection volume. If the rate is made constant, the volume ejected with each beat varies. If the volume is made constant, the rate of ejection varies. Results of the REMATCH Trial justified the use of LVADs. In this trial, patients with Class IV heart failure who were ineligible for heart transplant were randomly assigned to standard medical therapy *vs.* LVAD. Those receiving LVAD had significantly better one year (52% *vs.* 25%, P – 0.002) and trend towards better two year (23% *vs.* 8%, P – 0.08) survival *vs.* medical therapy, as well as better Quality of Life scores.

Unfortunately, the bulkiness of these devices was a bit dissatisfying. More importantly, the valves assuring unidirectional flow would degenerate over time, requiring replacement. This lead to the development of **laminar flow devices**. These consist essentially of a rotor (Heartmate II) or impeller (Heartware) which is electromagnetically made to spin. The external controller to which it is connected allows adjustment of the pump speed (rotations per minute, RPM) and monitors the energy required to accomplish this speed. The centrifugal (Heartmate II) or axial (Heartware) nature of these pumps obviated the need for valves. Clinical trials demonstrated these devices lead to higher survival and better quality of life (due to their smaller size and more quiet nature) than the first generation (pulsatile) devices. *First generation devices became obsolete, and are essentially nonexistent in clinical use today.*

To understand the adequacy of assistance being provided by laminar flow VADs, recognize that the parameters actually measured by the controller are the pump speed (RPM) and the energy required to achieve this speed (Power for Heartmate II, Watts for Heartware). **Flow is not** directly measured. It is calculated based on a nomogram derived from 'speed' and 'power' data (as well as hematocrit for Heartware). For any given speed, in general, an increase in required power indicates that a greater volume and/or viscosity of blood is going through the pump. If pump speed and patient hematocrit are not changing, power (or wattage) is therefore directly related to pump output. If hematocrit (blood viscosity) increases, some of the power is being used to move the more viscous blood rather than to move a volume of blood. Flow at any given RPM:power combination would therefore be overestimated unless this effect of increased blood viscosity were considered.

In general, then, **RPM** can be thought of as "inotropy". All other conditions being equal, increasing RPM will increase VAD output. "Stable" patients typically have a pump speed at which they optimally function. **RPM** is therefore typically not adjusted by anesthesiologists for patients undergoing outpatient surgery. The **"power" trend**, though, should be monitored as an indicator of pump output with consistent pump speed and hematocrit.

If pump power (flow) does begin to drop, it is **important** to distinguish between low pre-load and high afterload as an etiology. "Pulsatility Index" is a parameter that may help in this distinction. **Pulsatility Index** is a measure of the fluctuations in power utilized by the VAD to maintain pump speed averaged over 15 seconds. Power over such a time course is essentially a measure of blood volume presented to the VAD. A higher Pulsatility Index indicates that the VAD is being presented with a steady volume of blood supplemented with large "boluses" of volume throughout a 15 seconds period. These blood boluses are the result of blood being ejected by the native ventricle. Although its contractile function is poor, the native ventricle can usually still contract to some degree. The volume of blood ejected by each contraction depends both on the contractile function of the native ventricle and the volume it contains. Though native function does not change rapidly, the volume within the ventricle can. For any given patient, then, an increase in the pulsatility index suggests an increase in left ventricular distention and an increase in preload to the LVAD.

A **drop** in pulsatility index suggests native LV ejection is dropping. This could be due either to a change in LV volume or contractility. **LV volume** can drop either because the total intravascular volume is low or because the RV is failing. Measurement of a trend in central venous pressure (CVP) can help with this distinction, as CVP will drop if total intravascular volume is down and rise if RV is failing. **RV failure** can be due to overaggressive volume resuscitation or to overaggressive pump speed. In either case, the ventricular septum is shifted towards the left ventricle, decreasing the contractile efficiency of both ventricles. In a previously stable patient undergoing elective minor surgery, such a shift in the position of the ventricular septum is more likely to result from overaggressive volume resuscitation.

In a previously stable patient undergoing elective surgery, LV contractility would not be expected to change unless a dysrhythmia or worsening ischemia were to develop. Either of these could suddenly compromise the effectiveness of a ventricle with severely compromised baseline contractile function. An EKG may help screen for this. As with RV failure, LV failure could also result from a shift in the position of the interventricular septum. Because of ventricular interdependence, a shift in septal positioning decreases the effectiveness of contraction of both ventricles. As stated previously, RV failure can shift the septum to the left and cause biventricular failure. This could be suggested by a rise in CVP and improvement with the initiation of inotropic support. Alternatively, insufficient LVAD speed could lead to LV dilation and a rightward shift of the ventricle. Though less likely in a patient previously stable patient admitted from home for elective surgery, this could be suggested by a low CVP which fails to respond to volume resuscitation. Echocardiographic visualization of the position of the interventricular septum would lead to a more definitive exclusion or confirmation of this diagnosis.

Caring for the Patient with VAD

Intraoperative Care

PRE-OP INFORMATION: Ask patient: **1)** their typical power/flow range for their set RPM; **2)** to show you how they change the batteries on their VAD (and practice yourself in front of patient); **3)** if there are any (patient) positions that cause problems for their VAD function. Determine: **1)** ease of locating pulse and of obtaining blood pressure noninvasively; **2)** ease of obtaining pulse oximetry; Understand: **1)** In the case of an LVAD, understand the function of chambers and valves on native right side of heart. The ability of the right heart to fill the left heart/LVAD. If RV function is poor, inotropic support for RV function may be necessary.

INTRA-OP: Rhythm monitor; defibrillator; Doppler and sphygmomanometer (for bp); possible arterial catheter and/or CVP; available inotrope(s) (epinephrine, dopamine, dobutamine and/or milrinone), vasopressor(s) (phenylephrine, norepinephrine and/or vasopressin); consider echo (TTE or TEE).

Systemic flow generated by the LVAD can be supplemented by cardiac output generated by native ventricle. When this occurs, pulsatile arterial flow can be appreciated. The anesthesiologist should plan for the magnitude of this pulsatility to decrease after exposure to anesthetics. The contribution from a severely dysfunctional ventricle being exposed to the venodialating and myocardial depressant effects of anesthetics is unpredictable. Monitors dependent on arterial pulsatility, such as noninvasive bp cuffs and arterial saturation monitors, can be unreliable. As the pulse pressure narrows, noninvasive blood pressure cuffs may begin providing only a mean pressure. It may also fail to detect any blood pressure. A Doppler probe and sphygmomanometer can often achieve an arterial pressure when a noninvasive blood pressure cuff in ineffective. Arterial saturation monitors can similarly be effective even when noninvasive blood pressure cuffs fail. For short duration cases without anticipated significant changes in blood pressure or volume, this combination is often adequate. For longer cases or more complex cases, though, <u>arterial catheters are probably prudent</u>. Their placement can be facilitated with <u>ultrasound Doppler</u>. Once placed, they allow for hands-free blood pressure monitoring as well as access to arterial blood samples. Obtaining mean arterial pressure with Doppler flow and sphygmomanometer can be time consuming and distracting. Pulse oximetry can also become inconsistent as native heart output changes.

<u>Most VAD patients are susceptible to dysrhythmias and have defibrillators in place</u>. The process leading to dysfunction of one ventricle often affects, to some degree, the other ventricle. Function of this ventricle is therefore likely quite sensitive to dysrhythmias. Monitoring for, and readiness to treat, dysrhythmias is important. Though an LVAD can likely function adequately without any support from the native left ventricle, it does require a functioning right ventricle to assure adequate filling. **EKG monitoring** <u>as well as available antidysrhythmics and defibrillators is therefore prudent</u>.

<u>The effect of patient positioning on VAD function should be repeatedly evaluated.</u> VAD filling can be mechanically compromised by seated positioning or pressures placed upon the chest and upper abdomen. Patients to be positioned any way other than supine (*i.e.* prone, seated, lateral decubitus) are particularly at risk of this. <u>Verifying that the patient's power/flow does not change when in the surgical position for 5 min is reassuring</u>. The cables connecting the VAD to its external monitor, as well as the area around their entrance into the skin, should be padded to minimize the chance of their injuring the patient. Caution to avoid pulling on these cables during patient positioning is also important.

One approach to evaluating a drop in pulsatility index would be to check the CVP. If it is low, give volume. If CVP is high, consider inotropes. If these maneuvers fail, check ventricular septum (ECHO) and consider changing pump speed.

CONCLUSION

This chapter attempts to show how an understanding of the fundamentals of cardiovascular physiology – preload, afterload, contractility, pressure work, volume work – guide in the management of patients with specific disease states such as aortic stenosis and insufficiency, mitral stenosis and insufficiency, hypertrophic cardiomyopathy, as well as those with systolic and diastolic heart failure. A brief introduction to ventricular assist devices is included as well.

CONSENT FOR PUBLICATION

Not applicable.

CONFLICT OF INTEREST

The author declares no conflict of interest, financial or otherwise.

ACKNOWLEDGEMENT

Declared none.

REFERENCES

[1] Sherrid MV, Chu CK, Delia E, Mogtader A, Dwyer EM Jr. An echocardiographic study of the fluid mechanics of obstruction in hypertrophic cardiomyopathy. J Am Coll Cardiol 1993; 22(3): 816-25.
[http://dx.doi.org/10.1016/0735-1097(93)90196-8] [PMID: 8354817]

[2] Moss AJ, Hall WJ, Cannom DS, *et al.* MADIT-CRT Trial Investigators. Cardiac-resynchronization therapy for the prevention of heart-failure events. N Engl J Med 2009; 361(14): 1329-38.
[http://dx.doi.org/10.1056/NEJMoa0906431] [PMID: 19723701]

[3] Andersen MJ, Hwang SJ, Kane GC, *et al.* Enhanced pulmonary vasodilator reserve and abnormal right ventricular: pulmonary artery coupling in heart failure with preserved ejection fraction. Circ Heart Fail 2015; 8(3): 542-50.
[http://dx.doi.org/10.1161/CIRCHEARTFAILURE.114.002114] [PMID: 25857307]

[4] Bonow RO, Carabello BA, Chatterjee K, *et al.* 2006 Writing Committee Members; American College of Cardiology/American Heart Association Task Force. 2008 Focused update incorporated into the ACC/AHA 2006 guidelines for the management of patients with valvular heart disease: a report of the American College of Cardiology/American Heart Association Task Force on Practice Guidelines (Writing Committee to Revise the 1998 Guidelines for the Management of Patients With Valvular Heart Disease): endorsed by the Society of Cardiovascular Anesthesiologists, Society for Cardiovascular Angiography and Interventions, and Society of Thoracic Surgeons. Circulation 2008; 118(15): e523-661.
[PMID: 18820172]

ADDITIONAL MATERIAL USED FOR THIS WORK

Kerbaul F, Rondelet B, Demester JP, *et al.* Effects of levosimendan *versus* dobutamine on pressure load-induced right ventricular failure. Crit Care Med 2006; 34(11): 2814-9.
[http://dx.doi.org/10.1097/01.CCM.0000242157.19347.50] [PMID: 16971854]

Fuchs F, Smith SH. Calcium, cross-bridges, and the Frank-Starling relationship. News in physiological sciences : an international journal of physiology produced jointly by the International Union of Physiological Sciences and the American Physiological Society 2001; 16: 5-10.
[http://dx.doi.org/10.1152/physiologyonline.2001.16.1.5]

Barnes J, Dell'Italia LJ. The multiple mechanistic faces of a pure volume overload: implications for therapy. Am J Med Sci 2014; 348(4): 337-46.
[http://dx.doi.org/10.1097/MAJ.0000000000000255] [PMID: 24781435]

Cannegieter SC, Rosendaal FR, Wintzen AR, van der Meer FJ, Vandenbroucke JP, Briët E. Optimal oral anticoagulant therapy in patients with mechanical heart valves. N Engl J Med 1995; 333(1): 11-7.
[http://dx.doi.org/10.1056/NEJM199507063330103] [PMID: 7776988]

Douketis JD, Spyropoulos AC, Spencer FA, Mayr M, Jaffer AK, Eckman MH, *et al.* Perioperative management of antithrombotic therapy: Antithrombotic therapy and prevention of thrombosis, 9th ed: American college of chest physicians evidence-based clinical practice guidelines. Chest. 2012; 141: pp. (2 Suppl)e326S-50S.

Whitlock RP, Sun JC, Fremes SE, Rubens FD, Teoh KH. Antithrombotic and thrombolytic therapy for valvular disease: Antithrombotic Therapy and Prevention of Thrombosis, 9th ed: American College of Chest Physicians Evidence-Based Clinical Practice Guidelines. Chest. 2012; 141: pp. (2 Suppl)e576S-600S. Epub 2012/02/15

Mebazaa A, Nieminen MS, Filippatos GS, *et al.* Levosimendan *vs.* dobutamine: outcomes for acute heart failure patients on beta-blockers in SURVIVE. Eur J Heart Fail 2009; 11(3): 304-11.
[http://dx.doi.org/10.1093/eurjhf/hfn045] [PMID: 19158152]

Mattera GG, Lo Giudice P, Loi FM, *et al.* Istaroxime: a new luso-inotropic agent for heart failure. Am J Cardiol 2007; 99(2A): 33A-40A.
[http://dx.doi.org/10.1016/j.amjcard.2006.09.004] [PMID: 17239702]

Micheletti R, Palazzo F, Barassi P, *et al.* Istaroxime, a stimulator of sarcoplasmic reticulum calcium adenosine triphosphatase isoform 2a activity, as a novel therapeutic approach to heart failure. Am J Cardiol 2007; 99(2A): 24A-32A.
[http://dx.doi.org/10.1016/j.amjcard.2006.09.003] [PMID: 17239701]

Rocchetti M, Besana A, Mostacciuolo G, *et al.* Modulation of sarcoplasmic reticulum function by Na+/K+ pump inhibitors with different toxicity: digoxin and PST2744 [(E,Z)-3-((2-aminoethoxy)imino)androst-ne-6,17-dione hydrochloride]. J Pharmacol Exp Ther 2005; 313(1): 207-15. [(E,Z)-3-(-2-aminoethoxy)imino)androstane-6,17-dione hydrochloride].
[http://dx.doi.org/10.1124/jpet.104.077933] [PMID: 15576469]

Rocchetti M, Alemanni M, Mostacciuolo G, *et al.* Modulation of sarcoplasmic reticulum function by PST2744 [istaroxime; (E,Z)-3-((2-aminoethoxy)imino) androstane-6,17-dione hydrochloride)] in a pressure-overload heart failure model. J Pharmacol Exp Ther 2008; 326(3): 957-65.
[http://dx.doi.org/10.1124/jpet.108.138701] [PMID: 18539651]

Alemanni M, Rocchetti M, Re D, Zaza A. Role and mechanism of subcellular Ca^{2+} distribution in the action of two inotropic agents with different toxicity. J Mol Cell Cardiol 2011; 50(5): 910-8.
[http://dx.doi.org/10.1016/j.yjmcc.2011.02.008] [PMID: 21354172]

CHAPTER 4

Neuroanesthesia

Punita Tripathi*

Johns Hopkins Medical Institutions, Baltimore, Maryland, USA

Abstract: Neuro-anesthesia involves the anesthetic management of neurosurgical patients based on pathophysiology of the central nervous system and the effects of anesthetic agents on the CNS. The anesthetic goal is to avoid secondary injury to the brain and limit the possibility of neurologic deficits in the postoperative period. It is also to provide a rapid wakeup (where appropriate), at the end of the case in order to test for any deficits. Awake craniotomy is used to increase lesion removal from the brain and also minimizing the damage caused to the eloquent cortex. A working scalp block is mandatory for the success of an awake craniotomy.

Keywords: Arnold Chiari, Awake Craniotomy, Cerebral Aneurysm, CNS Tumors, Infratentorial Tumors, Ischemic Cerebrovascular Disease, Malformation, Neuroanesthesia, Scalp Block, Supratentorial Tumors, Traumatic Brain Injury.

INTRODUCTION

Neuro-anesthesia [1 - 4] involves the anesthetic management of neurosurgical patients based on the physiology and pathophysiology of the central nervous system (CNS) and the effects of the anesthetic agents on the CNS. The team involved in the care of neurosurgical patients consists of neurosurgeons, neuro-anesthesiologists, neurologists, neuromonitoring team, neuro critical care team and the nurses.

Goal of the neuro anesthesiologists is to work closely with the surgeons to provide optimum operating conditions for the surgeons while keeping the patient anesthetized, pain free and immobile during the surgery while providing good blood flow and oxygenation to the brain and spinal cord, also providing good neuromonitoring conditions intraoperatively. At the end of surgery, the goal is to provide a quick wake up, so the surgeon is able to do a satisfactory neuro-assessment. It is a specialty where more importance is attached to waking the patients than in putting them to sleep.

* **Corresponding author Punita Tripathi:** Johns Hopkins Medical Institutions, Baltimore, Maryland, USA; Tel: (410) 550-0100; E-mail: ptrip2@jhmi.edu

Amballur D. John (Ed.)

The preoperative, intraoperative and the postoperative goals are to avoid secondary insults to an already injured brain. It is a specialty where the knowledge and expertise of the anesthesiologist can directly influence the patient outcome (Figs. **1 - 3**).

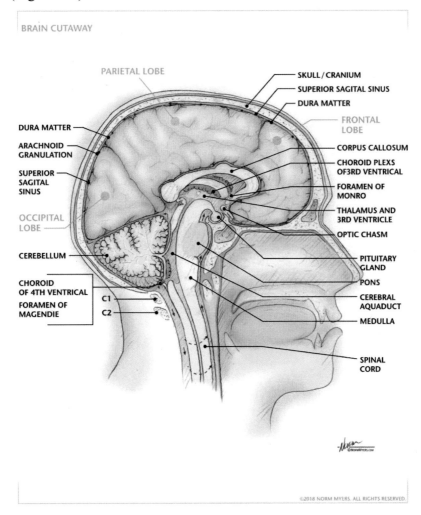

Fig. (1). Brain Structures Cutaway. Image provided by Norm Myers.

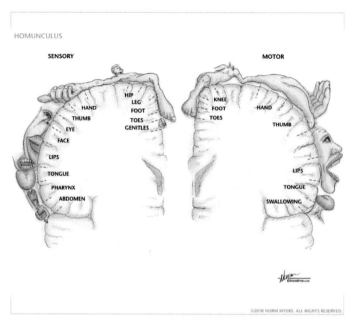

Fig. (2). Homunculus. Image provided by Norm Myers. Reference/Source: This drawing is based on Homunculus (Topographic) Diagram after Wilder Penfiend and Theodore Rasmussen, Montreal Neurological Institute, McGill University, Montreal, Quebec, Canada – ©1950 by Macmillin Publishing Company.

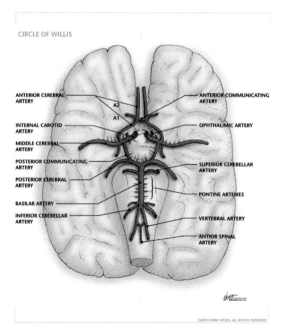

Fig. (3). Circle of Willis. Image provided by Norm Myers.

Secondary Insults to Brain

Intracranial – increased intracranial pressure, seizures, vasospasm and herniation.

Systemic – hypercapnia, hypoxemia, hypo or hypertension, hypo or hyperglycemia, hypoosmolality, shivering or hyperthermia.

Monro-Kellie doctrine or hypothesis – According to this hypothesis, the central nervous system and its accompanying fluids are enclosed in a rigid container whose total volume tends to remain constant. An increase in the volume of one component (*e.g.*, brain, blood, or cerebrospinal fluid) will elevate pressure and decrease the volume of one of the other elements. The ability to compensate for the presence of intracranial mass depends on the volume of the mass and its rate of growth. The compensatory mechanisms to accommodate this mass are:

Early (limited capacity) – shift of blood from intracranial to extra cranial compartment

Late (large capacity) – cerebrospinal fluid (CSF) displacement

Exhausted compensatory mechanism – rapid rise in intracranial pressure (ICP), impaired cerebral circulation, brain herniation which is the end stage of compensation.

PREOPERATIVE CONSIDERATIONS

Patients presenting for neurosurgical procedures maybe undergoing an elective procedure or may present for emergent or urgent surgery. These emergent surgeries may include procedures such as unstable neck with polytrauma, extradural hematomas and ruptured aneurysms. For the urgent cases, a preoperative assessment is very brief but for elective cases routine preoperative evaluations as for any patient should (Tables **1 - 2**) be done.

Patients presenting for neurosurgical procedure can have a wide range of symptomatology. Patients may be asymptomatic (incidental findings on CT scan) or may present with seizures, altered level of consciousness, cranial nerve abnormalities, motor or sensory deficits, speech abnormalities, visual impairment. AVM or aneurysm may present as the "worst headache of my life".

Table 1. Glasgow Coma Scale.

Eye:	1 – No eye opening 2 – Opens eyes to painful stimuli 3 – Opens eyes to voice 4 – Opens eyes spontaneously
Verbal:	1 – Make no sounds 2 – incomprehensible sounds 3 – Inappropriate words 4 – Confused, disoriented speech 5 – Oriented, converses normally
Motor:	1 – No movement 2 – Extensor posturing 3 – Flexor posturing 4 – Moves limbs away from pain 5 – Grabs hand afflicting pain 6 – Follows commands ©2018 A.D. JOHN

Table 2. Hunt-Hess Classification.

Grade 1	Asymptomatic, mild headache, slight nuchal rigidity
Grade 2	Moderate to severe headache, nuchal rigidity, cranial nerve palsy (CN III, VI)
Grade 3	Lethargy, confusion, or mild focal deficit
Grade 4	Stupor, moderate to severe hemiparesis, decerebrate rigidity
Grade 5	Decerebrate rigidity, moribund appearance ©2018 A.D. JOHN

It is important to document any neurological history – type of trauma, functional status before and after trauma, level of consciousness, gross movement of limbs, cardio respiratory status, and seizure activity.

Peripheral nervous system involvement may include weakness of arm legs, sensory loss, bladder and bowel dysfunction may be present with sacral nerve root compression. Documentation of pre-existing deficits is important in spine cases.

Chronic subdural hematoma may present as hemi paresis, s/s of meningeal irritation maybe seen such as headaches, photophobia and stiff neck. Outflow obstruction of CSF may present with evidence of raised ICP.

TIA (transient ischemic attack) and stroke – TIA lasts for few minutes to 24 hours and if it lasts for more than 24 hours, it is called a stroke. The knowledge of the type of TIA gives an idea of vascular areas at risk – Amaurosis fugax indicates ophthalmic artery is involved, indicating an ipsilateral carotid artery disease, transient weakness of face and arms associated with difficulty with speech indicates contra lateral middle cerebral artery involvement, leg weakness only may indicate ischemia of contra lateral anterior cerebral artery, posterior circulation (basilar and vertebral artery) involvement may present as dizziness, vertigo, hoarseness, dysarthria and dysphagia.

Functioning pituitary tumors may present as acromegaly (prognathism, large tongue deepening of voice, large hand and feet). It may be associated with difficult intubation. Cushing's disease present as moon facies, proximal myopathy, central obesity, striae and hirsutism.

Past relevant medical history should be elicited and documented. Optimizing any coexisting disease is important. Cardiac complications are a major source of morbidity and mortality and should be optimized.

Past history of surgery, aneurysm coiling, hydrocephalus as a child, radiation or chemotherapy should be included in the preoperative.

Social history of drug and alcohol intake must be included preoperatively.

Fasting status – It is important to remember that for the trauma patient it is the time from the last oral intake to trauma which represents the duration of fasting.

Symptoms of elevated ICP – can present with subtle symptoms like headaches worse in morning and worse with straining, nausea, vomiting and confusion usually occurs before obtundation. CT scan may show a midline shift of more than 0.5 cm. with expanding cerebral ventricles, cerebral edema or hydrocephalus.

Herniation Syndromes (Fig. 4)

Brain herniation commonly occurs when there is an increase in ICP. It denotes the end point of compensatory mechanism.

Subfalcine (<u>under the falx</u>) – associated with effacement of ipsilateral lateral ventricles and midline shift of the falx. This usually <u>results in</u> loss of movement and sensation in lower extremities.

Transtentorial (<u>through the tentorial notch</u>) – Brain tissues are pushed through the tentorial notch into the posterior fossa. They maybe descending, which is a lesion pushing down leading to pressure on the brain stem. The ascending type of transtentorial herniation occurs when an infratentorial leison pushes up through the tentorium (ascending). It usually <u>presents with</u> an enlarged ventricle because of aqueduct obstruction. A subtype of transtentorial herniation is **uncal herniation** which causes unilateral shift of uncus, a temporal lobe structure under the tentorium which <u>may lead to</u> anisocoria, ptosis and lateral deviation of eye.

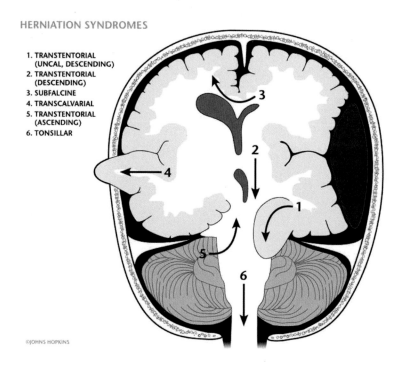

HERNIATION SYNDROMES

1. TRANSTENTORIAL
   (UNCAL, DESCENDING)
2. TRANSTENTORIAL
   (DESCENDING)
3. SUBFALCINE
4. TRANSCALVARIAL
5. TRANSTENTORIAL
   (ASCENDING)
6. TONSILLAR

Fig. (4). Brain Herniation Syndromes. Image provided by Punita Tripathi, M.D., Johns Hopkins.

Tonsillar (through the foramen magnum) – This occurs due to increased pressure in posterior fossa or transmitted increase in pressure from supratentorial space. It causes the cerebellar tonsils to herniate inferiorly through the foramen magnum. It is associated with decerebrate posturing, respiratory and cardiac irregularities and death.

Transcalvarial (through a defect in the skull) – It is usually associated with severe head injury or surgical opening in the cranial vault.

Cushing's triad is used as an indicator of elevated ICP before the actual measurement of ICP. The hall marks of **Cushing's triad** are hypertension, bradycardia and respiratory irregularities.

Informed consent for patients who are very sick with impaired consciousness is taken from the next of kin. Surgery labeled as a Level 1 is the exception where no consent is needed. Consent for anesthesia should include consent for invasive lines and consent for postoperative intubation and ventilation where applicable. Next of kin can give consent in unconscious patients. Telephone consent can be taken with the signature of a witness. In case of the conscious patients, communication with the patient is necessary about the wakeup at the end of the case so they are mentally prepared to move their hands and legs for the neurological check, which the surgeon is likely to be a part of at the end of the case.

Preoperative Medications

All medications especially those started by the neuro-surgeons should be continued to avoid any postoperative complications. These include steroids (decadron), anti-seizure medications (keppra or phenytoin). Chronic steroids may lead to diabetes and stress dose maybe needed at induction.

Anticonvulsant increases the metabolism of steroidal muscle relaxant.

ASA and NSAIDS cause platelet dysfunction.

Patients should continue to get calcium channel blockers if started preoperative to prevent vasospasm.

Anxiolytics, hypnotics and narcotics are used sparingly in neurosurgical cases.

Aspirin, heparin or warfarin that the patient has been prescribed for TIA's should be continued.

Medications used to reduce gastric acidity (ranitidine) and speed gastric emptying (metoclopramide) may be used before induction in emergent cases.

Antibiotics – All patients to undergo surgery get cefazolin 2 gms. intravenous 30 minutes before incision. It is usually repeated every 4 hours. Patients who are allergic to cefazolin are given Clindamycin 600 mg IV.

Allergies – patients with spina bifida who have had multiple bladder catheterizations have a high incidence of latex allergy.

Laboratory

CBC, platelet count (risk of bleeding), hemoglobin baseline should bleeding occur, WBC elevated secondary to steroid use or infections.

Electrolytes, as baseline as electrolyte disturbances fairly common secondary to intracranial pathology and use of diuretics and mannitol, glucose elevated secondary to stress response and steroids, calcium disturbances common in malignancies.

Coagulation tests, as baseline.

LFTs, as baseline, phenytoin may lead to hepatotoxicity.

ECG may indicate underlying cardiac disease and show electrolyte abnormalities which may lead to arrhythmias. It may show changes after catecholamine release secondary to intracranial hemorrhage which may be confused with myocardial infarction. It is thought that the ST-T changes on ECG are secondary to hypothalamic ischemia leading to increased catecholamine production.

Echocardiogram in patients with impaired cardiac functions or those with valvular disease, detection of patent foramen ovale in patients having surgery in sitting position, to rule out clot in the atrial appendage.

CT scan for evidence of intracranial bleeds, mass and mass effects (midline shift).

Communication with Surgeon

Always talk to the surgeon about the surgical side and site, positioning for surgery, temporary occlusion *versus* induced hypotension for aneurysm, intraoperative angiogram, invasive lines (a vascular tumor or an incision that will include sinus will need a central line). Discussion about medications and doses that will be given intra-operatively should be mentioned at this time. It is also important to discuss plans for postoperative care.

MONITORING

Noninvasive Monitoring

ASA standard monitors – ECG lead 2 for arrhythmia detection and V5 for ischemia detection.

Noninvasive blood pressure, neuromuscular blockade, end-tidal CO_2, oxygen saturation *via* pulse oximeter

Urinary output, temperature probe.

All patients get two large bore IVs.

Invasive Monitoring

Arterial line – All neurosurgical cases get an arterial line except for the v-p shunts and simple lumbar spine surgeries. In sitting craniotomy blood pressure should be measured at the level of the head as pressure measured at level of heart will underestimate the pressure perfusing the brain.

ABG and electrolytes, glucose should be sent for a prolonged case.

Central lines are indicated in any case with high risk of air embolism as in sitting craniotomies, tumor invading the sinus or if the surgical approach is through the sinus. Insert double lumen central line with one lumen dedicated for extraction of air if needed.

Cordis should be inserted for vascular tumors or scoliosis surgery with high anticipation of blood loss.

Precordial Doppler – We use it for the sitting craniotomies and if the surgical approach involved the venous sinuses. Precordial Doppler is very sensitive and IV push of drugs can cause the mill wheel murmur! Doppler is placed after patient is in the operative position. The site for the precordial Doppler placement is usually in the middle third of the sternum on the right side. Position is confirmed by injecting agitated saline through the central line or through peripheral line which should produce the classic mill wheel murmur.

Neuromonitoring

<u>Somato sensory evoked potential (SSEP)</u> monitors the integrity of sensory pathway. It is affected by inhaled anesthetic agents. It is indicated for cerebral aneurysm, tumors involving brain stem, major spine surgeries, and cervical spine fractures.

<u>Brain stem auditory evoked response (BAER)</u> resistant to influence of anesthetic agent and can be recorded with high dose inhalation anesthetics. It is indicated for tumors of 8th cranial nerve, vestibular nerve tumors and pontine brain stem tumors.

<u>Motor evoked potential (MEP)</u> recorded over muscles of hand or foot in response to depolarization of motor cortex. It monitors the integrity of motor pathway. It cannot be recorded in presence of complete neuro-muscular blockade.

<u>Cortical mapping</u> indicated in epilepsy surgery and arteriovenous malformation (AVM's).

<u>Electro encephalogram (EEG)</u> used during carotid endarterectomy (CEA), cerebral aneurysm surgery where temporary clipping is used, cerebral protection, extra cranial –intracranial bypass procedures, monitoring cranial nerve function-used for surgery in posterior fossa and lower brain stem.

Cranial nerve function monitoring is done in surgery involving posterior fossa and lower brain stem.

Intracranial Pressure Monitoring (ICP)

Monitoring the ICP allows for optimization of cerebral perfusion pressure (CPP). CPP is calculated as the difference between the mean arterial pressure (MAP) and the ICP. This helps in preventing brain herniation by promptly starting treatment for raised ICP. Normal ICP is about 10 mmHg.

Methods commonly used to measure ICP include ventriculostomy catheter, subarachnoid bolt, epidural sensor and intraparenchymal monitor. The advantage of ventriculostomy catheter is that it can be used to drain CSF.

Fluid and Blood

There is no place for dextrose containing fluid in neurosurgical patients as hyperglycemia might aggravate neurological damage. Isotonic crystalloid (normal saline) or colloids are used. Slightly hypotonic ringers lactate may be used. Hypertonic saline 3% may be beneficial in small quantities (may cause hypernatremia in larger quantities).

Since most patients get mannitol or lasix or both, electrolyte dysfunction may be present. Intra cranial pathology by itself can cause electrolyte abnormalities. In patients with low hematocrit less than 30%, with ongoing blood loss, blood transfusion may be necessary.

INDUCTION OF ANESTHESIA

Goal to have a smooth induction and limit the hypertensive response to laryngoscopy and intubation, prevent secondary insult to already injured brain. This is achieved by avoiding hypercapnia, hypoxemia, hypotension or hypertension, hypo or hyperglycemia, seizure or hyperthermia and hypo osmolality.

These goals can be achieved by preoxygenation for 3-5 minutes followed by lidocaine 1-2 mg/kg, fentanyl 1-2 microgm/kg, propofol 1.5-2mg/kg and after making sure that ventilation is easy nondepolarizing muscle relaxant rocuronium 0.6-1.2 mg/kg is generally used. Persistent depolarizing muscle relaxant succinylcholine 1-2 mg/kg reserved for patients with difficult intubation, bad reflux disease or if neuro monitoring colleagues would desire a pre-positioning neuro-monitoring data in cases of unstable spine. Mild hyperventilation is started with bag mask before manipulation of the airway for intubation. Controlled ventilation is started with goal of keeping $PaCO_2$ about 30 mmHg. Hemodynamic support with sympathomimetic drugs may be needed to prevent a drop in blood pressure so that CPP is not compromised.

The endotracheal tube is secured with tincture benzoin and paper tape re-enforcing with opsite (tegaderm) to avoid accidental extubation. We use umbilical tape to secure the tube in bearded patients and in some patients secured the tube by wiring it to the gums if needed. Using lubrication on the eyes and using opsite to prevent any cleaning solution from going into the eyes are important. Controlled ventilation is started to maintain $PaCO_2$ between 30 and 35 mmHg. Use of PEEP is not recommended as it could impair cerebral venous drainage thus increasing the ICP.

Position and Padding

During craniotomy, the patient's head is placed in a three pin Mayfield skull clamp. Pinning, is a very stimulating part of the surgery. Deepening the depth of anesthesia by giving propofol 0.5-1.0 mg/kg. IV, fentanyl 1-3 mcg/kg. IV or remifentanil 0.5 mcg/kg. IV and increasing the isoflurane to about 1.0 MAC for the duration of pinning is helpful. Antihypertensives short acting esmolol 0.5 mg/kg. IV can also be used. Remember that pin insertion and removal can cause air embolism. A high index of suspicion is needed for diagnosis.

For the prone positioning, in spine cases, the prone pillow is used routinely, making sure the eyes are protected at all times and there is no undue pressure on them. For the park bench and sitting positions avoid extreme flexion or extension of the neck, maintaining more than two fingers space between chin and nearest bone so as to facilitate venous drainage. For lateral positioning a soft shoulder roll (axillary roll) is used on contralateral shoulder to prevent brachial plexus injury.

Supratentorial tumors and vascular leisons are usually done in supine and lateral position. Resection of infratentorial and posterior fossa tumors require either sitting or prone position. **Parkbench** position is lateral position with the body rolled slightly forward, with head rotated to look at the floor. The park bench position allows the surgeon full access to the posterior fossa without increasing the risk of air embolism significantly.

Pad any region susceptible to pressure, abrasion or movement injury. Mild knee flexion decreases back strain.

MAINTENANCE OF ANESTHESIA

Goal is to provide good operating conditions for the surgeon, prevent brain tension, neuroprotection and provide good neuromonitoring conditions. These are achieved by providing adequate depth of anesthesia, good nociception, adequate paralysis, hyperventilation to maintain $PaCO_2$ between 26-30 mmHg.

Choice of technique is controversial – intravenous or volatile anesthetic agent.

The decision to use inhalational anesthesia *versus* the intravenous anesthesia is dictated by underlying physiology, comfort level of the provider or institutional protocols. At our institution we use volatile anesthesia technique. Advantage- it is easy to control and provides predictable wakeup. Disadvantage- Cerebral blood flow (CBF) and cerebral metabolic rate of oxygen ($CMRO_2$) uncoupling occurs.

Isoflurane increases the CBF despite hypocapnia, so it is used in low concentration MAC of 0.5-0.6. It also provides good conditions for SSEP monitoring at that MAC without causing awareness. Sevoflurane 1-1.2% has the advantage of maintaining autoregulation at normocapnia. Remifentanil a short acting opioid is used at our institution. It is esterase metabolized, highly lipid soluble with a half-life of about 3-10 minutes. Remifentanil infusion is run throughout the case at a doses of 0.05-0.2 mcg/kg/min. Keeping the patient paralyzed as long as the patient is pinned by monitoring the twitches and maintaining two twitches at all time is recommended. This makes it easy for the neuromonitoring team to be able to monitor MEPs without difficulty. Monitoring the twitches separate from the neuro- monitoring team is best. There should be good communication between the neuromonitoring team and anesthesia team. The paralytic agent used by us to maintain paralysis is rocuronium 5-10 mg IV, vecuronium can also be used.

Propofol has many theoretical advantages – There is a tightly coupled decrease of cerebral blood flow along with the decrease in cerebral metabolic rate. The ability to reduce cerebral blood volume (CBV), reduces intracranial pressure (ICP) and ability to preserve both autoregulation and vascular reactivity is beneficial. However, it is not always possible to demonstrate these benefits clinically.

The detrimental effects of nitrous oxide are well documented in neurosurgery. It increases CBV by causing vasodilatation even at 0.5 MAC and therefore increases ICP. Postoperative tension pneumocephalus may occur secondary to nitrous oxide trapped in subdural space.

Steroids commonly prescribed by the neurosurgeons as a single dose of Decadron 10 mg IV. It reduces cerebral edema, but a single dose of Decadron 10 mg can also cause increase in blood glucose concentration in non-diabetic patients. Adverse effect of high blood glucose concentration in neurosurgical patient is well documented.

Before bone flap removal mannitol is given 0.25-1 gm/kg., 7.5% Hypertonic Saline NaCl 3-5 ml/kg can also be given. Mannitol is associated with increased urine output, electrolyte disturbances, increased lactate level and decrease in serum sodium. Hypertonic saline increased serum sodium, caused less urine output and less electrolyte disturbance. They were comparable at achieving brain relaxation.

For seizure prophylaxis levetiracetam (Keppra) and/or phenytoin (Dilantin) are commonly used.

Drugs used to prevent nausea vomiting are ondansteron 4 mg. IV 30 minutes before end of case. Decadron is also an antiemetic.

In a prolonged case blood glucose are routinely monitored to avoid hyperglycemia. It is recommended to keep serum glucose below 200 mg/dl.

Measures to Decrease the ICP

Positioning – 30 degrees head up positioning facilitates cerebral venous drainage and decreases ICP Hyperventilation to keep $PaCO_2$ between 26-30 mmHg, no PEEP

Osmotic diuretics in the form of mannitol 0.25-1 gm./kg., loop diuretic like furosemide can be used if unresponsive to mannitol

Hypertonic saline in small amounts (hyper-natremia if used in large quantities)

Steroids in form of decadron 10 mg IV for tumors to decrease brain edema

CSF drainage – through the ventriculostomy drain inserted in the lateral ventricle by the surgeons or by lumbar spinal catheter inserted by the anesthesiologist

Avoid bucking at emergence due to light anesthesia

Seizure prophylaxis

Blood pressure control

INTRAOPERATIVE COMPLICATIONS IN NEUROSURGERY

Unintended Wake-up During Neurosurgery

It is a catastrophic complication and can be minimized with vigilance.

There are several factors that make the neurosurgical patients more prone to this complication. The surgical procedures in the brain have periods of intense stimulation (pinning, skin incision, duramater incision) followed by periods of no stimulation and lack of pain (brain itself). Our neuromonitoring colleagues usually desire 0.6 MAC for monitoring SSEP and want two twitches to monitor MEP. Due to the neurosurgical colleagues' desire to do a prompt wakeup for neurological examination at the end of the procedure, longer acting agents and higher dose of anesthetics are avoided. Also these patients are on antiseizure medications which cause enzymatic induction of P450 system leading to quick metabolism of neuromuscular blocking agents. The patients may also be taking benzodiazepines chronically which may lead to tolerance.

The most important factor to prevent this complication is by paying close attention to anesthetic depth, level of stimulation and following the neuromuscular blockade by peripheral nerve stimulation.

Emergence (Early *versus* Late Emergence)

The goal of emergence in neuroanesthesia is a speedy recovery to allow for a quick neurological assessment at the end of the case. An early detection of neurological complications is important so an early intervention can be performed by the surgeons. It also provides a baseline for subsequent neurological examination. The goal is also to have a calm co-operative patient at the end of surgery who responds to and follows verbal commands.

Aims for emergence is to avoid factors leading to increase in ICP (coughing, intratracheal suctioning, fighting against the ventilator or increase in airway pressure).

Advantages of an early emergence – It allows for a quick neurologic exam and early surgical intervention if needed, less catecholamine surge and hypertensive response due to endotracheal tube, early surgical recovery and decreased costs.

Disadvantages – risk of hypoxemia, hypercarbia during early post-operative period.

Indication for Late Emergence

Preoperative intubated, obtunded patients who is unable to protect their airway

Intraoperative events like prolonged surgery, bleeding more than anticipated for that surgery, repeat surgery, surgery with long vascular clipping times, extensive retractor pressure

The presence of other associated injuries like chest injuries, facial fractures, anticipated brainstem or cranial nerve damage. If late emergence is chosen it should be discussed with the surgeon. In such a case adequate sedation and analgesia should be planned preferably by short acting agents.

The disadvantages of late emergence are less neurologic monitoring at the end of case, delay in treatment of pain, more hypertension and catecholamine release.

Criteria Met for Early Emergence

- Preoperative awake patient
- No catastrophic event intra-operatively
- All extubation criteria met, patient reversed without any inhalational anesthesia on board.
- Patient should be awake and able to follow simple commands and move their extremities.

Differential Diagnosis of Delayed Emergence

Anesthetic causes – use of any long acting opioids, patients should be completely reversed, inhalation anesthetic agent should be completely gone from the system

Non anesthetic causes – intraoperative seizure, cerebral edema, intracranial hematoma (rule out by CT scan), pneumocephalus, vessel occlusion/ischemia, metabolic or electrolyte disturbances, tumor size greater than 3 cm, midline shift more than 3 mm, frontal lobe tumor or posterior fossa tumors and cerebral edema.

Reversal of Anesthesia and Extubation

Almost all cases are awake at the end of surgery to have a good neurological examination, the patient may or may not be extubated. It is recommended to wait to reverse the patients only after pins are out. The extubation criteria should be met for the patient to be extubated. Remember to look at all the intraoperative events prior to deciding to extubate the patient. If the brain is swollen, substantial blood loss has occurred or the patient was not conscious to begin with, then it is appropriate not to extubate the patient. Also involve the surgeon in your decision not to extubate. It is recommended for the attending to be present in the operating room 30 minutes prior to the end of case in order to make sure that safe extubation occurs.

Transfer to Neurosurgical ICU or Post Anesthesia Care Unit

Ideally the patients are extubated in the operating room, which allows for immediate assessment of neurologic function. The patient is usually transported to NSICU with transport monitors, Ambu bag, intubation equipment and emergency drugs. Make sure the oxygen tank is full. Unless contraindicated patient is transported in a 30 degrees head up position. A full report is given to the PACU or ICU nurse.

IMPORTANT ISSUES WITH DIFFERENT NEUROSURGICAL PROCEDURES

Traumatic Brain Injury (TBI)

Traumatic brain injury is defined as a jolt to the head or penetrating injury to head that disrupts the function of the brain. It often involves adolescents, young adults and those older than 75 years.

Results of the Corticosteroid Randomization After Significant Head Injury (CRASH) trial indicates that there is higher risk of death and severe disability in patients getting corticosteroids after brain injury. Investigators concluded it should not be routinely used in treatment of brain injury.

Classification of severe head injury is based on <u>Glasgow Coma Scale (GCS)</u>. The prognosis after head injury depends on the type of lesion sustained, age of patient and the severity of injury defined by GCS.

Evidence based guidelines for management of severe TBI was updated in 2007. The extensive review of literature recommends three standards based on Class 1 evidence and several guidelines based on Class 2 evidence (Table **3**).

Recommendations from Guidelines for Management of Severe Traumatic Brain Injury (TBI)

Burr hole is often indicated for cranial decompression in traumatic brain injury. Goal is to improve functional outcome by surgery (evacuation of hematoma, craniotomy) or medical therapy to avoid prevention of secondary brain injury.

Patients can have associated cervical spine injury and are considered full stomach. If associated with spine injury tracheal intubation is performed with manual in line stabilization, bimanual cricoid pressure. Glide scope maybe used.

Two types of surgical **hematomas** – <u>subdural hematomas</u> result from torn bridging veins and <u>epidural hematomas</u> are usually from an arterial bleed, commonly the middle meningeal artery. These surgeries improved patient survival and prevent secondary brain injury, if an early surgical evacuation is performed.

Management of Elevated ICP

- Hyperventilation – $PaCO_2$ of less than 30 mmHg
- Diuretic – Mannitol in dose of 0.25 to 1 g/kg infused over 20 min. It can be re-dosed at 3 to 6 hours interval

- Posture – 30 degree head up tilt
- Corticosteroids – to decrease brain edema is avoided in head injury patients as it worsens outcome

Table 3. Approaches to Postoperative Analgesia. Adapted from (Bullock RM, Chestnut RM, Clifton GL, *et al.*: Guidelines for management of severe traumatic brain injury. J Neurotrauma 2000;17:449-554; Robertson CS: Management of cerebral perfusion pressure after traumatic brain injury. Anesthesiology 2001;95:1513-1517;) and (Guidelines for the management of severe traumatic brain injury, 3rd. The Brain Trauma Foundation, American Association of Neurological Surgeons; Congress of Neurological Surgeons. J Neurotrauma 2007;24:S1-106).

Standards Based on Class 1 Evidence • Intracranial pressure (ICP) normal avoid prolonged hyperventilation therapy ($PaCO2<25mmHg$) • Steroids are not recommended for improving outcomes or decreasing cerebral edema • Prophylactic use of anticonvulsants does not prevent late post-injury seizures
Standards based on Class 2 Evidence • All regions should have organized trauma care system • Immediately correct hypotension (SBP<90mmHg) and hypoxia (SaO2<90% or PaO2<60mmHg) • Indication for ICP monitoring include GCS score of 3 to 8 with abnormal CT findings or two or more of these adverse features: age>40yrs, posturing and SBP<90mmHg. • Initiate treatment for ICP at threshold above 20mmHg • Cerebral perfusion pressure (CPP) target to lie between 50-70mmHg. Attempts to maintain CPP above 70mmHg avoided because of increased risk of Adult respiratory distress syndrome (ARDS) • Avoid using prophylactic hyperventilation (PaCO2<25 mmHg) during first 24hours after severe TBI. • Mannitol is effective for controlling raised ICP after severe TBI in doses 0.25-1gm/kg. • High dose barbiturate therapy considered in hemodynamically stable, salvageable patients who have severe TBI and whose intra cranial hypertension is refractory to maximum medical and surgical ICP lowering therapy. • Provide nutritional support (140% of resting energy expenditure in patients without respiratory paralysis and 100% of resting energy expenditure in patients with respiratory paralysis) using enteral or parenteral formula containing at least 15% calories as protein by day 7 after major injury. ©2000, 2007 BULLOCK, CHESTNUT, CLIFTON

CENTRAL NERVOUS SYSTEM TUMORS

WHO Grading of CNS Tumors (Table 4)

Of the newly diagnosed brain tumor <u>80% are primary and supratentorial</u> (gliomas 35%, meningiomas about 32%, pituitary adenomas 8%), <u>20% are infratentorial</u>, and <u>12% are metastatic</u> or secondary. Of the <u>metastatic</u> tumor half are from lung cancer and the rest are from cancer of breast, colon, kidney or melanomas.

Table 4. World Health Organization Grading System.

WHO Grading of CNS Tumors	
Grade I Tumor	• Benign = non-cancerous • Slow growing • Cells look almost normal under a microscope • Usually associated with long-term survival • Rare in adults
Grade II Tumor	• Relatively slow growing • Sometimes spreads to nearby normal tissue and comes back (recurs) • Cells look slightly abnormal under a microscope • Sometimes comes back as a higher grade tumor
Grade III Tumor	• Malignant = cancerous • Actively reproduces abnormal cells • Tumor spreads into nearby normal parts of the brain • Cells look abnormal under a microscope • Tends to come back, often as a higher grade tumor
Grade IV Tumor	• Most malignant • Grows fast • Easily spreads into nearby normal parts of the brain • Actively reproduces abnormal cells • Cells look very abnormal under a microscope • Tumor forms new blood vessels to maintain rapid growth • Tumors have areas of dead cells in their center (called necrosis)

©WHO

Supratentorial Tumors

Patient's symptoms are from local or generalized evidence of raised intracranial pressure. The main anesthetic goal is to avoid secondary brain damage. Seizures are common presenting symptoms.

Intraoperative problems – Due to massive hemorrhage, seizure, air embolism (incidence increased with head up position or when venous sinuses are traversed). Steroids are given to decrease cerebral edema, antiseizure medications for seizure prophylaxis, mannitol to decrease brain swelling are commonly used.

Infratentorial Tumors

They are usually tumors of the floor of fourth ventricle, pineal gland tumor, pontomedullary junction, cerebellopontine angle tumors. Acoustic neuromas are the most common infratentorial tumors in adults.

Infratentorial space is a confined space. The brain tolerates tumor poorly leading to symptoms early on. The tumor may involve the brainstem (with cardiovascular and respiratory center). The cardiovascular response may include bradycardia and hypotension or tachycardia with hypertension. It may include ventricular dysrhythmias. Cranial nerve dysfunction of 9th, 10th and 12th may lead to loss of control of upper airway.

Sedative premedication should be used with caution. Resection of the tumor involves unusual positioning (sitting, park bench) of patient for surgery leading to increased incidence of air-embolism, pressure point injury, skin tears, brachial plexus injury. Extreme neck flexion should be avoided as it can lead to quadriplegia. Other peripheral nerve injuries may occur. Cranial nerve dysfunctions may present with dysphagia, chronic aspirations secondary to loss of airway reflexes.

Venous air embolism (VAE) – can occur whenever the pressure in the vessel is sub-atmospheric. Incidence in sitting position as much as 40%, prone or lateral position 15%

Paradoxical air embolism – 25% of general population has probe patent foramen ovale (PFO)

Prevention of VAE- Good surgical technique, high level of PEEP more than 10 cm (controversial), volume loading, hypoventilation (as a consequence of higher cerebral blood flow, controversial)

Treatment- Alert the surgeon, if N_2O is used discontinue immediately, aspirate the central line, give cardiovascular support, compress the jugular veins bilaterally, change patient position (head down) to prevent ongoing VAE, left lateral decubitus position if possible. The surgeon uses saline to flood the operative field, cautery or bone wax used to prevent further air being entrapped.

Intraoperative problems – surgery at or near brain stem may lead to significant cardiovascular response, stimulation of floor of fourth ventricle, medullary reticular formation or trigeminal nerve may result in hypertension along with bradycardia. Vagus n. stimulation may lead to bradycardia. Alert the surgeons.

Postoperative problems – hydrocephalus due to obstruction of ventricular outflow is common cause of increase intracranial pressure (ICP)

Intracranial Aneurysm and Cerebral Arteriovenous Malformation (AVM)

Types – saccular (less than 2.5 cm), giant (10 cm) incidence 5%, fusiform, mycotic, traumatic after severe head injury

Location – 90% occur in the anterior circulation. Gender – female predominantly have internal carotid-post communicating aneurysms whereas <u>men</u> predominantly have anterior communicating artery location and middle cerebral artery bifurcation. 10% occur in posterior circulation, commonly at basilar apex.

Incidence – 1 per 10,000, commonly present in sixth decade. Men outnumber women until 50years of age, women predominate after that. About 20% will have more than one aneurysm. One patient in six will die of subarachnoid hemorrhage (SAH) within minutes. Of the patient admitted 25% will die and 50% will recover completely. It is common in those with connective tissue disorders or those with polycystic kidney disease and Ehlers Danlos syndrome. Cerebral injury, infections and tumors may be associated with aneurysm formation. Other <u>risk factors</u> are hypertension, smoking, and drug abuse (cocaine). Family history is an independent risk factor for SAH.

AVM's incidence in general population 2% – 4%, the annual rate of rupture is 2%.

Symptoms – "worst headache of my life", malaise, irritability, combative and uncooperative

Signs – impaired consciousness, nuchal rigidity, photophobia, focal neurological deficits, seizure, nausea, vomiting, hypertension, fluid, and electrolyte imbalance

Surgical intervention

Early – aneurysm clipping occurs if surgery done in first 24-48 hours after SAH. It has the advantage of preventing any rebleeds, it also leads to a decrease in incidence of vasospasm, reduction in medical complication and hospitalization cost.

Late – surgical intervention occurs in about 2 weeks.

Prevention of Rebleed After SAH

- Control of blood pressure
- Maintain cerebral perfusion pressure
- Adequate control of pain anxiety
- Adequate control of seizures
- Prophylaxis against hypovolemia and vasospasm
- Early surgical or endovascular obliteration of aneurysm
- Treatment with <u>calcium channel blocking drugs</u> to prevent vasospasm
- Treatment of vasospasm – <u>Triple-H therapy</u> (hypertension, hypervolemia and hemodilution). It is the accepted treatment to prevent the progression from vasospasm induced mild ischemia to infarction.

<u>Complications of triple H therapy</u> includes rebleeding leading to hemorrhagic infarction, cerebral edema, intracranial hypertension, hypertensive encephalopathy, pulmonary edema, myocardial infarction, congestive heart failure, coagulopathy.

Majority of aneurysms are treated with a metal clip placed on the base for which controlled hypotension is used. In recent times use of a temporary clip to isolate the aneurysm from the surrounding circulation is used. It allows the surgeon to manipulate the aneurysm without fear of rupture. The disadvantage of the temporary clipping is that it can result in focal cerebral ischemia.

Several neuroprotective interventions have been described. Mild hypothermia (33 degree centigrade) or pharmacological interventions both have been described. Both these have not been associated better neurologic outcomes. A longer temporary clip time (more than 20 minutes) was associated with less favorable outcomes. Once the aneurysm is clipped or ablated, it is desirable to increase the mean arterial pressure (MAP) to help increase the collateral perfusion and avoid ischemia.

Preoperative intra cerebral embolization of large feeding vessels of very vascular tumors and AVM's decreases bleeding and facilitates resection.

In the event of an aneurysm rupture there could be massive bleeding intraoperative, massive brain swelling can occur. Intraoperative barbiturates or propofol may be used for neuroprotection. Adenosine, a purine nucleoside which slows conduction through the atrioventricular node can be used in case of rupture during surgery to facilitate aneurysm clipping. The suggested dose is 0.4 mg/kg. Pacing pads may need to be placed as 4% of patients may need temporary pacing after use of adenosine.

Clinical Signs of Vasospasm

- Progressive impairment of level of consciousness
- Appearance of new focal neurologic deficits more than 4 days after initial SAH, not associated with structural or metabolic cause
- Onset sudden or insidious
- Associated with headache, meningismus and fever

Predictors of Mortality After Subarachnoid Hemorrhage

- Poor neurologic condition on hospital admission
- Older patient
- Preexisting illness
- Elevated blood pressure

- CT scan shows evidence of thick clot in the brain substance or ventricle
- Repeat hemorrhage
- Basilar aneurysm

Anesthesia for AVM Repair

- Flow characteristics – low-pressure high-low shunts, they are unlikely to rupture during acute episode of hypertensive response to laryngoscopy, that are frequently associated with aneurysm. However high pressure vascular channels, especially in veins that have fibromuscular thickening and incompetent elastic lamina are prone to rupture.
- Location supratentorial (70-90%), inratentorial (10-30%), deep brain structure (5-18%).
- Maybe associated with aneurysm in more than 50% patients.
- Associated with Osler Weber Rendu disease, Sturge Weber syndrome.
- One must be prepared for massive persistent blood loss and postoperative cerebral swelling.

Aneurysm Coiling

Endovascular approach is used to secure both intact aneurysm and those associated with SAH. The coiling was indicated for the aneurysms that are not anatomically favorable for surgical intervention such as posterior cerebral circulation or aneurysm where the neck is narrow relative to the dome. Since anesthesiologist are at a distance from the patient slack of monitoring and intravenous lines should be maintained. The pain associated is confined to the sheath placement so narcotics should be limited.

Access to the arterial circulation is through a sheath placed in the femoral artery. Immobilization to the point of holding respiration for short period is necessary for the success of the procedure. Controlled respiration also helps to reduce motion artifact and improve the image quality. Anticoagulant therapy is important component of endovascular therapy.

Contrast reaction can range from direct cardiac depression to anaphylactoid reaction. Contrast nephropathy can occur. Risk factors for nephropathy are diabetes, large dye load during prolonged procedure, dehydration, pre-existing renal dysfunction and concurrent administration of other nephrotoxic agents.

Anesthesia technique may range from local, sedation or general anesthesia. If general anesthesia is not used the patient should be able to lie still for a few hours and also be able to follow commands. If sedation is to be used it should be light sedation so that neurological checks can be possible on the patient and there is minimum respiratory artifact from an obstructed airway. In case of patients with an increased risk for vasospasm such as those with SAH, it is necessary to maintain a higher blood pressure to provide adequate cerebral perfusion.

Aneurysm rupture during procedure can be catastrophic and has an incidence of 3-5%. Rupture is associated with massive Cushing's response (bradycardia) or cardiac arrest. If possible the ruptured aneurysm should be packed with coils and it may be necessary to reverse any heparin with protamine. Maintaining a good cerebral perfusion pressure is desirable.

ISCHEMIC CEREBROVASCULAR DISEASE

Carotid Endarterectomy (CEA)

The management goals for CEA is protecting the heart and brain by preventing any ischemic event to either organ. This is achieved by maintaining strict hemodynamic stability.

A significant proportion of strokes are due to stenosis of carotid artery leading to disability. Randomized controlled trials have confirmed the benefits of carotid endarterectomy (CEA). These are older patients with several risk factors like CAD, HTN, DM, tobacco use.

Surgical guidelines for CEA- the selected candidate should have symptomatic transient ischemic attack (TIA) with 70% to 99% stenosis of the artery. The stenosis should be surgically accessible and the patient should be stable medically and neurologically. There is a perioperative risk of stroke and death in about 4%-7% of cases undergoing CEA.

They can be performed under general or regional anesthesia safely. Regional anesthesia includes superficial or deep cervical plexus block. Superficial cervical plexus block is done by injecting LAA along the posterior border of sternocleidomastoid muscle. Deep cervical plexus block is a paravertebral block of C2 to C4 nerve roots. Goals for anesthesia for CEA are prevention of cerebral ischemia through maintenance of adequate cerebral perfusion pressure and prevention of myocardial ischemia by avoiding acute rise in blood pressure and heart rate both intraoperative and postoperative. Advantages of regional anesthesia are superior neurologic monitoring as the patient is awake, rapid recovery from surgery and shorter hospitalization. Disadvantages includes that the awake patient has an unprotected airway. It is stressful to manage complications (stroke, loss of airway, disinhibition or local anesthetic toxicity) in an awake patient.

Other important consideration in these patients are central nervous system protection by glycemic control, maintain normocarbia and keep blood pressure within 20% of baseline. Postoperative – frequent CNS assessment, blood pressure control, hematoma/airway, nerve injury

Carotid Angioplasty and Stenting (CAS)

In recent years, Carotid angioplasty and stenting have gained momentum and are the leading alternative to CEA. Two recent trials –The Stenting and Angioplasty with Protection in Patients at High Risk for Endaretrectomy (SAPPHIRE) and recent Carotid Revacularization Endarterectomy *versus* Stenting Trial (CREST) have helped to form the practice guidelines for extracranial stenosis management. SAPPHIRE study concluded that CAS was not inferior to CEA in regards to adverse events and major strokes in high-risk surgical candidates. It showed lower incidence for myocardial infarction in these candidates. CREST results indicate there was no difference in primary end points between CEA and CAS after 4 years. However, there was a slight increase in stroke in CAS group and a slight increase in myocardial infarction in CEA group. All patients presenting for CEA should be maintained on regimen of ASA and/or clopidogrel in order to decrease the risk of TIA and stroke.

Contraindications to CEA

- Complete internal carotid artery occlusion
- Previous stroke on ipsilateral side with significant sequelae
- Comorbidities deemed too risky for CEA
- Tracheostomy
- Neck irradiation
- Prior neck dissection
- Prior vocal cord paralysis

Indications for CAS

- Previous CEA
- Contralateral carotid artery occlusion
- Previous neck dissection or radiation to neck
- Require concurrent major cardiac or aortic surgery
- Inability to extend the neck
- Contralateral laryngeal n palsy
- Tracheostomy

Contraindications for CAS

- Abnormal vessel anatomy

- Diffuse carotid disease
- Unacceptable high medical risk

NEURO ENDOCRINE TUMORS

Pituitary micro adenomas, adenomas which may be intrasellar or extend into the cranium superiorly (involving the optic chiasm) or extend laterally into the cavernous sinus (involving the intrasphenoid carotid artery, 3rd, 4th, 5th ophthalmic and maxillary division and the 6th cranial nerves). These tumors can be functioning and nonfunctioning tumors. Usual presentation as headaches, visual field defect, galactorrhea, amenorrhea or infertility.

Transsphenoidal approach involves intraoperative injection of epinephrine containing local anesthetic agent to nasal mucosa. It may lead to hypertension, arrhythmias or myocardial ischemia. Advantage of this approach is that there is no scar, less damage to frontal lobe or olfactory apparatus, lower incidence of diabetes insipidus and shorter hospital stay. Disadvantage of this approach includes potential for CSF leak, meningitis, blood loss which may be difficult to control, may require packing of the cavernous sinus.

Transfrontal approach, the advantage of this approach is direct visualization of optic chiasm and other structure, surgeon can easily access suprasellar tumors.

Disadvantage includes higher morbidity than trans-sphenoidal approach, diabetes insipidus more likely.

Epilepsy, Surgical Intervention

Most patients with epilepsy are well managed medically but 5 to 15% of patients with epilepsy have intractable seizures and cannot be managed medically. About 13% of these patients are candidates for resection of epileptogenic focus. Partial seizures are treated with some form of temporal lobectomy. Awake craniotomy is performed to preserve functionally important areas at risk for damage like the Wernicke's area for speech and the motor area. These patients are on a variety of antiepileptic drugs for a prolonged time. Adverse effect of antiepileptic drugs is dose dependent and are associated with long term therapy.

Spinal Cord Tumors

These tumors can be primary or metastatic in origin. Lesions located on the upper cord are more damaging physiologically. The choice of anesthesia will be dictated by location and severity of the lesion. The risk of hyperkalemia with use of succinylcholine is increased as with any spinal injury. Patients may show evidence of spinal shock. They maybe at increased risk of air embolism, as surgical site is above the level of the heart in the prone position. It is usually associated with blood loss. Positioning – prone, type and cross match, neuromonitoring

ARNOLD CHIARI MALFORMATION

It is caused by a downward displacement of the cerebellar tonsils into the spinal canal. It may be associated with other malformation like syringomyelia, spina bifida, and hydrocephalus. These defects develop during fetal development. The etiology is thought to be genetic or maternal diet lacking in some nutrient. Less commonly thought to be due to injury or infection. Incidence is 1 in 1000 births, but maybe more common as the diagnostic imaging is showing it more commonly.

Types

Type 1 – commonly seen in children and is due to cerebellum extending through foramen magnum, without involving the brain stem. It is the only type that can be acquired.

Type 2 – seen in children with spina bifida. It is also called the classic Chiari malformation. It is associated with extension of both cerebellar and brain stem tissue extending through the foramen magnum.

Type 3 – It is associated with herniation of cerebellum and brain stem through the foramen magnum. A part of the 4th ventricle may also protrude.

Type 4 – It is associated with incomplete or underdeveloped cerebellum.

Signs and symptoms Patients complain of neck pain, dizziness, problems with balance, muscle weakness, numbness or other abnormal feelings in arms and leg, vision problems, swallowing difficulties, ringing in the ears, hearing loss, vocal cord paralysis, vomiting insomnia, depression, headaches worse on straining.

Type 3 and 4 are rare and associated with gross herniation of cerebellum and severely malformed brain stem.

Treatment

No treatment needed in asymptomatic cases. Surgery is needed to correct or halt the progression of damage to the central nervous system. The surgical procedure may include suboccipital decompression of the posterior fossa, with or without duraplasty, with stabilization of craniocervical junction by occipitocervical fusion with autogenous bone graft, restoration of CSF flow, ablation and drainage of syringomyelia where applicable.

CERVICAL SPINE FUSION, SCOLIOSIS AND MULTILEVEL LAMINECTOMIES, INSTRUMENTATION AND FUSION

Airway management – Awake fibreoptic intubation is used in traumatic spine injury or unstable spine. Manual inline stabilization for glidescope intubation can be used in some cases. Intraoperative risk of recurrent laryngeal n injury (5%), sympathetic chain injury, esophageal injury, carotid artery or jugular vein injury may lead to massive blood loss. Rapid emergence to be able to facilitate neurologic examination at the end of case is recommended.

Anterior cervical discectomy and fusion (ACDF) – Anterior approach provides good access to vertebral bodies and tranverse processes of C2-7. Right approach is associated to with increased damage to recurrent laryngeal nerve but decreases the damage to thoracic duct. Fusion rate is greater with autograft from iliac bone. Smooth emergence to prevent graft dislodgement is important. Postoperative dysphagia is common secondary to traction on esophagus.

Intraoperative issues – Blood loss may be an issue as cancellous bones can bleed, decreased lung compliance because of chest wall and abdominal compression in the prone position. VAE may be possible. Direct pressure on the orbit may lead to blindness. Stretching or direct pressure to nerves may lead to nerve injury. Pressure point injuries are common. Some surgeons may like to do a wake up test during the procedure.

Neuromonitoring

SSEP is not affected if MAC of inhalation anesthesia used is kept between 0.5-0.6. For MEP monitoring keep 2 twitches at all time, especially at time of instrumentation. Wakeup at end of surgery so as to be able to document the ability to move extremities and follow simple commands is desired. Postoperative extubation may or may not be performed depending on all factors.

Epidural hematoma in postoperative period is a rare but devastating complication. Early diagnosis and evacuation may prevent irreversible damage to spinal cord. Permanent postoperative visual loss is rare but devastating complication.

VENTRICULOPERITONEAL SHUNT AND ENDOSCOPIC VENTRICULOSTOMY

Hydrocephalus – Two types

In **communicating hydrocephalus,** the obstruction occurs at the point of CSF absorption and all the ventricles lateral, third and fourth ventricles are dilated on CT scan, herniation syndromes are not seen. In **noncommunicating hydrocephalus**, the obstruction occurs within the ventricular system resulting in some of the ventricle to dilate out of proportion to the rest; herniation syndrome may then be seen. It presents with evidence of raised ICP due to overproduction of CSF or impaired drainage. **Normal pressure hydrocephalus** seen in elderly may present with gait disturbances or headaches. Shunt malfunction and revision can be seen in small percentage coming to the OR. Other shunts being performed are ventriculo-atrial shunt and the ventriculo-pleural shunts to drain the CSF. Complications- aspiration risk as they are prone to increased nausea and vomiting due to rise in ICP, latex allergy seen in those with history of myelomeningocele, surgical trauma (rapid decompression may lead to rupture of bridging veins, intrathoracic trauma due to tunneling of shunt) and venous air embolism (placement of ventriculoatrial shunt). Endoscopic ventriculostomy is performed to relieve noncommunicating hydrocephalus by making a perforation on the floor of the third ventricle with an endoscope. Benefits – no foreign material is left in the patient. Complications – bradycardia can occur in 40% of patients, can damage structures near floor of 3rd ventricle, lead to arrhythmias, asystole, hypertension and hemorrhage.

POSTOPERATIVE COMPLICATIONS

Signs That Should Trigger Immediate Response

- Decrease in level of consciousness
- Pupillary abnormalities
- Development of focal deficits
- Increased ICP
- Extreme agitation and repeated vomiting

Delayed Emergence from Anesthesia

Delayed emergence from anesthesia is a stressful problem for both the surgeons and anesthesiologists. It may lead to expensive and often unnecessary neuro-radiologic testing. The reasons are multifactorial. They are anesthesia related (the longer acting anesthetic agents used), surgery related (brain retraction, frontal pathology, surgical excision, posterior fossa tumors), medication administered and drug interaction (both preoperative and intraoperative), the disease process (seizure) and electrolyte or metabolic causes.

Major Predictors of Delayed Emergence:

- Tumor size greater than 30 mm

- Midline shift more than 3 mm
- Cerebral edema
- Frontal and posterior cranial fossa tumors associated with highest incidence
- Cerebral hematomas exceeding 2-3 cm in size
- Large lobar hematomas
- Temporary occlusion of cerebral artery leading to ischemic-reperfusion cerebral injury after restoration of blood flow
- Preoperative decreased level of consciousness

Postoperative Paralysis and Nerve Injury

Postoperative paralysis is a devastating complication, may first manifest in the PACU. Central paralysis must be differentiated from peripheral. Quick diagnosis is critical as immediate surgical intervention as in case of epidural hematoma may prevent long term sequel. Peripheral neuropathies are less likely to need urgent surgical interventions.

Pressure Injury, Skin Lesions, and Corneal Abrasion

These occur at a higher frequency in neurosurgical cases. The skin lesions are due to adhesive tape or pressure over an ECG electrode. They are not life threatening but may cause discomfort to the patients. The pressure injuries are due to the positioning of the patient. Corneal abrasion may present with foreign body sensation, tearing, blurring or photophobia to the eye. Prevention is important and an ophthalmologic consult may be called if needed.

Upper Airway Complications

Residual anesthetic should be ruled out if it occurs in the immediate postoperative period. Damage to the cranial nerves or their nuclei can lead to difficulty maintaining the airway. These may include posterior fossa tumor resection, skull base tumor resection, carotid endarterectomy. Cranial nerve 5th, 7th, 9th, 10th and 12th are important in maintaining airway integrity. Cranial nerve 9th and 10th damage can lead to swallowing difficulties. Damage to 12th cranial nerve can lead to poor control of tongue. Damage to vagus nerve can lead to vocal cord paralysis. Other reasons for airway obstruction could be postoperative swelling of the tongue in cases which have prolonged surgery in the prone position or where massive fluid exchange has occurred. Hematoma formation after carotid endarterectomy may lead to tracheal deviation and difficult intubation.

Hypertension

As many as 80% of patient undergoing elective craniotomy may have hypertensive episodes in the postoperative period. They should be promptly evaluated and treated. If left untreated may lead to hemorrhage from the surgical field. In patients with increased intracranial pressure, hypertension must be treated to lower the ICP without decreasing the cerebral perfusion pressure (CPP) which may cause cerebral ischemia. Labetolol an alpha and beta blocker is a good choice in neurosurgical patients because of its rapid onset of action, easy titrability and no effect on ICP. Esmolol may be used where short duration of action may be needed. Hydralazine (arterial dilator) and nifedipine (calcium channel blocker) can be used but are difficult to titrate and can increase ICP. Nicardipine given by infusion allows rapid control.

Postoperative Seizure:

The incidence of seizures in postoperative period is about 3% and about 70% occur within 6 hours. Seizures are <u>more likely to occur</u> if involved surgical site is the sensory or motor cortex. The incidence is higher in patients with a history of preexisting seizure. Prevention is crucial as they may cause complications like aspiration, hypoxemia, increased ICP and intracranial bleed. The commonly used anti-seizure medications are

Phenytoin – It is a sodium channel blocker, undergoes hepatic metabolism, loading dose is 18-20 mg/kg IV, maintenance dose 3-5 mg/kg IV

Phenobarbital – It prolongs chloride channel conductance, undergoes hepatic metabolism and renal excretion, loading dose 20 mg/kg and maintenance dose 2-4mg/kg/day IV.

Levetiracetam (Keppra) – It binds to synaptic vesicle protein 2A, undergoes renal metabolism, dosage in less than 65 yrs 500-1000 mg every 12 hours IV, in patients more than 65 yrs old 250-500 mg every 12 hours IV. Ongoing seizure activity in the postoperative period, maintaining a patent airway and oxygenation are essential. This is followed by medications to arrest the seizure activity immediately.

Drugs commonly used are midazolam (1-5 mg IV) increases chloride channel conductance, propofol (25-50 mg IV) incremental doses till seizure stops, acts by inhibiting the NMDA receptors. Neuromuscular blockage will stop the motor activity but will not halt the seizure activity.

Arrhythmias

Arrythmias occuring in the postoperative period maybe due to hypoxemia, hypercarbia, acid-base disturbances, electrolyte abnormalities, preexisting organic heart disease, myocardial ischemia, stress and postoperative pain. The arrhythmia may range from benign to lethal, so it is important to identify the cause and treat them.

Postoperative Pain

Multimodal analgesic regimen seems to be more successful as it helps to reduce the narcotic side effect. Narcotics, short acting fentanyl is usually used initially as bolus followed by PCA, acetaminophen 500 mg to 1000 mg IV, scalp infiltration with IV bupivacaine 0.25% with 1:200,000 of epinephrine decreased the pain scores and reduces the dose of narcotics used by patients. Pain is usually undertreated in neurosurgical patients to avoid sedation and can lead to chronic pain syndromes.

Postoperative Nausea and Vomiting

Prevention is important, ondansteron 4 mg IV, decadron 4 mg IV. Postoperative promethazine (phenergan) 12.5-25 mg IV, prochlorperazine (Compazine) 5-10 mg IV may also be used. Refractory nausea and vomiting may denote intracranial pathology with rise in ICP.

POSTOPERATIVE COMPLICATIONS ASSOCIATED WITH SPECIFIC NEUROSURGICAL PROCEDURES

Carotid Endarterectomy

These could include stroke (2-10%), cranial nerve damage, myocardial ischemia or infarction, hemorrhage, hypertension (more than 60%) or hypotension. Hemorrhage at the operative site may lead to distortion of airway with difficult reintubation.

Posterior Fossa Craniotomies

Bleeding and edema in the posterior fossa craniotomies is poorly tolerated as it may lead to brain stem compression or ischemia. Cranial nerve 4th to 12th maybe involved leading to loss of airway integrity. Acute hydrocephalus can occur because of obstruction of CSF flow from edema or blood clots. They need to be treated emergently with ventriculostomy (lifesaving) or ventricular shunt.

Pituitary Tumor Resection

Inability to breathe through the nose because of nasal packs is a common cause of distress for the extubated patients. CSF leak may lead to meningitis. In transphenoidal resection of pituitary tumor, the intrasellar cavity maybe packed with fat or muscle which may cause chiasmal compression leading to visual field defect. Endocrinal abnormalities may manifest as adrenal insufficiency. This may require perioperative replacement of hydrocortisone 100 mg IV every 6 hours. Patients with Cushing's disease may have hyperglycemia, hypokalemia and hypertension. Diabetes insipidus may occur in the postoperative period.

Spinal Surgeries

Evaluation of new neurologic deficit in the postoperative period may indicate an epidural hematoma, which may need quick diagnosis and surgical evacuation to prevent long term sequel. Hemodynamic instability may be seen in the quadriplegic patients in the PACU. Postoperative visual loss is a dreaded but rare complication after major spinal surgery.

AWAKE CRANIOTOMY [5 - 7]

Indication for Doing an Awake Craniotomy

The two major indications for doing an awake craniotomy are:

- Intraoperative neurological testing which allows for optimal tumor resection with minimal postoperative neurological deficits in lesions located close to motor cortical area, sensory cortical areas and those responsible for speech both Broca's area and Wernicke's area.
- Resection of epileptic foci close to vital areas of the brain especially those responsible for speech and motor activity

The indications for awake craniotomy has extended from procedures necessitating functional mapping to improve perioperative outcomes, minimize resource utilization in cases of stereotactic brain biopsy, ventriculostomy and resection of small brain lesion. Patients are highly motivated and eager to maximize the chance of cure with minimum postoperative neurological deficits.

Anesthetic Goals

The anesthetic goals for awake craniotomy is to provide adequate analgesia, amnesia, airway protection, hemodynamic stability during the painful portion of the procedures with restriction of movement. This is followed by period when an alert cooperative patient is needed who is able to follow commands and speak during the intraoperative neurological mapping and assessment. It is generally well tolerated. Success of the technique depends on a careful selection of patients, knowledge of neuro-anesthesia techniques, an effective scalp block, and a dedicated sedation protocol. It is important to be prepared to manage the airway under emergent conditions.

Benefits of an Awake Craniotomy

These include greater extent of resection with better preservation of language function, shorter ICU stay, and shorter hospitalization thereby reducing costs, decrease in use of invasive monitors without compromising patient care. Associated with decreased postoperative anesthetic complications (nausea and vomiting) and decreased risk of permanent deficit. One retrospective comparison found no difference in seizure-free outcomes after awake resections *versus* those done under general anesthesia.

Contraindications

A claustrophobic patient with high level of anxiety not amenable to treatment or psychological preparation.

Tumors requiring prone positioning, tumors with extensive dural invasion (significant pain on resection) and inability to cooperate because of profound dysphasia, confusion or language barrier are absolute contraindication for this procedure.

Relative contraindications include complicated airway, morbidly obese, severe gastric reflux, decreased pulmonary reserve, mentally retarded patients, young children and very large tumors.

Preoperative Preparation and Evaluations

It is same as for any surgical case, preoperative evaluation for anesthesia with cooperation between the surgical and anesthesia teams. A meeting with the anesthesiologist assigned to the case is important to allay some of the anxiety that the patient may have. A step by step discussion of sequence of events and the duration of the procedure and what to expect usually is helpful. Most patients are highly motivated, when they know the reason for doing the surgery awake. It is important to assess for difficult intubation, obstructive sleep apnea, risk of aspiration, and the ability to maintain good oxygenation and carbon-di-oxide elimination during unprotected spontaneous ventilation. Preoperative one must determine that the patient does not suffer from claustrophobia, uncontrolled anxiety, post nasal drip or uncontrolled gastro esophageal reflux (diabetes mellitus or obesity). The patient should be able to breath adequately in lateral position and able to take part in complex and subtle neurological testing. Medical optimization of any condition is important. As always preoperative assessment should include neurological examination and documentation of baseline status, any evidence of raised ICP need to be documented. Assessment of risk factors for sedation failure should be done in the preoperative visit namely history of alcohol and drug abuse, chronic pain disorders, low tolerance to pain and anxiety, psychiatric disorders, language barrier are some of the factors. Since we use nasopharyngeal airway for maintaining a patent airway for the case, examination of external nares and airflow through them is important.

Positioning and Padding

Since the patient has to be immobile for a long duration, pillows should be placed behind the patient's back, between the legs and under the arms. Warming blankets should be placed so as to keep the patient warm in the cold operating room. Positioning should allow for some freedom of movement of extremities. The placement of surgical drapes should allow for maximum visibility of the face by the anesthesiologists. The patient is positioned in supine, semi lateral or lateral position. It is important to make sure that the axis of head neck and the body is aligned so as not to impede venous drainage and thereby increase the ICP. The neck should be somewhat extended, as a flexed neck may lead to airway obstruction. Access to the surgical field, airway, speech, sight, and facial expression must all be made possible without causing the patient to feel claustrophobic. The patient must remain in rigid pin fixation and lie motionless on an operating table for several hours so it is important to keep the pressure point padded and protected for patient comfort. Egg crates and axillary rolls are commonly used if the patient is in semi-lateral position.

Expanded Role of the Anesthesiologist

During an awake craniotomy, the role of the anesthesiologist broadens from clinician to encompass the role of coach, confidant, and interpreter. In addition to making frequent inquiries about the wellbeing of a patient, the anesthesiologist must remain vigilant about their primary job of monitoring the patient. At the same time anesthesiologist facilitates patient communication with the surgeon and provides encouragement and reassurance to the patient.

Anesthetic Management

A variety of anesthetic techniques have been described for an awake craniotomy. The two general techniques in the literature are asleep-awake-asleep (AAA) and monitored anesthetic care (MAC), with sedation. MAC provides a better smoother transition from asleep to awake states so we follow it at our institution.

Premedication

It has to be individualized for every patient. The primary goal of premedication is to achieve anxiolysis without over sedation. Secondary goals include prevention of nausea, seizure, reflux, pain, hemodynamic instability, or other adverse effects. Anxiety – good psychological preparation and preoperative visit by the anesthesiologist is better than any medication. If anxiolytics are to be used, short acting benzodiazepines, midazolam 1-2 mg. IV should be given in the immediate preoperative period. Short acting narcotics such as fentanyl 25-50 mcg. IV maybe helpful. Over sedation should be avoided. Antibiotics should be given 30 minutes prior to the incision. Anticonvulsants should be continued in the preoperative period. Levetiracetam (keppra) and or phenytoin (dilantin) are used by our neurosurgeons. Steroids are used to decrease brain edema. It is also an antiemetic. Nausea and vomiting – antiemetic is used pre-emptively to reduce the risk. Drugs that can be used are ranitidine, metoclopramide, ondansetron, dexamethasone and scopolamine patch. Use of 5% lidocaine ointment for nasopharyngeal tube insertion along with Afrin nasal spray (pseudoephedrine) is used. Afrin acts as a vasoconstrictor and lidocaine is a local anesthetic agent.

Monitoring

Noninvasive monitors – ASA standard monitoring, $ETCO_2$ (aim is to determine respirations rather than accurate end tidal CO_2), urinary output, body temperature, BIS monitor (BIS Index is kept at or more than 60). Invasive monitors – arterial catheter for continuous blood pressure monitoring is used in all cases, central venous catheters are inserted where large blood loss is anticipated or where craniotomy in sitting position is to be performed or where peripheral access cannot be found. Two peripheral IV lines are recommended. One line should be dedicated for intravenous anesthetic agent and analgesic to prevent inadvertent bolus. Ringers lactate is infused 3-4 ml/kg/hour for maintenance.

Intraoperative

Goals are to maintain sufficient depth of anesthesia and adequate analgesia for pinning, skin incision and craniotomy. Our protocol is to wake up our patients prior to duramater incision so that even if the patient moves slightly during the sleep-awake period the duramater is intact. Local anesthetic agents are used for scalp block and duramater incision. Aim is to achieve full consciousness during electrical mapping and functional testing, adequate airway management without hypoxia or hypercarbia and having comfortable patient for the duration of surgery. Several techniques are used to maintain airway patency. A soft nasopharyngeal airway insertion (unsecured airway), LMA (partially secured airway) and endotracheal intubation (secured airway). At our institution we insert a soft nasopharyngeal airway to maintain airway patency. The incidence of coughing straining is more in cases of airway instrumentation at the time of waking the patient up for testing.

INDUCTION AND MAINTENANCE OF ANESTHESIA

Craniotomy

Usually lasts for 1.5-2 hours. Propofol intravenous bolus for nasopharyngeal tube insertion. The loading dose ranges from 1-2 mg/kg and the continuous infusion is started at 150 mcg/kg/min and is titrated down to about 75 mcg/kg/min with the addition of 50% nitrous oxide in oxygen and volatile inhalational agent (sevoflurane) to a MAC of about 0.7. This is added through a 7.0 endotracheal tube connector connected to the nasopharyngeal airway, which is then connected to the anesthesia circuit. It is important to know that the MAC value displayed may not be accurate as it is not a fully sealed circuit. Fentanyl (1-2 mcg/kg) is given intravenously before doing the scalp block for pinning. The patient breathes spontaneously throughout the case. Assisted ventilation through the bag is recommended if the $ETCO_2$ goes very high and sedation need to lighten. Mannitol 0.25-1 gm/kg IV is given at the request of the surgeon. Occasionally loop diuretics furosemide IV maybe given. Urinary catheter and invasive monitoring (A-line and/or CVP) is usually inserted after induction.

The use of different agents during this part prevents the side effect associated with one agent. Propofol leaves residual EEG footprint characterized by high frequency, high amplitude beta activity that can obscure abnormal activity being sought in the cortical surface. Excessive or potent narcotics will lead to decreased respiratory rate leading to carbon-di-oxide retention and increased brain swelling. Dexmedetomidine infusion is known to delay patient responsiveness when trying to wake up in some cases. Sevoflurane in high doses may lead to emergence excitement, which is especially dangerous in a patient with pins. Nitrous oxide in 50% dose allows for some analgesia and amnesia where needed (Table **5**).

Scalp Block

The scalp block is an anatomical block and not a ring block. All 14 of the nerves need to be blocked. A ring block will require large volumes of local anesthetic agents which will increase the risk of toxicity. A working scalp block is important for the success of the procedure. Analgesia with local anesthetic agent is performed by the surgeons or the anesthesiologists. It includes blocking supraorbital, supratrochlear, zygomatico-temporal, auriculotemporal, greater occipital, lesser occipital nerves and greater auricular nerve on both sides. Also infiltration at the point of pinning and at incision site is important. Success of surgery is greatly dependent on the adequacy of the block otherwise the patient may become restless, uncooperative and will need higher dose of sedatives and analgesics which may interfere with cortical mapping. Also with the higher dose of anesthesia it is likely that the patient may become dis-inhibited. The skin is cleaned with chlorhexidine, use of sterile glove and 25 gm needle is recommended.

Table 5. Anesthetic Agents used – Pros and Cons.

Agent	Advantage	Disadvantage
Propofol dose bolus 1-2mg/kg, infusion 50-150mcg/kg/min	- Rapid onset and recovery - Decreased CBF, ICP, CMR02 - Antiemetic, amnesic properties, anticonvulsant	- Rapid onset and recovery cumulative effect
Sevoflurane	- Rapid onset and emergence, decreased CMR02 - Less of airway irritation	- Potential to increase CBF, in concentration over 1.5MAC, excitation on emergence
Fentanyl dose bolus 1mcg/kg, infusion 0.01mcg/kg/min	- Short acting, potent analgesic, does not cause apnea, can be reversed	- May interfere with mapping if not well titrated
Nitrous oxide 50% in healthy pts does not alter regional CBF and CMRO2	- 50% of nitrous reduced the dose of both propofol and sevoflurane – rapid onset and recovery	- Pnemocephalous not an issue because of sufficient time for it to wash out
Local anesthetic agents	- Less expensive, ability to examine neurological status	- Toxicity in seizure prone patients
Remifentanil dose 0.02-0.2mcg/kg/min	- Quick onset of action, may cause apnea	- Poorly tolerated in elderly, hypotension, bradycardia
Dexmedetomidine dose bolus 0.1-0.5mcg/kg/hr infusion	- No resp. depression, no rise of ICP, may impair cognitive testing in some	- Hypotension, bradycardia

©2018 A.D. JOHN

Land Marks for an Effective Scalp Block (Fig. 5)

Supra-orbital Nerve – a branch of trigeminal nerve. It innervates the forehead, anterior part of the scalp and top part of the head. It is blocked by injected at the supraorbital foramen along the upper orbital margin.

Supra-trochlear Nerve – a branch of trigeminal nerve. It innervates the forehead and anterior part of the scalp. It can be blocked by medial extension of supra-orbital block.

Auriculo-temporal Nerve – a branch of trigeminal nerve. It innervates the temporal area, lower lip, lower face, auricle and the scalp above the auricle. It is blocked by infiltration over zygomatic process 1-1.5 cm anterior to ear at the level of tragus. The nerve is accompanied by the artery so aspirate

SCALP BLOCK

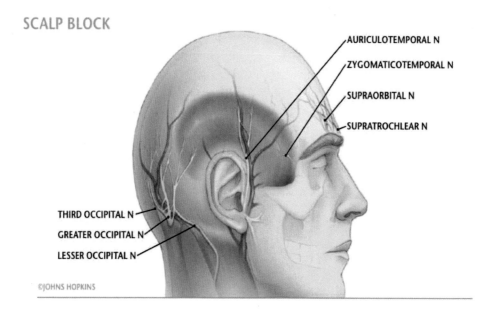

Fig. (5). Scalp Block. Image provided by Punita Tripathi, M.D., Johns Hopkins.

Zygomatico-temporal Nerve – a branch of Trigeminal nerve. It innervates a small area of the fore head and the temporal area. It lies midway between the auriculotemporal nerve and supra-orbital nerve; the nerve passes through the temporalis muscle to enter the temporalis fascia. So the local anesthetic agent needs to be infiltrated deep and superficial to the temporalis muscle.

Greater Occipital Nerve – It arises from second cervical spinal nerve. It innervates the skin around the posterior part of the scalp and can innervate the scalp at the top of the head and over the auricle. It lies halfway between the occipital protuberance and mastoid process 2.5 cm lateral to nuchal median line

Lesser occipital Nerve – branch of the second and third cervical spinal nerve. It innervates the scalp the scalp in the lateral third of the head posterior to the auricle. It lies 2.5 cm lateral to greater occipital nerve and can be blocked at that point.

Greater auricular Nerve – which is a branch of second and third cervical spinal nerve. The nerve can be blocked by injecting local anesthetic agent 2 cm.

posterior to the auricle at the level of the tragus.

For the scalp block to be effective a total of 14 nerves need to be blocked, the pinning site needs to be infiltrated (3 site for the Mayfield frame) and the incision site also need to be infiltrated.

Local Anesthetic for the Block

Ropivacaine 0.5% with 1:200,000 epinephrine is commonly used. A total of 60cc is used with about 2-3cc for each nerve and the remainder for the surgeons to infiltration at site of incision and site of pinning. As with any case dose is adjusted for the elderly and those with renal or hepatic disease.

Maximum dose of some local anesthetic agents commonly used

- Lidocaine without epinephrine – 3 mg/kg, with epinephrine 7 mg/kg
- Ropivacaine with or without epinephrine – 3-4 mg/kg
- Bupivacaine without epinephrine – 2 mg/kg, with epinephrine 2.5 mg/kg

It is important to keep track of the total dose of local anesthetics used by the surgeon and the anesthesiologists, making sure it does not exceed the maximum dose.

Electrophysiological Monitoring and Functional Mapping

May last for up to 3 hours. Communication with the patient is important at this time. The patient is reminded not to move or cough, especially when the patient is going through a short excitement phase as they wake up. Remind the surgeons to use local anesthetic agents specifically around dural vessels where the nerves are located. Intraoperative wake up test – We usually wake our patient prior to dural incision so that even if the patient inadvertently moves during the wakeup phase it does not cause any problems. Stop the propofol infusion 30 minutes before the electrophysiological testing. Stop the nitrous and the volatile anesthetic agent at least 15-20 minutes before the test. When the patient is fully awake, we leave the nasopharyngeal airway *in situ* unless the surgeon complains (gives nasal intonation to the voice).

A calm and quiet room is needed when the patient wakes up. Communication with the patient is very important at this time. The patient also needs to be reminded not to move or cough at this time, especially when the patient is going through a short excitement phase as they wake up intraoperative. Maximum amount of complications occurs at this time namely discomfort from immobility, nausea, vomiting, agitation and seizures. Focal motor or psychomotor seizures do not usually require treatment. It is important to quickly deal with any complication that occur at this time. Remind the surgeons to use local anesthetic agents specifically around dural vessels where the nerves are located. Neuro-monitoring personnel observe the patient and record deficits. Neurocognitive testing and mapping is done at this time. Awake testing may include some or all of the following – immediate or delayed memory, pattern recognition, discrimination of words or pictures, language in bilingual patients, motor movement in response to electrical stimulation, voluntary motor movement, muscle strength, electro cortico gram (ECoG), or EMG. Cortical stimulation for brain mapping localizes the eloquent areas of the brain by direct stimulation of the cerebral cortex by electrodes. Broca's area is needed for speech production and language processing. Wernick's area is needed for language comprehension. Motor and sensory cortex are also identified. Any alteration in speech or motor function is communicated to the surgeon at this time. Resection only begins after the cortex is functionally mapped by this process.

Resection of Tumor

This phase lasts for about 2 hours. At our institution we keep the patient lightly sedated for the remaining part of the case by using propofol (25-50 mcg/kg/min).

Post Resection Monitoring – Lasts about 15-20 minutes. Sedation dose may be reduced during this time.

Closure – Lasts for about 2 hours. Usually the scalp block performed by the surgeons remains effective, but the surgeon may have to re-inject local anesthetic agents.

Non-Pharmacologic Measures

Constant reassurance and encouragement throughout the procedure is very valuable for the success of the surgery. Keeping the operating room quiet is very helpful. Providing some ice chips or wet swaps, especially when the patient has been talking is helpful. Holding the patients hand or rubbing the fore head is very valuable to reassure the patient.

Intraoperative Complications

Problems that could be encountered and troubleshooting them are

1. A backup plan for securing the airway must be present at all times. The challenges of securing the airway in a patient with their heads pinned and with a craniotomy in progress needs to be well thought out. Securing the airway with a laryngeal mask airway (LMA) is easier than securing the airway with an orotracheal intubation.

2. Brain engorgement is a possible risk. It should be treated with head up position, hyperventilation, mannitol, loop diuretics, decrease venous pressure (head positioning is an important factor), and if needed CSF drainage. Other causes of brain swelling should be ruled out like hypoxemia, accidental over-hydration, acute intracerebral bleed, severe hypo or hypertension.

3. Patient agitation and movement – incidence about 4% are managed by altering the dose of sedative medications and making changes in a patient's immediate surroundings, such as temperature, amount of light, and padding. The incidence of conversion to general anesthesia occurs in 2-6%. Always rule out hypoxia and hypercarbia as a cause of agitation.

Anesthetic Agents Used – Pros and Cons

1. Nausea and vomiting – incidence 4% suspend the surgical procedure; give metoclopramide and $5HT_3$ antagonist; propofol if necessary, decadron is also an anti-emetic. Rule out hemodynamic instability. Prevention works better as once the vomiting center is stimulated it is hard to stop.

2. Convulsion – incidence 6-18%. Focal seizures do not need treatment and is self-limiting. Grand mal seizures need to be treated. They may be due to cortical stimulation, decreased levels of anticonvulsant in patient or as a result of local anesthetic toxicity. Surgeon need to stop cortical stimulation; using cold saline on brain surface to stop seizures, small dose of pentothal sodium, propofol, midazolam, or other sedative may be given intravenously. Secure the airway if seizures are intractable and risk of aspiration is present. At our institution Keppra is usually given at the beginning of the case. Dilantin may be added.

3. The incidence of venous air embolism in awake craniotomy patients is not more frequent than in craniotomy under general anesthesia. In the sitting or semi-sitting position, venous air embolism occurs with an incidence of 4-5%, as recorded by precordial Doppler. It is signaled by coughing. Maintaining hemodynamic stability and communicating with the neurosurgeon is important, so that they can apply bone wax and/or cautery. Changing the position of the operating table, head down position to prevent more entrapment of the air is important. Maintaining hemodynamic stability and if possible applying bilateral jugular venous pressure.

4. Loss of patient cooperation is usually due to inappropriate patient preparation, prolonged surgery, excessive or light sedation, insufficient analgesia and uncomfortable position. This may lead to conversion to general anesthesia if reassurance and other efforts fail.

5. Men would usually complain about the Foley catheter- use of lidocaine jelly at time of insertion has been shown to be very helpful in our practice.

6. Some patients will complain of headache – reassurance and if testing has been

done fentanyl 25 mcg can be given IV or local anesthetic agent infiltration by surgeons.

7. Blood pressure control – labetalol, esmolol, hydralazine, metoprolol all can be used intravenously

8. Dry mouth and thirst are frequent complaints by the patients. We usually provide swabs to help with this.

Transportation to neurosurgical ICU – The patient should have his head elevated slightly. Oxygen through face mask and on transport monitors. Always carry intubation equipment and resuscitation drugs during transport to the NSICU. Make sure that the oxygen tank is full and carry an Ambu bag.

Future Development

There is increasing evidence that awake craniotomy would be an appropriate technique for all supratentorial tumors. Although functional MRI are being used they are not always very accurate.

CONCLUSION

Neuroanesthesia is an extremely interesting and fascinating aspect of the anesthetic practice. It involves the anesthetic management of neurosurgical patients and requires the understanding of anatomy, pathophysiology, disease process, technical skill, and co-operation with a wider number of team members. The need for a successful interaction with a patient and their family is paramount. This chapter focuses on the care of the most common diseases encountered in neuroanesthesia: tumors, cerebral hemorrhage, intracranial pressure, cerebrovascular disease, and Chiari-malformations. Our approach to a successful awake craniotomy is discussed in detail. An understanding of the issues involved in Neuroanesthesia is requisite for a successful anesthetic practice.

CONSENT FOR PUBLICATION

Not applicable.

CONFLICT OF INTEREST

The author declares no conflict of interest, financial or otherwise.

ACKNOWLEDGEMENT

Declared none.

REFERENCES

[1] Newfield P, Cottrell JE, Eds. Handbook of Neuroanesthesia. 5th ed., LW&W.

[2] Miller RD, Ed. Miller's Anesthesia. 8th ed., Elsevier Health Sciences.

[3] Brambrink AM, Kirsch JR, Eds. Essentials of Neurosurgical Anesthesia and Critical Care. Springer.
     [http://dx.doi.org/10.1007/978-0-387-09562-2]

[4] Dinsmore J. Anaesthesia for elective neurosurgery. Br J Anaesth 2007; 99(1): 68-74.
     [http://dx.doi.org/10.1093/bja/aem132] [PMID: 17573395]

[5] Frost EA, Booij LH. Anesthesia in the patient for awake craniotomy. Curr Opin Anaesthesiol 2007;
     20(4): 331-5.
     [http://dx.doi.org/10.1097/ACO.0b013e328136c56f] [PMID: 17620841]

[6] Brydges G, Atkinson R, Perry MJ, Hurst D, Laqua T, Wiemers J. Awake craniotomy: a practice
     overview. AANA J 2012; 80(1): 61-8.
     [PMID: 22474807]

[7] Burnand C. Sebastialn J. Survey of Anesthesia for Awake Craniotomy. J Neurosurg Anesthesiol 2012;
     24: 249.

CHAPTER 5

MICU Issues

Jonathan E. Sevransky*, **Michael S. Lava** and **Russell D. Dolan**

Emory University School of Medicine, Atlanta, Georgia, USA

Abstract: In this chapter, we review c-ommon critical care medicine illnesses and syndromes, including epidemiology, diagnosis and treatment. Prominent topics discussed include: sepsis, ARDS, shock, GI bleeding, hypertensive emergency, acute kidney injury, toxidromes and exposures, and delirium.

Keywords: ARDS, Acute Kidney Injury, Alcohol Withdrawal, Critical Care, Cocaine Intoxication, Delirium, Ethylene Glycol, Gastrointestinal Bleed, Hypertensive Emergency, Intensive Care Unit, Isopropyl Alcohol, Methanol, Sepsis, Shock.

INTRODUCTION

Common illnesses seen in the medical ICU often complicate the course of patients in other ICUs. This chapter will review prevalent syndromes including ARDS and sepsis, as well as provide an overview of other common medical critical care illnesses.

Acute Respiratory Distress Syndrome (ARDS)

<u>ARDS is an acute inflammatory disease of the lungs, characterized by hypoxemia and bilateral infiltrates, and the need for positive pressure ventilation</u>. It is a frequent cause of acute respiratory failure, with the incidence of ARDS in the United States estimated to 190,000 patients annually [1, 2]. <u>Common causes</u> of ARDS include viral and bacterial pneumonia, non-pulmonary sepsis, aspiration and trauma. Pancreatitis, transfusions and drugs are also known causes [3].

The **pathophysiologic changes** seen in ARDS include <u>increased permeability, pulmonary edema due to a breakdown in the alveolar capillary membrane, increased dead space, and decreased lung compliance</u>. In the rare cases when pathology is available, a diffuse alveolar damage pattern, with hyaline membrane

---

* **Corresponding author Jonathan E. Sevransky:** Emory University School of Medicine, Atlanta, Georgia, USA; Tel: (404) 727-5630; E-mail: jonathan.sevransky@emoryhealth.org

Amballur D. John (Ed.)

formation is seen [4]. **ARDS, however, is a clinical diagnosis**.

In **2012, the Berlin Criteria** for ARDS provided a useful and validated revision to the previously used American and European Consensus Definitions. Patients who meet the following criteria fit the syndrome definition:

• Predisposing factor in the last week
• Bilateral opacities on CXR
• Edema not exclusively explained by volume overload

Severity of ARDS (Table **1**) is defined by the PaO_2/FiO_2 ratio with PEEP≥5, with increasing severity correlated to increasing mortality [2]. Importantly, both incidence and case fatality rates have decreased for ARDS in the past decade [3].

Table 1. Severity of ARDS in relation to PF Ratio and Morality. Provided by Jonathan E. Sevransky, M.D., Michael S. Lava M.D., and Russell D. Dolan: Emory University.

Severity	PF Ratio	Mortality
Mild	201-300	27%
Moderate	200-100	32%
Severe	<100	45% ©2018 J. SERVANSKY, EMORY UNIV.

Management of ARDS

The **management** of patients with ARDS is focused on treatment of the precipitating condition, lung protective mechanical ventilation, a fluid conservative strategy, and avoidance of nosocomial complications.

Lung protective ventilation is the most important intervention in the treatment of ARDS. The use of smaller tidal volumes coupled with decreased plateau pressures was shown to reduce mortality to 31% from 39.8% compared with higher tidal volumes and higher plateau pressures [5]. The clinician should start with a tidal volume of 6cc/kg, aiming to keep the plateau pressure under <30cm H_2O. Further reductions in tidal volume to 4cc/kg may be employed to reach this goal, and ventilator rate should be adjusted to maintain a pH >7.3. Failure to achieve this pH may lead to consideration of increasing the tidal volume if the pH cannot be maintained, as long as the plateau pressure remains ≤30cm H_2O.

For patients not in shock, a **fluid conservative strategy** increases ventilator free days (days alive but off the ventilator) without affecting 60 days mortality. Thus, limiting fluids in hemodynamically stable patients, and diuresing if volume overloaded are now part of standard therapy for patients with ARDS [6].

For patients with severe ARDS refractory to standard therapy, there are several potential rescue therapies that should be considered in addition to the standard therapies listed above. Patients with early severe ARDS (PaO$_2$/FiO$_2$ ratio≤150 with less than 48 hours on the ventilator) given cisatracurium for 48 hours instead of placebo had improved survival at 90 days [7]. In addition, patients with early severe ARDS (PaO$_2$/FiO$_2$ ratio ≤150 with less than 36hours on ventilator), treated with prone positioning for >16 hours day had a 28 days mortality of 16% compared to 33% with standard treatment [8]. Proning can either be done using staff to turn or by the use of a specialty bed. The rate of complications of proning, including loss of airway or catheters appears to be related to the experience of the staff in proning.

Other **salvage therapies** that may be considered include High Frequency Oscillatory Ventilation, Airway Pressure Release Ventilation, and the use of pulmonary vasodilators. Although each of these therapies may improve selected measures (iNO improves oxygenation for short periods of time), none have been shown to improve mortality [9, 10]. Transfer to an expert center for consideration of Extracorpreal Membrane Oxygenation (ECMO) is an alternative therapy in severe ARDS for patients who are early in their course and who do not respond to other proven therapies [11]. For now, its remains less clear whether the expert center or the ECMO itself is more important.

SHOCK

Shock is characterized by a mismatch of oxygen delivery and oxygen utilization at the cellular level leading to cellular injury [12]. 1/3 of ICU patients will develop shock during their stay [13]. Common clinical markers of shock include hypotension with a mean arterial pressure of less than 70, diminished end organ perfusion and lactic acidosis [12].

Classes of Shock (Table **2**) include hypovolemic shock, cardiogenic shock, obstructive shock and distributive shock. In practice, it is possible for more than one type of shock to co-exist [12], thus mandating a rational approach to identifying the cause and specific etiology of shock. With a suspected mixed shock state or unclear etiology of shock, placement of a pulmonary artery catheter can be considered, but the routine use of pulmonary artery catheters has not been shown to improve mortality in patients with shock [14].

Shock often necessitates placement of a central line to facilitate vasopressor use (Table **3**). Adjunctive testing with TTE or other measures to assess cardiac function may assist with narrowing the differential diagnosis [12]. Dynamic measures of volume status, such as stroke volume variation or passive leg raise may help guide volume resuscitation [15]. Immediate vasopressor use in conjunction with volume resuscitation is indicated in the setting of profound hypotension [12, 16, 17].

Table 2. Classification of Shock. Provided by Jonathan E. Sevransky, M.D., Michael S. Lava M.D., and Russell D. Dolan: Emory University.

Type of Shock	PVR	CVP	Cardiac Output	Etiology
Cardiogenic	⬆	⬆	⬆	Acute MI, Decompensated Heart Failure, Arrhythmias, Valvular Disorders and Myocarditis
Distributive	⬇	⬇	⬌/⬆	Sepsis, Anaphylaxis, Pancreatitis, <u>Post Operative</u> State
Hypovolemic	⬌/⬆	⬇	⬌/⬇	GI Bleeds, Diarrhea, Internal Bleeding
Obstructive ©2018 J. SERVANSKY, EMORY UNIV.	⬌/⬆	⬆	⬇	PE, Tampanode, Tension Pneumothorax

Table 3. Vasopressor treatment of shock. Provided by Jonathan E. Sevransky, M.D., Michael S. Lava M.D., and Russell D. Dolan: Emory University.

Norepinephrine
- First line pressor
- Alpha>Beta
- Vasoconstriction, mild chronotropic/inotropic effects
- Less arrhythmias than dopamine

Vasopressin
- Fixed Does (0.03-0.04U/Min)
- Allows lower dose of NE to be used

Epinephrine
- 2nd line pressor
- Beta>Alpha
- Increased chronotrop/inotropy
- Type B lactic acidosis
- Due to cellular metabolism, not end organ ischemia

©2018 J. SERVANSKY, EMORY UNIV.

In the setting of **cardiogenic shock**, <u>dobutamine is less likely than other inotropes to produce hypotension</u> [18]. A recent pragmatic trial suggested that the use of norepinephrine is preferred over dopamine for correction of lower MAP in cardiogenic shock [16]. For most patients, a target MAP is 65-70 [12]. In the setting of patients with preexisting poorly controlled hypertension, an increased MAP goal may lead to less acute kidney injury and need for renal replacement therapy. This increased MAP goal, however, does not lead to decreased mortality [19]. Low dose dopamine is not recommended for renal protection [20].

SEVERE SEPSIS AND SEPTIC SHOCK

Sepsis is <u>precipitated by an infection, and is a leading cause of morbidity and mortality in ICU's worldwide</u> [21]. Both the direct effects of infection, as well as some potential adverse effects of the host defense system may contribute to the high morbidity and mortality seen in patients with sepsis. <u>Early identification and treatment of patients with sepsis is crucial to prevent the consequences of sepsis, including shock, multisystem organ failure and death</u>.

660,000 cases of sepsis are seen in the US annually, with case fatality rates ranging from 18-29% [22 - 24]. **Sepsis**<u> remains a syndrome rather than a disease</u>, so it lacks a true biomarker, which complicates the early recognition of sepsis patients. Thus screening for sepsis requires an appropriate index of suspicion, and we **recommend** considering <u>both risk factors for sepsis</u> in addition to the syndromic criteria. Increasing age, male gender and race are important risk factors [25]. While the SIRS criteria are part of the 1992 consensus definition for sepsis, they are neither sensitive nor specific, and a new definition for sepsis will be available in early 2016 [26].

<u>Common sites of infection</u> leading to sepsis include the bloodstream, urinary tract or kidneys, lungs, bowel (*i.e.* peritonitis, appendicitis), meninges of the brain, skin (cellulitis) and iatrogenic causes (*i.e.* intravascular access devices and catheters). Sepsis cases due to <u>pneumonia and intra-abdominal infectious foci have a higher case fatality rate</u> than those arising from urinary tract infections (UTI's) [27].

Treatment of sepsis includes prompt identification of patients, early antibiotics directed at likely causative organisms, fluid resuscitation and hemodynamic support [28, 29]. For the majority of patients, crystalloids are preferred over colloids, and with the exception of patients with spontaneous bacterial peritonitis, there are no patient groups in which albumin or other colloids are clearly superior [30, 31]. Recent observational studies suggested a potential benefit to chloride poor crystalloids over chloride rich solutions, but this was not confirmed in a phase 2 clinical trial [32, 33]. After obtaining appropriate culture samples, <u>empiric broad-spectrum antibiotics directed at likely pathogens should be infused within 1</u>

hour of a patient developing hypotension, with inadequate or delayed coverage associated with increased mortality. Blood cultures, CXR and a urinalysis should be performed to look for source of sepsis, and closed space infections require drainage as soon as feasible [29].

Implementation of both early fluids and targeted antibiotics have been shown to lower mortality in septic patients [21]. However, when early antibiotics and fluids are effectively delivered, there appears to be no clear additional benefit to strategies designed to reach specific targets such as lactate clearance or $SCVO_2$ levels [22 - 24].

Survivors of sepsis and severe sepsis are at increased risk for hospital readmission, recurrent sepsis and increased mortality within 1year following discharge from an ICU setting compared to non-sepsis survivors [34]. At 90 days post-discharge, the most common diagnoses at readmission were recurrent sepsis, UTI, heart failure, pneumonia and acute exacerbations of previously existing COPD [35].

Gastrointestinal Bleeding

Gastrointestinal Bleeding (GIB) (Table **4**), including both upper and lower, is a commonly encountered critical illness. The presentation, workup and management of GIB is presented in the table below. In most cases, the source of bleeding is clinically identifiable on presentation. However, 10-15% of patients with hematochezia are found to have an upper GI source with findings of hypotension, resting tachycardia, and orthostasis [36]. Most patients with active bleeding are managed in an intensive care unit.

Table 4. Gastrointestinal Bleed Location, Workup and Management. Provided by Jonathan E. Sevransky, M.D., Michael S. Lava M.D., and Russell D. Dolan: Emory University.

Gastrointestinal Bleeding	
Upper GI Bleed	**Lower GI Bleed**
Upper GIB Presentation - Coffee Ground Emesis - Hematemesis - Melena	Lower GIB Presentation - Hematochezia
Workup - CBC, Chemistry with Liver Panel, Coags	
Management - 2 Large Bore IVís (16G or larger) - Volume resuscitation with Isotonic Crystalloids - Type and Screen/Cross - Transfusion – Hb goal of 7 - Correct Coagulopathy	
- EGD - PPI Drip	- EGD +/- Colonoscopy ©2016 J. SERVANSKY, EMORY UNIV.

In the United States, the annual incidence of upper GIB is 102 per 100,000 [37], with mortality ranging from 3-14% [38]. Targeting a transfusion goal of 7 is associated with decreased mortality and risk of further bleeding compared to a transfusion goal of 9 or 10. In the setting of unstable CAD (ie ongoing NSTEMI or STEMI), a transfusion goal of 9 may be appropriate, although there remains some controversy [39 - 42]. While some clinicians advocate the use of nasogastric lavage to clear blood clots or secretions that may interfere with endoscopy it has not been shown to impact outcomes in UGIB, and should only be used for clearly defined indications [39, 42, 43]. After adequate intravenous access is obtained (see Table for suggestions), a PPI infusion is recommended for patients with presumed active upper GI bleeding [39, 40, 44]. An early upper endoscopy EGD (≤24h) [42] facilitates both early diagnosis and potential intervention on upper GI bleeding.

In addition to the above standard UGIB management, variceal (or suspected) UGIB requires additional therapies. **Octreotide**, which decreases portal blood flow, should be started as a continuous infusion [45, 46]. Patients with variceal bleeding are at risk for massive hemorrhage with hemodynamic instability, and may require the use of a massive transfusion protocol that includes fresh frozen plasma (FFP) and platelets in a defined ratio along with packed red cell transfusion. To facilitate endoscopy and protect the airway, these patients oftenrequire intubation. An INR<1.5 should be targeted with FFP and vitamin K, and platelets should be administered to a goal of 50,000 [39].

As up to **20%** of patients with cirrhosis who have UGIBs are found to have infections, empiric antibiotics are essential, and appear to decrease mortality. At the current time a **quinolo**ne, or if severe cirrhosis exists, an extended spectrum cephalosporin such as**ceftriaxone**, is recommended empirically for 7 days [47, 48].

Lower GIB incidence is 20.5 per 100,000 annually [49]. 80-85% of LGIBs stop spontaneously, and mortality is lower than UGIB at 2-3% [36]. Of note, given the transient nature of LGIB, it is sometimes difficult to localize the site of bleeding, and repeated diagnostic testing often needs to be performed.

In the setting of a hemodynamically unstable LGIB, the patient is stabilized as above. An EGD is often performed first, to rule out a brisk upper GIB as a source. If no source of bleeding is found, and the patient continues to bleed, either radionuclide scanning or angiography is indicated in an effort to diagnose and in the latter instance embolize the source. If angiography is negative, a colonoscopy is pursued, assuming stability. If still unstable, the patient may be considered for emergent laparatomy [50].

Several features portend an aggressive LGIB (Table **5**), and these patients should be considered for ICU management if they have multiple risk factors [51]:

Table 5. Risk Factors for Aggressive LGIB. Provided by Jonathan E. Sevransky, M.D., Michael S. Lava M.D., and Russell D. Dolan: Emory University.

Hemodynamic Changes
Active Bleeding
Comorbid Disease
Advanced Age
Already admitted to the hospital for another reason
History of Diverticular Bleeds or Angiodysplasia
Aspirin use or Coagulopathy
Anemia
Elevated BUN
Leukocytosis

©2018 J. SERVANSKY, EMORY UNIV.

Hypertensive Emergency

Hypertensive emergency is defined as new or increased hypertension with the presence of end organ damage. The mechanism of action is thought to be a sudden increase in systemic vascular resistance, causing increased shear stress on arteries and endothelial injury [52, 53], leading to a vicious cycle of proinflammatory cytokine release [54]. Volume depletion from pressure-natriuresis leads to further up-titration of the renin-angiotensin-aldosterone axis [55].

Specific end organ damage may include acute MI, pulmonary edema due to diastolic or systolic heart failure, aortic dissection, and encephalopathy. Further, acute hypertensive nephrosclerosis may present as microscopic hematuria and elevated creatinine.

While end organ damage rarely develops at a blood pressure of less than 180/120, there is no absolute blood pressure cutoff. Rapid changes in blood pressure, especially in those who are normotensive at baseline, can produce end organ damage (*e.g.* pre-eclampsia).

While true hypertensive emergency mandates aggressive treatment with IV antihypertensive drips and ICU admission (Table **6**), elevated blood pressure without end organ damage (so called Hypertensive Urgency) should be treated moreconservatively, due to a rightward shift of the autoregulation curve. Treatment that leads to rapid drops to 'normal' blood pressure can create clinically significant ischemic events including strokes, MI's and renal insufficiency [55]. In true hypertensive emergency, mortality at 90 days has been reported to be as high as **11%** [56].

Initial treatment consists of rapid blood pressure lowering with a goal of decreasing the MAP by 10-20% in the first hour, and a subsequent 5-15% in the next 23hours. As noted above, more rapid declines in blood pressure may lead to hypoperfusion of the brain and other vital organs. One exception to this rule is for patients with aortic dissection, where the goal is to decrease the systolic blood pressure to 100-120 over the first 20minutes of care.

There are multiple intravenous options for rapid lowering of blood pressure. The best choice of agent depends on patient factors such as which end organ is affected as well as preexisting comorbidities.

Nitroprusside, while a very potent antihypertensive agent, has potential side effects including decreasing cerebral blood flow while simultaneously increasing ICP. It has also been shown to augment cardiac steal in cases of CAD [55], and increase perioperative mortality [57]. Further, cyanide toxicity can develop even at recommended doses, especially in patients with renal insufficiency and at higher doses [55]. For these reasons, this medication should only be used if the benefits outweigh the risks.

Nitroglycerin is a commonly administered antihypertensive agent with venodilatory effects at low doses but arterial dilatory effects at higher doses. Nitroglycerin is best used as an adjunct to other antihypertensives in the setting of ACS and pulmonary edema [55].

Hydralazine is often used as an intravenous push to lower blood pressure rapidly. Patient response to this medication is highly variable, it is difficult to titrate, and has a duration of action up to 12hours [55]. Given these qualities, it is not often the first choice to treat hypertensive emergencies, but may play a role in patients with renal injury and intolerance to other agents [55].

Nicardipine is a dihydropyridine calcium channel blocker that can be delivered as a titratable infusion and is thus often chosen to treat hypertensive emergencies. Both stroke volume and coronary output are increased, and cerebral ischemia is reduced with this agent [55, 58, 59]. This makes it a reasonable choice for many cases of hypertensive emergency, especially CAD and systolic heart failure [55]. Clearance is through the liver, thus unaffected by renal dysfunction [60].

Clevidipine is a newer dihydropyridine calcium channel blocker. It has a very fast onset and offset, making it a potentially useful agent for rapid and accurate titration. This agent also increases stroke volume. Further, it is cleared by plasma esterases, making it an option for patients with renal or hepatic dysfunction [61, 62].

Labetalol is a non selective beta blocker with some alpha activity [63]. It undergoes elimination hepatically [55], and has been found to maintain cardiac output, a concern for selective beta blockers [63]. Further, it has been found to maintain blood flow to cerebral, renal and coronary arteries. It can be used as both a push as well as a continuous infusion for rapid blood pressure control [55].

Esmolol is a cardioselective beta blocker with no alpha receptor activity and a short half life [64, 65]. It is useful in the setting of liver or renal dysfunction, as it is cleared by plasma esterases. Esmolol can lead to bradycardia and decreased cardiac output [55].

Table 6. Drugs for the Treatment of Hypertensive Emergency. Provided by Jonathan E. Sevransky, M.D., Michael S. Lava M.D., and Russell D. Dolan: Emory University.

Drug [55,60-62,64-66]	**Onset**	**Duration**	**Major Side Effects**
Nicardipine	5-15 min	4-6 hours	Headache, Tachycardia, Edema
Clevidipine	2-4 min	5-15 min	Headache, Nausea, Vomiting
Labetalol Nausea	2-5 min	2-18 hours	Orthostasis, Fatigue, Dizziness,
Esmolol Diaphoresis	1-2 min	10-30 min	Dizziness, Nausea, Vomiting, ©2018 J. SERVANSKY, EMORY UNIV.

ACUTE KIDNEY INJURY

Acute Kidney Injury (AKI) is a frequent complication of critical illness and is defined as a relatively rapid (within 48hours) increase in creatinine ($>/= .3$, or 150% increase), or drop in urine output (<.5cc/kg for 6 continuous hours) [67].

Between 36-67% of ICU patients will develop AKI and 5-6% of these patients require renal replacement therapy (RRT) [68 - 72]. Severity of kidney injury is correlated with mortality [68], and AKI requiring RRT is associated with mortality rates of up to 60% [73, 74].

Most cases of AKI in the ICU are multifactorial. Standard diagnostic workup for AKI includes urinalysis and renal ultrasound, and renal consultation is frequently useful. Identification of casts in the case of ATN and eosinophils in the case of AIN may aid in diagnosis. Treatment is generally aimed at supportive care, and prevention of further injury. Of note, while prerenal azotemia is not uncommon in the ICU, empiric fluid challenge in the setting of AKI is recommended only when there is evidence of a prerenal cause of azotemia [75]. A more positive fluid balance in AKI is associated with a worse prognosis [76].

The most common etiology of AKI in the ICU is **sepsis**, with up to 50% of septic patients developing AKI during their stay. Other common etiologies include cardiac surgery, rhabdomyolysis and trauma [70]. Intraabdominal hypertension (>12mmHg) puts patients at risk for development of AKI [77].

The intensivist should avoid nephrotoxins if possible in patients at risk, including those with preexising CKD, diabetes, hypertension, cardiovascular disease and liver disease [75]. Commonly used medications that may precipitate **AKI** include NSAIDS, aminoglycosides, penicillin, its derivatives, vancomycin, acyclovir, as well as intravenous contrast [69, 78].

Contrast dye is frequently used for important diagnostic tests in critically ill patients, and patients often have more than one risk factor for AKI. It is important that the intensivist consider the risk benefit ratio for such studies. Risk factors for contrast induced nephropathy (CIN) include diabetes, CKD, hypotension and hypovolemia [78]. Fluid loading with crystalloids such as normal saline decreases the risk of CIN [79 - 82]. Other prevention measures including N-acetyl cysteine, and sodium bicarbonate do not clearly demonstrate benefit [78].

Albumin administration has been shown to decrease the risk for AKI following large volume paracentesis and SBP, and should be routinely administered in these settings [83].

There is some evidence that use of a slightly higher mean arterial pressure (MAP ≥75) in patients with septic shock and preexisting hypertension may decrease the need for CRRT without affecting mortality [19]. Importantly, current evidence for 'renal dose' dopamine suggests no benefit in patients with septic shock or for patients at risk for renal failure [20, 84]. Some have proposed giving chloride poor solutions for volume resuscitation, but this strategy was not supported in a recent phase 2 clinical trial [32, 33].

Despite the best efforts at prevention of AKI, some patients will require the initiation of RRT. There is little data supporting early or aggressive dialysis in patients with acute kidney injury [85 - 87]. Continuous RRT in comparison to intermittent hemodyalysis may be practically easier to deliver without hemodynamic changes [75].

TOXIDROMES AND EXPOSURES

Cocaine Intoxication

Cocaine is a widely used substance of abuse, and frequently complicates admissions to the ICU. Upwards of 6 million people use cocaine consistently in the United States, most frequently in the 18-25year old age group [88]. Cocaine, whether through nasal inhalation, smoking, or intravenous use inhibits reuptake of catecholamines in the presynaptic terminal, which leads to a sympathomimetic toxidrome marked by hyperthermia, hypertension, tachycardia, mydriasis, seizures, as well as respiratory and cardiac depression (Table **7**). In addition, cocaine has a systemic procoagulant effect [88]. The **half-life** of cocaine is about 60minutes, but cocaine metabolites are active up to 24-36hours after ingestion and the mixing of cocaine and ethanol leads to an even longer lasting metabolite [89].

Clinically, cocaine may involve nearly every organ system:

Table 7. Manifestations of Cocaine Toxicity. Provided by Jonathan E. Sevransky, M.D., Michael S. Lava M.D., and Russell D. Dolan: Emory University.

Organ System	Major Manifestations of Cocaine
CNS	Delirium, Seizures, Stroke, Vasculitis
Cardiovascular	AMI, Arrhythmias, Chest Pain
Pulmonary	Status Asthmaticus, "Crack Chest," Barotrauma, Pulmonary Edema, Pulmonary Hemorrhage
Renal	Rhabdomyolysis, Renal Infarct
GI	Acute Ischemia, Ulceration, Perforation
Vascular	Arterial Thrombosis, Dissection ©2018 J. SERVANSKY, EMORY UNIV.

In the setting of acute intoxication, cocaine acts to directly impact the cardiac myocyte by slowing the amplitude and speed of its sodium gated action potential. This raises the risk of ventricular tachycardia and sudden death. "**Crack Chest**" appears to be a hypersensivity reaction to cocaine inhalation, and presents with fever, productive cough, wheeze, and diffuse infiltrates on imaging. Any form of cocaine ingestion may cause a non cardiogenic pulmonary edema, which presents similarly to ARDS, but has a shorter time course [88, 89]. Patients can also present with the effects of barotrauma, including pneumothorax and pneumomediastinum [88].

Treatment of cocaine ingestion is generally supportive. In the setting of seizures and hypothermia, endotracheal intubation and active cooling are indicated, along with close monitoring for arrhythmias. Chest pain is treated with nitrates and calcium channel blockers. The use of selective beta blockers remains controversial, but generally acceptable provided they are not used alone [89]. Oral ingestion can be treated with activated charcoal to decrease absorption, but hemodialysis is not effective in clearing cocaine [89].

Alcohol Withdrawal

Half of a million people experience some level of alcohol withdrawal in the United States annually [90]. Alcohol acts directly on GABA receptors, the main inhibitory neurotransmitter in the brain, and inhibits the release of glutamate. With chronic use of alcohol, habituation occurs, and the brain becomes less sensitive to the effects of GABA, and up-titrates glutamate receptors. With cessation of drinking and its inhibitory effects on the brain, an excitatory response occurs. The initial symptoms of alcohol withdrawal may be mild (anxiety, tremors, headaches and diaphoresis) and present 6-36 hours after the last drink [91]. **Withdrawal seizures** typically occur 12-48 hours after the last drink. They tend to be generalized, tonic-clonic seizures, and occur as either one event or a series of short seizures. Status epilepticus is rare in withdrawal, and alternative causes should be considered if it occurs. **Treatment** consists of benzodiazepine administration; if this fails, phenobarbital or propofol may be considered [92, 93]. Withdrawal seizures do not predict the development of other manifestations of cessation, including delirium tremens (DTs) [93]. Of note, patients with seizures related to alcohol withdrawal do not need long term anti-convulsant therapy.

Alcoholic hallucinosis, a distinct entity from DTs, tends to occur 8-48 hours after the last drink. Patients present with specific hallucinations and normal vital signs, without altered mental status [93].

Delirium tremens tends to occur 48-72 hours after the last drink [93]. Clinical findings include altered mental status, tachycardia, tachypnea, hypertension, fevers and agitation [93]. Patients tend to be hypovolemic due to insensible losses, and IVF resuscitation is needed. Hypokalemia and hypomagnesemia are common, putting patients at increased risk for arrhythmias. Tachypnea leads to a respiratory alkalosis and associated decrease in cerebral blood flow [93].

Basic **supportive care** for patients with DT's consists of aggressive monitoring, electrolyte repletion and IV fluid resuscitation. Thiamine and folate should be administered early in the course to correct likely vitamin insufficiencies, along with benzodiazepine administration, which counters the effect of withdrawal on GABA [93]. We recommend symptom triggered (as opposed to scheduled dosing) treatment using CIWAS (Clinical Institute Withdrawal Assessment for Alcohol Scale) or a similar scale to target administration of these agents. Such symptom triggered management of withdrawal has been shown to decrease the amount of benzodiazepine administered, and reduce length of stay [94]. DTs that are refractory to benzodiazepines can be managed using either phenobarbatal or propofol [93].

We **do not recommend** use of ethanol, which is difficult to titrate and not as effective as benzodiazepines. Further, antipsychotics have no pharmacologic overlap with alcohol, decrease the seizure threshold, and should not be used in isolation, but may be included as part of a treatment plan for the adjunctive therapy of agitated delirium. Dexmedetomidine or other alpha-adrenergic agents may additionally be considered as an adjunct to current therapy [93].

Toxic Alcohols

Toxic alcohol ingestion should be suspected in patients with an unexplained metabolic acidosis. The calculated serum osmolar gap is found using the formula: 2NA + Glu/18 + BUN/2.8 + ETOH/4.6. A gap of greater than ten is abnormal, and should prompt suspicion of toxic alcohol ingestion, including methanol and ethylene glycol. Isopropyl alcohol should be on the differential with a normal anion gap and an elevated osmolar gap [95].

Ethylene glycol is commonly found in antifreeze, while methanol is the active compound in paint removers. **Isopropyl alcohol** is found in rubbing alcohol. It is the metabolites of these compounds that are toxic, a concept essential in treatment.

The management of ethylene glycol and methanol exposure are similar. **Ethylene glycol**'s metabolites precipitate in renal tubules causing ATN. Further, they bind calcium, causing hypocalcemia and resultant myocardial dysfunction. Early in the course of ingestion, patients are inebriated, develop an anion gap metabolic acidosis with an osmole gap, and can have seizures secondary to cerebral edema. Later in the course, myocardial dysfunction and ATN develop. There are reports of delayed neurological sequelae in survivors. With **methanol**, initial findings include inebriation and ataxic gait. Anion gap metabolic acidosis with an osmole gap develops, and the quintessential finding of visual disturbance occurs.

The breakdown of both ethylene glycol and methanol into their toxic metabolites occurs *via* alcohol dehydrogenase. Inhibition of this pathway is therapeutically important. This can be done with either an ethanol drip, or preferably fomepizole, both of which competitively inhibit alcohol dehydrogenase. In cases of severe toxicity, adjunctive hemodialysis may be considered, but use of bicarbonate has not been shown to improve mortality.

Isopropyl alcohol ingestion presents with ketones in the urine, <u>sweet breath</u> and in the absence of an anion gap. An elevated osmole gap is present. Treatment consists of <u>hemodyalysis</u> [89].

DELIRIUM

Delirium is a <u>neurocognitive disorder characterized by a disturbance in attention, awareness and cognition</u> that develops over a relatively short period of time and fluctuates throughout the day [96]. <u>Delirium is prevalent in the ICU</u>, where it affects up to 31.8% of patients, and present as either increased or decreased levels of psychomotor activity (<u>hyperactive delirium and hypoactive delirium respectively</u>) [97]. Several tools have been validated to assist with the diagnosis of ICU delirium, including the <u>Confusion Assessment Method for the ICU (CAM-ICU) and the Intensive Care Delirium Screening Checklist (ICDSC)</u> [98]. Routine screening of patients to identify those with delirium will allow proper use of both pharmacologic and non-pharmacologic therapy to treat delirium.

<u>Delirium in adult ICU patients is associated with increased mortality, prolonged ICU and hospital length of stay as well as the development of post-ICU neurocognitive impairment</u> [98, 99]. Thus, consensus recommendations suggest avoidance of medications that may precipitate delirium, such as benzodiazepines. Medications such as <u>haloperidol and dexmedetomidine may be used for the treatment of agitated delirium</u>, but it is unclear whether use of these agents improve patient outcomes.

Better evidence exists for the use of non-pharmacologic treatment of delirium. For example, <u>early mobilization</u> of patients appears to both treat delirium as well as decrease the length of mechanical ventilation [100]. In addition, there appears to be an association between <u>improvement of sleep</u> and decreased delirium, and the use of sleep protocols appears to decrease the incidence of delirium [98, 101, 102]. A recent consensus statement recommends use of early mobilization, implementation of sleep protocols, use of atypical antipsychotic therapy to reduce delirium duration, and <u>continuous dexmedetomidine infusions (as opposed to benzodiazepine infusions) for sedation in delirious ICU patients</u> [98].

CONCLUSION

This chapter reviews common critical care illnesses and syndromes along with epidemiology, diagnostic criteria, and treatment. ARDS, sepsis, shock, GI bleeding, hypertensive emergencing, acute kidney injury, toxic exposures, and delirium are among the topics covered.

CONSENT FOR PUBLICATION

Not applicable.

CONFLICT OF INTEREST

The authors declare no conflict of interest, financial or otherwise.

ACKNOWLEDGEMENT

Declared none.

REFERENCES

[1] Rubenfeld GD, Caldwell E, Peabody E, *et al.* Incidence and outcomes of acute lung injury. N Engl J Med 2005; 353(16): 1685-93.
[http://dx.doi.org/10.1056/NEJMoa050333] [PMID: 16236739]

[2] Ranieri VM, Rubenfeld GD, Thompson BT, *et al.* Acute respiratory distress syndrome: the Berlin Definition. JAMA 2012; 307(23): 2526-33.
[PMID: 22797452]

[3] Matthay MA, Ware LB, Zimmerman GA. The acute respiratory distress syndrome. J Clin Invest 2012; 122(8): 2731-40.
[http://dx.doi.org/10.1172/JCI60331] [PMID: 22850883]

[4] Beasley MB. The pathologist's approach to acute lung injury. Arch Pathol Lab Med 2010; 134(5): 719-27.
[PMID: 20441502]

[5] Brower RG, Matthay MA, Morris A, Schoenfeld D, Thompson BT, Wheeler A. Ventilation with lower tidal volumes as compared with traditional tidal volumes for acute lung injury and the acute respiratory distress syndrome. N Engl J Med 2000; 342(18): 1301-8.
[http://dx.doi.org/10.1056/NEJM200005043421801] [PMID: 10793162]

[6] Wiedemann HP, Wheeler AP, Bernard GR, *et al.* Comparison of two fluid-management strategies in acute lung injury. N Engl J Med 2006; 354(24): 2564-75.
[http://dx.doi.org/10.1056/NEJMoa062200] [PMID: 16714767]

[7] Papazian L, Forel JM, Gacouin A, *et al.* Neuromuscular blockers in early acute respiratory distress syndrome. N Engl J Med 2010; 363(12): 1107-16.
[http://dx.doi.org/10.1056/NEJMoa1005372] [PMID: 20843245]

[8] Guérin C, Reignier J, Richard JC, *et al.* Prone positioning in severe acute respiratory distress syndrome. N Engl J Med 2013; 368(23): 2159-68.
[http://dx.doi.org/10.1056/NEJMoa1214103] [PMID: 23688302]

[9] Ferguson ND, Cook DJ, Guyatt GH, *et al.* High-frequency oscillation in early acute respiratory distress syndrome. N Engl J Med 2013; 368(9): 795-805.
[http://dx.doi.org/10.1056/NEJMoa1215554] [PMID: 23339639]

[10] Afshari A, Brok J, Møller AM, Wetterslev J. Inhaled nitric oxide for acute respiratory distress syndrome and acute lung injury in adults and children: a systematic review with meta-analysis and trial sequential analysis. Anesth Analg 2011; 112(6): 1411-21.
[http://dx.doi.org/10.1213/ANE.0b013e31820bd185] [PMID: 21372277]

[11] Peek GJ, Mugford M, Tiruvoipati R, *et al.* Efficacy and economic assessment of conventional ventilatory support *versus* extracorporeal membrane oxygenation for severe adult respiratory failure (CESAR): a multicentre randomised controlled trial. Lancet 2009; 374(9698): 1351-63.

[http://dx.doi.org/10.1016/S0140-6736(09)61069-2] [PMID: 19762075]

[12] Vincent JL, De Backer D. Circulatory shock. N Engl J Med 2013; 369(18): 1726-34.
      [http://dx.doi.org/10.1056/NEJMra1208943] [PMID: 24171518]

[13] Sakr Y, Reinhart K, Vincent JL, *et al.* Does dopamine administration in shock influence outcome?
      Results of the sepsis occurrence in acutely Ill patients (SOAP) study. Crit Care Med 2006; 34(3): 589-
      97.
      [http://dx.doi.org/10.1097/01.CCM.0000201896.45809.E3] [PMID: 16505643]

[14] Payen D, Gayat E. Which general intensive care unit patients can benefit from placement of the
      pulmonary artery catheter? Crit Care 2006; 10 (Suppl. 3): S7.
      [http://dx.doi.org/10.1186/cc4925] [PMID: 17164019]

[15] Pinsky MR. Functional hemodynamic monitoring. Crit Care Clin 2015; 31(1): 89-111.
      [http://dx.doi.org/10.1016/j.ccc.2014.08.005] [PMID: 25435480]

[16] De Backer D, Biston P, Devriendt J, *et al.* Comparison of dopamine and norepinephrine in the
      treatment of shock. N Engl J Med 2010; 362(9): 779-89.
      [http://dx.doi.org/10.1056/NEJMoa0907118] [PMID: 20200382]

[17] Myburgh JA, Higgins A, Jovanovska A, Lipman J, Ramakrishnan N, Santamaria J. A comparison of
      epinephrine and norepinephrine in critically ill patients. Intensive Care Med 2008; 34(12): 2226-34.
      [http://dx.doi.org/10.1007/s00134-008-1219-0] [PMID: 18654759]

[18] Karlsberg RP, DeWood MA, DeMaria AN, Berk MR, Lasher KP. Comparative efficacy of short-term
      intravenous infusions of milrinone and dobutamine in acute congestive heart failure following acute
      myocardial infarction. Clin Cardiol 1996; 19(1): 21-30.
      [http://dx.doi.org/10.1002/clc.4960190106] [PMID: 8903534]

[19] Asfar P, Meziani F, Hamel JF, *et al.* High *versus* low blood-pressure target in patients with septic
      shock. N Engl J Med 2014; 370(17): 1583-93.
      [http://dx.doi.org/10.1056/NEJMoa1312173] [PMID: 24635770]

[20] Bellomo R, Chapman M, Finfer S, Hickling K, Myburgh J. Low-dose dopamine in patients with early
      renal dysfunction: a placebo-controlled randomised trial. Lancet 2000; 356(9248): 2139-43.
      [http://dx.doi.org/10.1016/S0140-6736(00)03495-4] [PMID: 11191541]

[21] Miller RR III, Dong L, Nelson NC, *et al.* Multicenter implementation of a severe sepsis and septic
      shock treatment bundle. Am J Respir Crit Care Med 2013; 188(1): 77-82.
      [http://dx.doi.org/10.1164/rccm.201212-2199OC] [PMID: 23631750]

[22] Peake SL, Delaney A, Bailey M, *et al.* Goal-directed resuscitation for patients with early septic shock.
      N Engl J Med 2014; 371(16): 1496-506.
      [http://dx.doi.org/10.1056/NEJMoa1404380] [PMID: 25272316]

[23] Yealy DM, Kellum JA, Huang DT, *et al.* A randomized trial of protocol-based care for early septic
      shock. N Engl J Med 2014; 370(18): 1683-93.
      [http://dx.doi.org/10.1056/NEJMoa1401602] [PMID: 24635773]

[24] Mouncey PR, Osborn TM, Power GS, *et al.* Trial of early, goal-directed resuscitation for septic shock.
      N Engl J Med 2015; 372(14): 1301-11.
      [http://dx.doi.org/10.1056/NEJMoa1500896] [PMID: 25776532]

[25] Martin GS, Mannino DM, Eaton S, Moss M. The epidemiology of sepsis in the United States from
      1979 through 2000. N Engl J Med 2003; 348(16): 1546-54.
      [http://dx.doi.org/10.1056/NEJMoa022139] [PMID: 12700374]

[26] Kaukonen KM, Bailey M, Pilcher D, Cooper DJ, Bellomo R. Systemic inflammatory response
      syndrome criteria in defining severe sepsis. N Engl J Med 2015; 372(17): 1629-38.
      [http://dx.doi.org/10.1056/NEJMoa1415236] [PMID: 25776936]

[27] Levy MM, Fink MP, Marshall JC, *et al.* 2001 SCCM/ESICM/ACCP/ATS/SIS International Sepsis

Definitions Conference. Crit Care Med 2003; 31(4): 1250-6.
[http://dx.doi.org/10.1097/01.CCM.0000050454.01978.3B] [PMID: 12682500]

[28] Renaud B, Brun-Buisson C. Outcomes of primary and catheter-related bacteremia. A cohort and case-control study in critically ill patients. Am J Respir Crit Care Med 2001; 163(7): 1584-90.
[http://dx.doi.org/10.1164/ajrccm.163.7.9912080] [PMID: 11401878]

[29] Dellinger RP, Levy MM, Rhodes A, *et al.* Surviving Sepsis Campaign: international guidelines for management of severe sepsis and septic shock, 2012. Intensive Care Med 2013; 39(2): 165-228.
[http://dx.doi.org/10.1007/s00134-012-2769-8] [PMID: 23361625]

[30] Caironi P, Tognoni G, Masson S, *et al.* Albumin replacement in patients with severe sepsis or septic shock. N Engl J Med 2014; 370(15): 1412-21.
[http://dx.doi.org/10.1056/NEJMoa1305727] [PMID: 24635772]

[31] Finfer S, Bellomo R, Boyce N, French J, Myburgh J, Norton R. A comparison of albumin and saline for fluid resuscitation in the intensive care unit. N Engl J Med 2004; 350(22): 2247-56.
[http://dx.doi.org/10.1056/NEJMoa040232] [PMID: 15163774]

[32] Yunos NM, Bellomo R, Hegarty C, Story D, Ho L, Bailey M. Association between a chloride-liberal *vs.* chloride-restrictive intravenous fluid administration strategy and kidney injury in critically ill adults. JAMA 2012; 308(15): 1566-72.
[http://dx.doi.org/10.1001/jama.2012.13356] [PMID: 23073953]

[33] Young P, Bailey M, Beasley R, *et al.* Effect of a buffered crystalloid solution *vs.* Saline on acute kidney injury among patients in the intensive care unit: The SPLIT randomized clinical trial. JAMA 2015; 314(16): 1701-10.
[http://dx.doi.org/10.1001/jama.2015.12334] [PMID: 26444692]

[34] Prescott HC, Langa KM, Liu V, Escobar GJ, Iwashyna TJ. Increased 1-year healthcare use in survivors of severe sepsis. Am J Respir Crit Care Med 2014; 190(1): 62-9.
[http://dx.doi.org/10.1164/rccm.201403-0471OC] [PMID: 24872085]

[35] Prescott HC, Langa KM, Iwashyna TJ. Readmission diagnoses after hospitalization for severe sepsis and other acute medical conditions. JAMA 2015; 313(10): 1055-7.
[http://dx.doi.org/10.1001/jama.2015.1410] [PMID: 25756444]

[36] Farrell JJ, Friedman LS. Review article: the management of lower gastrointestinal bleeding. Aliment Pharmacol Ther 2005; 21(11): 1281-98.
[http://dx.doi.org/10.1111/j.1365-2036.2005.02485.x] [PMID: 15932359]

[37] Longstreth GF. Epidemiology of hospitalization for acute upper gastrointestinal hemorrhage: a population-based study. Am J Gastroenterol 1995; 90(2): 206-10.
[PMID: 7847286]

[38] van Leerdam ME. Epidemiology of acute upper gastrointestinal bleeding. Best Pract Res Clin Gastroenterol 2008; 22(2): 209-24.
[http://dx.doi.org/10.1016/j.bpg.2007.10.011] [PMID: 18346679]

[39] Barkun AN, Bardou M, Kuipers EJ, *et al.* International consensus recommendations on the management of patients with nonvariceal upper gastrointestinal bleeding. Ann Intern Med 2010; 152(2): 101-13.
[http://dx.doi.org/10.7326/0003-4819-152-2-201001190-00009] [PMID: 20083829]

[40] Hwang JH, Fisher DA, Ben-Menachem T, *et al.* The role of endoscopy in the management of acute non-variceal upper GI bleeding. Gastrointest Endosc 2012; 75(6): 1132-8.
[http://dx.doi.org/10.1016/j.gie.2012.02.033] [PMID: 22624808]

[41] Villanueva C, Colomo A, Bosch A, *et al.* Transfusion strategies for acute upper gastrointestinal bleeding. N Engl J Med 2013; 368(1): 11-21.
[http://dx.doi.org/10.1056/NEJMoa1211801] [PMID: 23281973]

[42] Laine L, Jensen DM. Management of patients with ulcer bleeding. Am J Gastroenterol 2012; 107(3):

345-60.
[http://dx.doi.org/10.1038/ajg.2011.480] [PMID: 22310222]

[43]   Huang ES, Karsan S, Kanwal F, Singh I, Makhani M, Spiegel BM. Impact of nasogastric lavage on outcomes in acute GI bleeding. Gastrointest Endosc 2011; 74(5): 971-80.
[http://dx.doi.org/10.1016/j.gie.2011.04.045] [PMID: 21737077]

[44]   Lau JY, Sung JJ, Lee KK, *et al.* Effect of intravenous omeprazole on recurrent bleeding after endoscopic treatment of bleeding peptic ulcers. N Engl J Med 2000; 343(5): 310-6.
[http://dx.doi.org/10.1056/NEJM200008033430501] [PMID: 10922420]

[45]   D'Amico G, De Franchis R. Upper digestive bleeding in cirrhosis. Post-therapeutic outcome and prognostic indicators. Hepatology 2003; 38(3): 599-612.
[http://dx.doi.org/10.1053/jhep.2003.50385] [PMID: 12939586]

[46]   Gotzsche PC. Somatostatin or octreotide for acute bleeding oesophageal varices. Cochrane Database Syst Rev 2000; (2): CD000193.
[PMID: 10796699]

[47]   Soares-Weiser K, Brezis M, Tur-Kaspa R, Leibovici L. Antibiotic prophylaxis for cirrhotic patients with gastrointestinal bleeding. Cochrane Database Syst Rev 2002; (2): CD002907.
[PMID: 12076458]

[48]   Garcia-Tsao G, Sanyal AJ, Grace ND, Carey W. Prevention and management of gastroesophageal varices and variceal hemorrhage in cirrhosis. Hepatology 2007; 46(3): 922-38.
[http://dx.doi.org/10.1002/hep.21907] [PMID: 17879356]

[49]   Longstreth GF. Epidemiology and outcome of patients hospitalized with acute lower gastrointestinal hemorrhage: a population-based study. Am J Gastroenterol 1997; 92(3): 419-24.
[PMID: 9068461]

[50]   Zuccaro G Jr. Management of the adult patient with acute lower gastrointestinal bleeding. Am J Gastroenterol 1998; 93(8): 1202-8.
[http://dx.doi.org/10.1111/j.1572-0241.1998.00395.x] [PMID: 9707037]

[51]   Strate LL, Orav EJ, Syngal S. Early predictors of severity in acute lower intestinal tract bleeding. Arch Intern Med 2003; 163(7): 838-43.
[http://dx.doi.org/10.1001/archinte.163.7.838] [PMID: 12695275]

[52]   Ault MJ, Ellrodt AG. Pathophysiological events leading to the end-organ effects of acute hypertension. Am J Emerg Med 1985; 3(6) (Suppl.): 10-5.
[http://dx.doi.org/10.1016/0735-6757(85)90227-X] [PMID: 3910062]

[53]   Wallach R, Karp RB, Reves JG, Oparil S, Smith LR, James TN. Pathogenesis of paroxysmal hypertension developing during and after coronary bypass surgery: a study of hemodynamic and humoral factors. Am J Cardiol 1980; 46(4): 559-65.
[http://dx.doi.org/10.1016/0002-9149(80)90503-2] [PMID: 6998270]

[54]   Funakoshi Y, Ichiki T, Ito K, Takeshita A. Induction of interleukin-6 expression by angiotensin II in rat vascular smooth muscle cells. Hypertension 1999; 34(1): 118-25.
[http://dx.doi.org/10.1161/01.HYP.34.1.118] [PMID: 10406834]

[55]   Marik PE, Rivera R. Hypertensive emergencies: an update. Curr Opin Crit Care 2011; 17(6): 569-80.
[http://dx.doi.org/10.1097/MCC.0b013e32834cd31d] [PMID: 21986463]

[56]   Katz JN, Gore JM, Amin A, *et al.* Practice patterns, outcomes, and end-organ dysfunction for patients with acute severe hypertension: the Studying the Treatment of Acute hyperTension (STAT) registry. Am Heart J 2009; 158(4): 599-606.e1.
[http://dx.doi.org/10.1016/j.ahj.2009.07.020] [PMID: 19781420]

[57]   Aronson S, Dyke CM, Stierer KA, *et al.* The ECLIPSE trials: comparative studies of clevidipine to nitroglycerin, sodium nitroprusside, and nicardipine for acute hypertension treatment in cardiac surgery patients. Anesth Analg 2008; 107(4): 1110-21.

[http://dx.doi.org/10.1213/ane.0b013e31818240db] [PMID: 18806012]

[58]   Lambert CR, Hill JA, Feldman RL, Pepine CJ. Effects of nicardipine on exercise- and pacing-induced myocardial ischemia in angina pectoris. Am J Cardiol 1987; 60(7): 471-6.
[http://dx.doi.org/10.1016/0002-9149(87)90288-8] [PMID: 3630928]

[59]   Lambert CR, Hill JA, Nichols WW, Feldman RL, Pepine CJ. Coronary and systemic hemodynamic effects of nicardipine. Am J Cardiol 1985; 55(6): 652-6.
[http://dx.doi.org/10.1016/0002-9149(85)90130-4] [PMID: 3976506]

[60]   Halpern NA, Sladen RN, Goldberg JS, *et al.* Nicardipine infusion for postoperative hypertension after surgery of the head and neck. Crit Care Med 1990; 18(9): 950-5.
[http://dx.doi.org/10.1097/00003246-199009000-00009] [PMID: 2203602]

[61]   Bailey JM, Lu W, Levy JH, *et al.* Clevidipine in adult cardiac surgical patients: a dose-finding study. Anesthesiology 2002; 96(5): 1086-94.
[http://dx.doi.org/10.1097/00000542-200205000-00010] [PMID: 11981147]

[62]   Ericsson H, Fakt C, Jolin-Mellgård A, *et al.* Clinical and pharmacokinetic results with a new ultrashort-acting calcium antagonist, clevidipine, following gradually increasing intravenous doses to healthy volunteers. Br J Clin Pharmacol 1999; 47(5): 531-8.
[http://dx.doi.org/10.1046/j.1365-2125.1999.00933.x] [PMID: 10336577]

[63]   Lund-Johansen P. Pharmacology of combined alpha-beta-blockade. II. Haemodynamic effects of labetalol. Drugs 1984; 28 (Suppl. 2): 35-50.
[http://dx.doi.org/10.2165/00003495-198400282-00004] [PMID: 6151890]

[64]   Gray RJ. Managing critically ill patients with esmolol. An ultra short-acting beta-adrenergic blocker. Chest 1988; 93(2): 398-403.
[http://dx.doi.org/10.1378/chest.93.2.398] [PMID: 2892647]

[65]   Lowenthal DT, Porter RS, Saris SD, Bies CM, Slegowski MB, Staudacher A. Clinical pharmacology, pharmacodynamics and interactions with esmolol. Am J Cardiol 1985; 56(11): 14F-8F.
[http://dx.doi.org/10.1016/0002-9149(85)90911-7] [PMID: 2864843]

[66]   Hardy YMJA. Hypertensive crises: Urgencies and emergencies. US Pharm 2011; 36(3).

[67]   Mehta RL, Kellum JA, Shah SV, *et al.* Acute Kidney Injury Network: report of an initiative to improve outcomes in acute kidney injury. Crit Care 2007; 11(2): R31.
[http://dx.doi.org/10.1186/cc5713] [PMID: 17331245]

[68]   Hoste EA, Clermont G, Kersten A, *et al.* RIFLE criteria for acute kidney injury are associated with hospital mortality in critically ill patients: a cohort analysis. Crit Care 2006; 10(3): R73.
[http://dx.doi.org/10.1186/cc4915] [PMID: 16696865]

[69]   Mehta RL, Pascual MT, Soroko S, *et al.* Spectrum of acute renal failure in the intensive care unit: the PICARD experience. Kidney Int 2004; 66(4): 1613-21.
[http://dx.doi.org/10.1111/j.1523-1755.2004.00927.x] [PMID: 15458458]

[70]   Uchino S, Kellum JA, Bellomo R, *et al.* Acute renal failure in critically ill patients: a multinational, multicenter study. JAMA 2005; 294(7): 813-8.
[http://dx.doi.org/10.1001/jama.294.7.813] [PMID: 16106006]

[71]   Uchino S, Bellomo R, Goldsmith D, Bates S, Ronco C. An assessment of the RIFLE criteria for acute renal failure in hospitalized patients. Crit Care Med 2006; 34(7): 1913-7.
[http://dx.doi.org/10.1097/01.CCM.0000224227.70642.4F] [PMID: 16715038]

[72]   Ostermann M, Chang RW. Acute kidney injury in the intensive care unit according to RIFLE. Critical care medicine 2007; 35(8): 1837-43. quiz 1852
[http://dx.doi.org/10.1097/01.CCM.0000277041.13090.0A]

[73]   Metnitz PG, Krenn CG, Steltzer H, *et al.* Effect of acute renal failure requiring renal replacement therapy on outcome in critically ill patients. Crit Care Med 2002; 30(9): 2051-8.

[http://dx.doi.org/10.1097/00003246-200209000-00016] [PMID: 12352040]

[74]   Bagshaw SM, Laupland KB, Doig CJ, *et al.* Prognosis for long-term survival and renal recovery in critically ill patients with severe acute renal failure: a population-based study. Crit Care 2005; 9(6): R700-9.
[http://dx.doi.org/10.1186/cc3879] [PMID: 16280066]

[75]   Dennen P, Douglas IS, Anderson R. Acute kidney injury in the intensive care unit: an update and primer for the intensivist. Crit Care Med 2010; 38(1): 261-75.
[http://dx.doi.org/10.1097/CCM.0b013e3181bfb0b5] [PMID: 19829099]

[76]   Payen D, de Pont AC, Sakr Y, Spies C, Reinhart K, Vincent JL. A positive fluid balance is associated with a worse outcome in patients with acute renal failure. Crit Care 2008; 12(3): R74.
[http://dx.doi.org/10.1186/cc6916] [PMID: 18533029]

[77]   De Waele JJ, Malbrain ML, Kirkpatrick AW. The abdominal compartment syndrome: evolving concepts and future directions. Crit Care 2015; 19: 211.
[http://dx.doi.org/10.1186/s13054-015-0879-8] [PMID: 25943575]

[78]   Pazhayattil GS, Shirali AC. Drug-induced impairment of renal function. Int J Nephrol Renovasc Dis 2014; 7: 457-68.
[PMID: 25540591]

[79]   Hogan SE, L'Allier P, Chetcuti S, *et al.* Current role of sodium bicarbonate-based preprocedural hydration for the prevention of contrast-induced acute kidney injury: a meta-analysis. Am Heart J 2008; 156(3): 414-21.
[http://dx.doi.org/10.1016/j.ahj.2008.05.014] [PMID: 18760120]

[80]   Meier P, Ko DT, Tamura A, Tamhane U, Gurm HS. Sodium bicarbonate-based hydration prevents contrast-induced nephropathy: a meta-analysis. BMC Med 2009; 7: 23.
[http://dx.doi.org/10.1186/1741-7015-7-23] [PMID: 19439062]

[81]   Navaneethan SD, Singh S, Appasamy S, Wing RE, Sehgal AR. Sodium bicarbonate therapy for prevention of contrast-induced nephropathy: a systematic review and meta-analysis. Am J Kidney Dis 2009; 53(4): 617-27.
[http://dx.doi.org/10.1053/j.ajkd.2008.08.033] [PMID: 19027212]

[82]   Brar SS, Shen AY, Jorgensen MB, *et al.* Sodium bicarbonate *vs.* sodium chloride for the prevention of contrast medium-induced nephropathy in patients undergoing coronary angiography: a randomized trial. JAMA 2008; 300(9): 1038-46.
[http://dx.doi.org/10.1001/jama.300.9.1038] [PMID: 18768415]

[83]   Sort P, Navasa M, Arroyo V, *et al.* Effect of intravenous albumin on renal impairment and mortality in patients with cirrhosis and spontaneous bacterial peritonitis. N Engl J Med 1999; 341(6): 403-9.
[http://dx.doi.org/10.1056/NEJM199908053410603] [PMID: 10432325]

[84]   Holmes CL, Walley KR. Bad medicine: low-dose dopamine in the ICU. Chest 2003; 123(4): 1266-75.
[http://dx.doi.org/10.1378/chest.123.4.1266] [PMID: 12684320]

[85]   Palevsky PM, Zhang JH, O'Connor TZ, *et al.* Intensity of renal support in critically ill patients with acute kidney injury. N Engl J Med 2008; 359(1): 7-20.
[http://dx.doi.org/10.1056/NEJMoa0802639] [PMID: 18492867]

[86]   Bellomo R, Cass A, Cole L, *et al.* Intensity of continuous renal-replacement therapy in critically ill patients. N Engl J Med 2009; 361(17): 1627-38.
[http://dx.doi.org/10.1056/NEJMoa0902413] [PMID: 19846848]

[87]   Payen D, Mateo J, Cavaillon JM, Fraisse F, Floriot C, Vicaut E. Impact of continuous venovenous hemofiltration on organ failure during the early phase of severe sepsis: a randomized controlled trial. Crit Care Med 2009; 37(3): 803-10.
[http://dx.doi.org/10.1097/CCM.0b013e3181962316] [PMID: 19237881]

[88]   Shanti CM, Lucas CE. Cocaine and the critical care challenge. Crit Care Med 2003; 31(6): 1851-9.

[http://dx.doi.org/10.1097/01.CCM.0000063258.68159.71] [PMID: 12794430]

[89]   Mokhlesi B, Leikin JB, Murray P, Corbridge TC. Adult toxicology in critical care: Part II: specific poisonings. Chest 2003; 123(3): 897-922.
[http://dx.doi.org/10.1378/chest.123.3.897] [PMID: 12628894]

[90]   Kosten TR, O'Connor PG. Management of drug and alcohol withdrawal. N Engl J Med 2003; 348(18): 1786-95.
[http://dx.doi.org/10.1056/NEJMra020617] [PMID: 12724485]

[91]   Etherington JM. Emergency management of acute alcohol problems. Part 1: Uncomplicated withdrawal. Can Fam Physician 1996; 42: 2186-90.
[PMID: 8939320]

[92]   McKeon A, Frye MA, Delanty N. The alcohol withdrawal syndrome. J Neurol Neurosurg Psychiatry 2008; 79(8): 854-62.
[http://dx.doi.org/10.1136/jnnp.2007.128322] [PMID: 17986499]

[93]   Sarff M, Gold JA. Alcohol withdrawal syndromes in the intensive care unit. Crit Care Med 2010; 38(9) (Suppl.): S494-501.
[http://dx.doi.org/10.1097/CCM.0b013e3181ec5412] [PMID: 20724883]

[94]   Daeppen JB, Gache P, Landry U, *et al.* Symptom-triggered *vs.* fixed-schedule doses of benzodiazepine for alcohol withdrawal: a randomized treatment trial. Arch Intern Med 2002; 162(10): 1117-21.
[http://dx.doi.org/10.1001/archinte.162.10.1117] [PMID: 12020181]

[95]   Mokhlesi B, Leiken JB, Murray P, Corbridge TC. Adult toxicology in critical care: part I: general approach to the intoxicated patient. Chest 2003; 123(2): 577-92.
[http://dx.doi.org/10.1378/chest.123.2.577] [PMID: 12576382]

[96]   Sachdev PS, Blacker D, Blazer DG, *et al.* Classifying neurocognitive disorders: the DSM-5 approach. Nat Rev Neurol 2014; 10(11): 634-42.
[http://dx.doi.org/10.1038/nrneurol.2014.181] [PMID: 25266297]

[97]   Salluh JI, Wang H, Schneider EB, *et al.* Outcome of delirium in critically ill patients: systematic review and meta-analysis. BMJ 2015; 350: h2538.
[http://dx.doi.org/10.1136/bmj.h2538] [PMID: 26041151]

[98]   Barr J, Fraser GL, Puntillo K, *et al.* Clinical practice guidelines for the management of pain, agitation, and delirium in adult patients in the intensive care unit. Crit Care Med 2013; 41(1): 263-306.
[http://dx.doi.org/10.1097/CCM.0b013e3182783b72] [PMID: 23269131]

[99]   Pandharipande PP, Girard TD, Jackson JC, *et al.* Long-term cognitive impairment after critical illness. N Engl J Med 2013; 369(14): 1306-16.
[http://dx.doi.org/10.1056/NEJMoa1301372] [PMID: 24088092]

[100]   Balas MC, Vasilevskis EE, Olsen KM, *et al.* Effectiveness and safety of the awakening and breathing coordination, delirium monitoring/management, and early exercise/mobility bundle. Crit Care Med 2014; 42(5): 1024-36.
[http://dx.doi.org/10.1097/CCM.0000000000000129] [PMID: 24394627]

[101]   Barr J, Kishman CP Jr, Jaeschke R. The methodological approach used to develop the 2013 Pain, Agitation, and Delirium Clinical Practice Guidelines for adult ICU patients. Crit Care Med 2013; 41(9) (Suppl. 1): S1-S15.
[http://dx.doi.org/10.1097/CCM.0b013e3182a167d7] [PMID: 23989088]

[102]   Kamdar BB, King LM, Collop NA, *et al.* The effect of a quality improvement intervention on perceived sleep quality and cognition in a medical ICU. Crit Care Med 2013; 41(3): 800-9.
[http://dx.doi.org/10.1097/CCM.0b013e3182746442] [PMID: 23314584]

CHAPTER 6

SICU Update

Sheri Berg* and **Edward A. Bittner**

Massachusetts General Hospital, Harvard Medical School, Boston, Massachusetts, USA

Abstract: Since the field of critical care is constantly changing, it is important for anesthesiologists to stay knowledgeable of these changes in order to provide optimal care to critically ill patients in the perioperative period. The purpose of this chapter is to provide an update for clinicians on ICU issues relevant to clinical practice. Topics which will be discussed include: modes of mechanical ventilation, renal replacement therapy, antibiotic prophylaxis, nutritional support, sedation management, transport of patients, and transfer of care.

Keywords: Airway Pressure Release Ventilation, Antibiotic Prophylaxis, Continuous Renal Replacement Therapy, Drug Resistant Organisms, High Frequency Oscillatory Ventilation, In Hospital Transport, Inverse Ratio Ventilation, Noninvasive Ventilation, Nutritional Support, Pressure Controlled Ventilation, Pressure Support Ventilation, Renal Replacement Therapy, Refeeding Syndrome, Sedation, Surgical Site Infections, Transfer of Care, Volume Controlled Ventilation.

INTRODUCTION

Among the foremost experts on Surgical Critical Care, the following chapter by Doctors Sheri Berg and Edward Bittner [Massachusetts General Hospital Review of Critical Care Medicine, by Sheri M. Berg, MD and Edward A. Bittner, MD, PhD, ©2014 Lippincott Williams & Wilkins] represents essential knowledge for the nonintensivist on Surgical Critical Care.

The field of critical care is constantly changing. It is important for anesthesiologists to stay knowledgeable of these revolutions in order to provide optimal care to critically ill patients in the perioperative period. The purpose of this chapter is to provide an update for clinicians on ICU issues relevant to clinical practice. Topics which will be discussed include: modes of mechanical ventilation, renal replacement therapy, antibiotic prophylaxis, nutritional support,

* **Corresponding author Sheri Berg:** Massachusetts General Hospital, Harvard Medical School, Boston, Massachusetts, USA; Tel: (617)-726-2000; E-mail: SBERG1@mgh.harvard.edu

Amballur D. John (Ed.)

sedation management, transport and transfer of care.

MODES OF MECHANICAL VENTILATION

Introduction

Most patients undergoing general anesthesia for surgical procedures require mechanical ventilation. One of the biggest challenges facing clinicians providing mechanical ventilatory support today, is managing the balance between providing adequate gas exchange and avoiding lung injury associated with positive pressure ventilation. Patients with respiratory failure need adequate tissue oxygenation and acid-base balance; however, over-distension, alveolar collapse and reopening, and high oxygen exposure can injure the lungs. The challenge to impart "lung protective ventilation" is made even more difficult by the fact that lung injury is often heterogeneous and thus, what may benefit gas exchange in one region (*e.g.*, higher pressure) may worsen injury in another.

Modern anesthesia ventilators are becoming increasingly sophisticated. They possess the ability to provide high performances in delivering accurate and precise specifically desired volumes and pressures, including assisted ventilation modes. It is therefore important that anesthesiologists become familiar with the most commonly used intraoperative ventilation modes, as well as their potential pitfalls. Although there is no clear evidence to support the advantage of any single mode of ventilation, protective mechanical ventilation with low tidal volume and low levels of positive end expiratory pressure (PEEP) should be considered for all patients undergoing surgery [1, 2].

Modes of mechanical ventilation have traditionally been divided into "pressure" or "volume" controlled modes; however the definitive lines between these modes are becoming continually blurred by increasingly complex methods of ventilation. A more modern classification scheme describes ventilatory modes based on three characteristics – the **trigger** (flow *versus* pressure), the **limit** (what determines the size of the breath), and the **cycle** (what actually ends the breath) [3]. In both volume controlled (VCV) and pressure controlled (PCV) ventilation, time is the cycle, the difference being in how the time to cessation is determined. Pressure support ventilation (PSV), by contrast, has a flow cycle. For ease of discussion, the ventilatory modes will be divided into volume controlled, pressure controlled, and other modes.

Volume-Controlled Ventilation

With **volume controlled ventilation** (VCV), a preset volume of gas is delivered to the patient over a set period of time. Once that volume of gas has been delivered, the flow stops and passive expiration occurs. The most widely used breath delivery mode with VCV is constant (square wave) inspiratory flow. With VCV, the patient is guaranteed to receive the set volume, but airway pressure will increase in response to factors that restrict the delivery of that volume of gas, such as decreased lung or chest wall compliance or increased airway resistance thereby potentially exposing the patient to the risk of high airway pressures. Pressure will vary in volume-targeted modes of ventilation; therefore careful monitoring and assessment of respiratory system compliance and resistance are required.

PRESSURE-CONTROLLED VENTILATION

With **pressure-controlled ventilation (PCV)**, the circuit is pressurized to a set peak inspiratory pressure as soon as the inspiratory valve opens. This pressure is then maintained for the duration of the set inspiratory time. Gas flow is initially high and then diminishes over the course of the inspiratory phase of the breath (decelerating flow pattern). Thus, with PCV, the alveoli remain fully inflated for a longer portion of the inspiratory phase, enhancing both gas exchange and lung inflation, and can achieve equal volumes with lower inflating pressures [4]. The potential for lung recruitment through increased mean airway pressure makes this an attractive mode in patients with large shunt fractions. This mode requires that the exhaled volumes and minute ventilation are monitored to ensure that adequate ventilation is being delivered in the face of changes in compliance or resistance. Despite its benefit in lower peak air way pressures, the impact on lung mechanics, gas exchange, and risk of barotrauma is variable and PCV has not been proven superior to other modes of mechanical ventilation. Implementation of PCV requires a practical understanding of the relationship between flow, time, and pressure.

Inverse Ratio Ventilation

Inverse Ratio Ventilation (IRV) is a subtype of PCV, in which inflation time is prolonged [5]. With IRV an inspiratory to expiratory (I:E) ratio of.1:1, 2:1, or 3:1 may be used (normal I:E is 1:2). This lowers peak airway pressures but increases mean airway pressures, which may result in improved oxygenation. IRV is most commonly used in patients with ARDS and refractory hypoxemia. Reduced venous return and cardiac output are downsides of IRV.

Airway Pressure Release Ventilation

Airway pressure release ventilation (**APRV**- also known as "Bi-level", "Bi-phasic" and "BiPAP") has recently been introduced into clinical anesthesia practice [6]. APRV is a <u>time cycled,</u> <u>pressure targeted</u> form of ventilatory support that uses an I:E ratio of up to 4:1 or 5:1). The potential advantages of this approach are similar to those of other long inspiratory time (IRV) strategies. Specifically, the long inflation phase recruits the more slowly filling alveoli and raises mean airway pressure without increasing tidal volume or applied PEEP (although intrinsic PEEP can develop with short expiratory or deflation periods). Patients are able to spontaneously ventilate at both low and high pressures, although typically most (or all) ventilation occurs at the higher pressures. In the <u>absence of attempted breaths, APRV and IRV are identical</u>. As in IRV, hemodynamic compromise is a concern in APRV. Additionally, application of APRV typically requires increased sedation.

Pressure Support Ventilation

With **pressure support ventilation (PSV)**, the ventilator supports spontaneous breathing by applying pressure to the airways in conjunction with the patient's supported breaths. Once a breath is initiated, the ventilator pressurizes the airway to a given inspiratory support pressure which is usually from 5-10cm H_2O. Each PSV assisted breath is terminated according to a preset decrease in flow or after a specific duration. PSV is particularly useful for patients maintained with spontaneous respiration under general anesthesia. <u>PSV reduces the patient's work of breathing during spontaneous respiration and counters the reduction in functional residual capacity</u>, which occurs with the concurrent usage of inhalational agents. By applying pressure to the airway immediately upon sensing a patient breath, PSV enhances inspiratory flow and provides improved gas distribution within the lungs. This enhanced gas distribution results in a lower peak airway pressure, which is quite advantageous when laryngeal mask airways (LMAs) are used [7]. Lower pressures result in less gas leakage around the LMA seal. Unlike controlled ventilation, PSV is usually well tolerated during light levels of anesthesia. PSV mode serves to facilitate a deeper plan of anesthesia while augmenting spontaneous respiration. Some ventilators have an apnea backup feature to provide ventilator breaths when there is a lack of spontaneous effort from the patient.

High Frequency Oscillatory Ventilation

High frequency oscillatory ventilation (HFOV) uses very <u>high breathing frequencies</u> (120-900 breaths per minute in the adult) <u>coupled with very small tidal volumes</u> (often less than 1ml/kg at the alveolar level) to provide gas exchange in the lungs. <u>Gas transport involves mechanisms such as Taylor dispersion, coaxial flows, and augmented diffusion</u> [8]. The device used to deliver HFOV in adults, uses a "to-and-fro" piston mechanism to vibrate a fresh bias flow of gas delivered at or near the tip of the endotracheal tube. As HFOV supplies substantial mean airway pressures, but applies very little pressure or volume fluctuations in the alveolus, it is sometimes termed "CPAP with a wiggle" [9]. The <u>potential advantages to HFOV</u> are two-fold. <u>First</u>, the very small alveolar tidal pressure swings minimize cyclical overdistension and derecruitment. <u>Second</u>, a high mean airway pressure can also prevent derecruitment. Mean pressures used during HFOV often exceed the 30-35cm H_2O threshold that is employed during conventional ventilation.

<u>Clinical experience</u> with various high frequency ventilation techniques has been <u>most extensively studied in the neonatal and pediatric populations</u>, where general consensus has arisen that high frequency ventilation appears to improve long-term clinical outcomes. There is less experience with high frequency techniques with regards to outcomes in adults. Small trials of HFOV over the last two decades have suggested possible beneficial outcomes. Two recent large randomized trials in moderate-severe ARDS failed to show any benefit [10, 11]. However, these studies have been criticized since both of them were conducted by a large number of centers who lacked sufficient previous experience with HFOV and over two thirds of the patients studied were in shock at the time of entry into the study. Clearly, if there is a role for HFOV use going forward, it should be reserved for trials in centers with experienced practitioners and for patients who have proven to be refractory to conventional management.

NONINVASIVE VENTILATION

Non-invasive ventilation (**NIV**) refers to techniques allowing respiratory support without an artificial airway. **Two types of NIV** are commonly used: <u>continuous positive airway pressure (CPAP)</u> and <u>positive pressure ventilation</u> (<u>NPPV</u>) which delivers two levels of positive pressure (pressure support ventilation + positive end-expiratory pressure). NIV may be used to prevent (prophylaxis) or to manage (treat) acute respiratory failure in hopes of possibly avoiding intubation. <u>NIV exerts its main effects on the pulmonary and cardiovascular systems</u>. Through the application of a positive end-expiratory pressure (PEEP), with or without a pressure support during inspiration, NIV restores lung volumes by opening atelectatic areas (which commonly occurs postoperatively), increases alveolar ventilation, and reduces the work of breathing. By reopening atelectatic areas, NIV can also prevent postoperative pneumonia. Additionally, NIV may have beneficial effects on the cardiovascular function, *via* lowering left ventricular afterload and therefore improving cardiac output [12].

There is a growing amount of data on NIV efficacy and safety in postoperative patients. Evidence suggests that NIV, as a prophylactic or curative treatment, is an effective strategy to reduce intubation rates, nosocomial infections, intensive care unit and hospital lengths of stay, and morbidity and mortality in postoperative patients [13, 14]. NIV has also been applied intraoperatively in settings that do not strictly require general anesthesia [15]. Moreover, NIV support allows for light sedation to increase patient comfort. Larger studies are required to demonstrate NIV efficacy in this complex setting.

Renal Replacement Therapy

Introduction

The general term **renal replacement therapy** (**RRT**) is used to describe the group of currently available approaches to "artificial" mechanical support of renal function. **RRT** includes traditional <u>intermittent hemodialysis</u> (<u>IHD</u>), <u>peritoneal dialysis</u> (PD), and a <u>variety of other intermittent and continuous therapies</u>. Most anesthesiologists are familiar with intermittent modes of dialysis and their implications in the perioperative care setting. However, the use of continuous RRT therapies to support the patient with renal failure is common in the critically ill patient. Therefore, anesthesiologists should understand the clinical indications for CRRT, the variety of approaches that are available for CRRT, and the implications of CRRT on anesthetic and perioperative management.

PRINCIPLES OF RENAL REPLACEMENT THERAPY

Regardless of the type of RRT employed, the <u>principles of dialysis are similar</u>. Three general methods are used to facilitate dialysis which are based on allowing water and solute transportation through a semipermeable membrane from the body into the dialysis fluid [16]. With **_diffusion_**, solutes move across a semipermeable membrane by concentration gradients (from higher solute concentrations to lower solute concentrations). With **_ultrafiltration_**, water is moved across a semipermeable membrane by osmotic pressure. With **_convection_**, water is moved across a semipermeable membrane by a transmembrane pressure gradient (similar to ultrafiltration) but solutes are "dragged" with the water; (small-molecular-weight substances such as blood urea nitrogen, creatinine, and potassium). When the ultrafiltration rate is increased to provide convection clearance of solutes, this is known as hemofiltration.

RRT Subtypes

Continuous renal replacement therapies (CRRT), **intermittent hemodialysis (IHD)**, and **Sustained low-efficiency dialysis (SLED)** are the <u>principal RRT modalities that are used in the critical care setting</u> [17]. CRRT modalities more closely approximate normal physiology with slow correction of metabolic derangements and removal of fluid. Therefore, CRRT is commonly thought to be better tolerated in the critically ill and/or hemodynamically unstable patient. SLED, sometimes referred to as extended dialysis, is considered a 'hybrid' of IHD and CRRT. SLED is administered using conventional dialysis technology but typical sessions run for 8-12 hours using blood and dialysis flows that are intermediate to those prescribed in IHD and CRRT. Despite the apparent advantages of continues modalities, there is an absence of clear evidence that these apparent physiologic advantages translate into a decrease in ICU or hospital mortality.

CRRT may be administered as **hemodialysis** (continuous venovenous hemodialysis, CVVHD), **hemofiltration** (continuous venovenous hemofiltration, CVVH) or a **combination** of these (continuous venovenous hemodiafiltration, CVVHDF) [18]. Although the specific method of delivering the therapy varies, all forms of CRRT include an extracorporeal circuit with a hemofilter and semipermeable membrane connected to the patient *via* a catheter in either the arterial or venous circuit. Fluid removal is determined by the hydrostatic pressure gradient across the hemofilter. Large volumes of fluid can be removed using this approach. Fluid balance is controlled by providing replacement fluid through the system; electrolytes and acid base balance are controlled by the electrolyte and bicarbonate concentration in the replacement fluid.

Indications for CRRT

CRRT is used most commonly to manage the critically ill patient with acute renal failure. The therapy is used to manage uremia associated with renal failure, treat hyperkalemia, control metabolic acidosis in patients with either a renal tubular acidosis or lactic acidosis, and to optimize fluid balance. CRRT may also used for management of problems not directly associated with renal failure, including therapy for pulmonary edema or congestive heart failure, in the septic patient to optimize cytokine clearance, and in patients with severe respiratory failure in which mechanical ventilatory support alone does not control their acid base imbalance. CRRT has also been used in patients with cerebral edema to optimize overall fluid balance without compromising cerebral blood flow [19].

PERIOPERATIVE CONSIDERATIONS WITH CRRT

Preoperative

For the patient who is receiving CRRT, the preoperative assessment must take into account for certain specific elements regarding the therapy. Many critically ill patients receiving CRRT, are hemodynamically unstable requiring vasopressor or inotropic therapy, have multi-system failure, and are receiving mechanical ventilatory support. In addition to the usual considerations for the management of the critically ill patient, the preoperative assessment of the patient receiving CRRT should clarify the indications for the therapy, the goals, and whether the goals have been met. <u>An initial concern for the anesthesiologist is the status of the patient's fluid, electrolyte, and acid base balance</u>. <u>The anesthesiologist must assess the metabolic status</u> of the patient undergoing CRRT; therefore the preoperative assessment should include an evaluation of the <u>coagulation status</u> of the patient. This is in part because of the implications of renal failure on coagulation (*e.g.*, platelet function) and whether or not the patient is receiving anticoagulants to prevent CRRT filter and circuit clotting. While heparin is most commonly used as an anticoagulant, and generally administered before the filter to minimize the systemic effects, the <u>impact on clotting can be unpredictable</u>. For some patients, alternative anticoagulants are used, including citrate. Finally, the <u>patient's temperature trend</u> should be evaluated preoperatively as there is a considerable amount of heat that is lost through the extensive extracorporeal circuit. Consequently, patients receiving CRRT are often hypothermic; some even require a warming blanket to maintain normothermia. It is rare that a patient receiving CRRT has a fever, so if the temperature is elevated, the likelihood of infection is high and may require evaluation before elective surgery.

CRRT will usually be discontinued before transfer to the operating room for most of these patients who require surgery. To facilitate management once CRRT has been discontinued requires an understanding of the process and careful planning. The CRRT pump and filter are separated from the access catheter and the circuit is discarded. When this occurs, the catheter should be flushed with a heparinized solution (unless heparin is contraindicated) before capping it off to ensure that it remains patent. Before using the catheter again, the heparin should be aspirated from it. In order to determine the best management for the patient when CRRT is discontinued, the <u>anesthesiologist should review the CRRT orders</u> to clarify the fluid goals for the therapy, the amount of replacement fluid provided each hour, as well as the specific electrolytes and bicarbonate that has been included in the replacement fluid. <u>Based on this review, a plan</u> for managing fluids, electrolytes, and acid-base balance can be developed for the intraoperative period.

Intraoperative

The primary advantage of using CRRT during surgery is related to fluid management in the patient. <u>Patients who receive CRRT during surgery are less edematous and may have smaller fluid shifts after major surgical procedures as compared to patients who receive conventional fluid management</u>. If the CRRT is to be initiated or continued intraoperatively, the anesthesiologist must either be familiar with use of the equipment or have the ability to "troubleshoot" problems that arise or must have additional personnel and resources available to support the system. In many institutions, an ICU nurse who is physically present in the OR for the duration of the procedure manages CRRT. In other cases, someone familiar with the equipment and therapy will be available on call to provide advice and assistance to the anesthesiologist. If CRRT is used during the surgical procedure, the cannula used for the therapy must be easily accessible to the anesthesiologist. Although femoral catheters are occasionally used for CRRT, it is more common to use internal jugular catheters as they provide beneficial flow characteristics and are on site in the operating room. Internal jugular catheters are easily monitored for evidence of kinking and malpositioning, which can help decrease the risk of the circuit clotting off.

Postoperative Considerations

When CRRT is used in the postoperative period, the clinicians who are now managing the therapy must be cognizant of the intraoperative course. The flows and replacement fluid composition must be carefully titrated to account for intraoperative fluid shifts, blood loss, and ongoing alterations in intravascular volume. Moreover, the patient must be closely monitored for evidence of postoperative coagulopathy and electrolyte abnormalities. **CRRT** should also be considered as a therapeutic option in the postoperative period for the patient with gross fluid overload that leads to compromised gas exchange or impaired pulmonary function.

Adverse Effects

Understanding the potential complications associated with CRRT should facilitate prevention of possible difficulties and early identification which should reduce morbidity. Complications of vascular access, including infection and vascular injury, are a common concern with CRRT [20]. Arterial puncture, hematoma, hemothorax, and pneumothorax are the most common complications reported. Arteriovenous fistulas, aneurysms, thrombus formation, pericardial tamponade, and retroperitoneal hemorrhage, albeit less common, have also been described. During therapy, close monitoring of the CRRT machine's performance, the patient's hemodynamics, and electrolytes are required to prevent complications. Common problems during therapy include hypotension, arrhythmias, fluid-balance and electrolyte disturbances, hypothermia, and bleeding issues from anticoagulation. Continuous renal-replacement therapy can result in clinically significant hypokalemia and hypophosphatemia, which may lead to severe detrimental effects on the patient if left uncorrected. Hypothermia can be mitigated with the use of a blood or fluid warmer. Another challenge during CRRT is the appropriate dosing of drugs with antibiotics as a particular concern.

Doses of antibiotics that are too low can result in inadequate treatment of sepsis; doses that are too high can lead to systemic exposure and toxicity. To ensure efficacy and prevent toxicity, following drug dosing guidelines is suggested and monitoring of levels is recommended when possible.

Areas of Uncertainty

A number of **areas of uncertainty** exist regarding the use of CRRT. These include the appropriate indications and timing of therapy, the ideal method of treatment, the benefits of convection over diffusion, the safest and most effective anticoagulant, and the most appropriate dose [21]. The potential effects of CRRT on renal recovery and the long-term need for long-term dialysis are unknown. It is unclear whether optimization of renal replacement therapy may modulate the high mortality associated with AKI. Recent trials indicated that continuous renal replacement therapy does not confer a survival advantage as compared to intermittent hemodialysis. Furthermore, there is no evidence to support a more intensive strategy of renal replacement therapy in the setting of AKI.

APPROPRIATE ANTIBIOTIC COVERAGE

Introduction

Surgical site infections (SSI) are a major contributor to morbidity and mortality in perioperative care. **Risk** for SSI is multifactorial and includes a combination of patient-related, procedure-related, and microbial factors. Although sterile surgical technique is extremely important to the prevention of SSIs, wound contamination occurs with every incision. Adherence to evidence-based preventative measures related to appropriate antimicrobial prophylaxis can decrease the rate of SSI [22]. Anesthesiologists play a prominent role in the prevention of SSIs through a variety of practices, including timing and selection of preoperative antibiotic administration, maintenance of perioperative normothermia, hyperoxia and normoglycemia, encouraging smoking cessation, and hand washing [23].

It is critical for anesthesiologists to recognize and appreciate the detrimental impact of intensive care unit (ICU)-acquired infections. Researchers and national committees have developed and continue to cultivate evidence-based guidelines to control ICU infections. To limit the incidence of ICU-acquired infections, aggressive infection control measures must be implemented and enforced. A multifaceted approach, including infection prevention committees, antimicrobial stewardship programs, daily reassessments-intervention bundles, identifying and minimizing risk factors, and continuing staff education programs, are essential.

Given the breadth of topics, the focus of this chapter will be on the selection, dosing, and duration of antibiotics in the perioperative setting for patients undergoing routine surgery, for patients with a compromised immune status, and in the setting of resistant organisms. In addition, brief discussion of additional prophylactics measures of hand-washing and central line management will be provided. A number or excellent recently published reviews on perioperative prophylaxis provide the basis for this section [24, 25].

Antibiotic Selection

While the <u>anesthesiologist</u> may not be the primary prescriber of prophylactic antibiotics, they <u>should be knowledgeable and involved</u> in the selection of appropriate prophylactic antibiotics. <u>Optimal antimicrobial agents</u> for prophylaxis should be bactericidal, nontoxic, inexpensive, and active against the typical pathogens that can cause surgical site infection postoperatively. Surgical site infections are commonly the result of skin flora contamination of the wound, including Staphylococcus and Streptococcus. When the surgical procedure involves hollow viscera, such as the intestine, gram negative bacteria and anaerobes also become an important source of SSI. The prophylactic regimen in patients undergoing surgery should include an agent effective against the most likely infecting organisms, but do not need to eradicate every potential pathogen. <u>The choice of prophylactic antibiotics should be based on the local anti-biogram</u>. Recommended regimens vary with the type of surgery (cardiovascular, orthopedic, colorectal, *etc*.) and wound classification (clean, clean contaminated). Patients undergoing dirty or contaminated procedures (*e.g.*, repair of a perforated colon) generally do not require antimicrobial prophylaxis because they already are receiving specific antibiotic treatment for an established infection.

Recognizing <u>patients who require modified antibiotic therapy</u>, such as those with a documented penicillin allergy and patients colonized with methicillin resistant Staphylococcus aureus (MRSA), is an important part of perioperative care. Patients will often report symptoms attributed to penicillin use that do not represent true allergic reactions. A focused history can help to identify those patients with true allergies who require a modification to their antibiotic regimen. When an allergy prevents beta-lactam antibiotic therapy and prophylaxis is directed against gram-positive cocci, clindamycin or vancomycin is an acceptable alternative.

Dosing of Antibiotics

To ensure that adequate serum and tissue concentrations of antimicrobial agents for prophylaxis of SSIs are achieved, antimicrobial specific pharmacokinetic and pharmacodynamic properties and patient factors must be considered when selecting a dose. In general, doses of prophylactic agents should maintain adequate levels of drug in serum and tissue for the interval during which the surgical site is open. The dosing of many antimicrobials in adults is not based on body weight, because it is safe, effective, and more convenient to use standardized doses for most of the adult patient population. Such standardized doses avoid the need for calculations and reduce the risk for medication errors. However, in obese patients, especially those who are morbidly obese, serum and tissue concentrations of some drugs may differ from those in normal-weight patients. Conclusive recommendations for weight-based dosing for antimicrobial prophylaxis in obese patients cannot be made because data demonstrating clinically relevant decreases in SSI rates from the use of such dosing strategies instead of standard doses in obese patients are not available in the published literature. It has not been determined whether the patient's ideal body weight or total (*i.e.*, actual) body weight should be used. In theory, using the ideal body weight as the basis for dosing a lipophilic drug (*e.g.*, vancomycin) could result in subtherapeutic concentrations in serum and tissue, and the use of actual body weight for dosing a hydrophilic drug (*e.g.*, an aminoglycoside) could result in excessive concentrations in serum and tissue.

While the optimal cefazolin dose has not been established in obese patients, a few pharmacokinetic studies have investigated the cefazolin concentrations in serum and tissues during surgical procedures. Doubling the normal dose of cephalosporins or making fewer adjustments based on renal dysfunction may produce concentrations in obese patients similar to those achieved with standard doses in normal weight patients. Considering the low cost and favorable safety profile of cefazolin, increasing the dose to 2g for patients weighing more than 80kg and to 3g for those weighing over 120kg has been recommended [25].

Timing of Antibiotic

The **timing** (initiation and duration) of antibiotics are important not only in preventing SSIs, but also in decreasing adverse events such as the selection of multidrug-resistant organisms. To maximize their effectiveness, intravenous perioperative prophylaxis should be administered within 30-60minutes before the surgical incision. Antimicrobial prophylaxis should be of short duration to decrease toxicity and antimicrobial resistance and to reduce cost. Vancomycin and fluoroquinolone infusions should be started 90-120 minutes before surgical incision, as their administration is usually takes at least 1hour. An exception to this rule is applies with oral administration of antimicrobial agents before colonic and urologic procedures. With regards to orthopedic surgical procedures, antimicrobial administration should be completed before the tourniquet is inflated.

Additional antibiotic doses may need to be administered intraoperatively for prolonged procedures or with antimicrobial agents with short half-lives. There is no documented benefit of antibiotics after wound closure in the reduction of surgical site infections. In general the duration of antibiotic prophylaxis for most procedures should not exceed 24 hours. Guidelines from the Society of Thoracic Surgeons recommend that antibiotic prophylaxis be continued for 48 hours after the completion of cardiothoracic surgery due to the effects of cardiopulmonary bypass on immune function and antibiotic pharmacokinetics [26]. Antibiotics given for implantation of a pacemaker or defibrillator should be discontinued within 24 hours of surgery. There is no evidence to support extending antibiotic administration until drains are removed. More prolonged postoperative antimicrobial prophylaxis should be discouraged because of the possibility of added antimicrobial toxicity, selection of resistant organisms, and unnecessary expense.

MRSA

The increasing prevalence of **methicillin-resistant Staphylococcus aureus** (MRSA) has resulted in a reevaluation of the role of vancomycin for surgical prophylaxis [27]. **MRSA** and **coagulase-negative staphylococci**have become the primary pathogens associated with SSIs in cardiothoracic, vascular, orthopedic, and neurosurgical operations. MRSA SSIs have been associated with increased mortality, length of hospital stay, and costs compared with SSIs due to other organisms, including methicillin susceptible S. aureus (MSSA). In addition Community acquired MRSA strains have noticeably increased in the United States during the past decade and are becoming prevalent among MRSA strains in hospitals.

Vancomycin has been commonly recommended as either a primary or adjuvant agent for perioperative prophylaxis in patients who are presumed or known to have Staphylococcus colonization, in institutions where a "high" prevalence of MRSA exists, and when a surgical procedure involves a prosthetic joint insertion, sternotomy, or vascular graft insertion. While several systematic reviews have concluded that no clear benefit in clinical effectiveness or cost-effectiveness has been demonstrated for the routine prophylaxis use of vancomycin compared with cephalosporins, most of these studies were conducted before the increasing prevalence of MRSA and do not reflect current clinical situations. Available data do not clearly define a threshold constituting a high rate of MRSA infection that can be applied to all institutional situations. Furthermore, studies from institutions with perceived high rates of MRSA have not provided consistent evidence that vancomycin is superior to cefazolin for reducing surgical site infections. In one study, patients who received vancomycin prophylaxis were more likely to develop SSI from MSSA compared with those who received cefazolin. The decision to use vancomycin for prophylaxis should consider local rates of MRSA infection, surgical risk, and include consultation among surgeons and infectious disease physicians. There is currently no evidence to suggest that using a combination of multiple prophylactic antibiotics or administering prophylactic antibiotics for an increased duration is of benefit for reducing MRSA infections [28].

<u>Implementation of a MRSA prevention bundle may significantly reduce MRSA SSIs</u>. However, the effect of preoperative identification and treatment of MRSA carriers on the incidence of surgical site infections is controversial. Guidelines from the Society of Thoracic Surgeons recommend routine administration of topical mupirocin (Bactroban) for all patients undergoing cardiovascular procedures in the absence of documented tests negative for MRSA. The American Academy of Orthopedic Surgeons advises that patients at risk of colonization by MRSA or MSSA be screened and decolonized preoperatively. Populations at risk of MRSA colonization may include patients recently discharged from a hospital or long-term care facility, patients with previous MRSA colonization or infection, patients with chronic hemodialysis, and intravenous drug users.

Prophylaxis for Other Drug Resistant Organisms

Improvements in the treatment of critically ill patients have resulted in their prolonged survival in a debilitated state. These patients often receive repeated courses of antibiotics and become colonized with multiresistant pathogens during their stay in the intensive care unit. As a result, surgical wound infections can become very difficult to treat. In addition to <u>MRSA, *Klebsiella* spp.</u> with multiple resistances is a common cause of septicemia and can be associated with cephalosporin use. *Acinetobacter* spp. and <u>vancomycin-resistant enterococci</u> are other pathogens of increasing prevalence that can cause infections resistant to all readily available antibiotics. The prevalence of infection with multidrug resistant pathogens is increasing [29].

Clinicians caring for critically ill patients have an important role in reducing infection by application of appropriate prophylactic measures. These <u>prophylactic measures</u> include hand washing, universal precautions for infection control, source isolation, and restrictive antibiotic policy [30]. Bundled-preventive approaches should be applied during insertion of intravascular lines, specifically central venous lines. Application of appropriate skin preparation and/or dressings with antiseptics is important. Although new antimicrobial agents currently in trials may be effective in the long term, the future for ensuring control of these resistant pathogens is dependent on prophylaxis and appropriate antibiotic treatment.

PERIOPERATIVE CONSIDERATIONS FOR NUTRITIONAL SUPPORT CRITICALLY ILL PATIENTS

Introduction

Nutrition is a vital, yet often overlooked aspect of perioperative care. This is particularly relevant in the critically ill surgical patient where malnutrition is common due to the effects of increased catabolism coupled with gastrointestinal symptoms, therapeutic restrictions, anorexia, depression, and other medical/surgical factors. Critically ill patients may be unable to feed volitionally by mouth for periods ranging from days to months. Unless they are provided with macronutrients in the form of enteral or parenteral nutrition, they accumulate nutritional deficits that are associated with adverse outcomes. Nutrition support is now considered an essential component of the management strategy of critically ill patients. Data from observational studies suggest wide variations in the ICU feeding practices, resulting in a large proportion of ICU patients receiving inadequate nutritional support [31]. This section focuses on general aspects of perioperative nutrition, providing data on the harm of inappropriate feeding, as well as informing the best methods of providing artificial nutrition in clinical practice.

Consequences of Inappropriate Feeding

Both underfeeding and overfeeding can have deleterious effects on the critically ill patient. Malnutrition in the perioperative period of critically ill patients is associated with muscle weakness, increased risk of infections, impaired wound healing, and prolonged time to convalescence. Starvation for a period as short as 48 hours and poor nutritional status can already predispose the patient to the re-feeding syndrome. It is likely that many patients are malnourished as a result of prolonged starvation before ICU admission. The **re-feeding syndrome** is the result of re-initiation of enteral or parenteral feeding in a previously malnourished patient [32]. Complications of this syndrome include electrolyte abnormalities (hypophosphatemia, hypokalemia, and hypomagnesemia) along with sodium and fluid retention potentially leading to heart failure, respiratory failure, and death. Severe hypophosphatemia, in particular, is an early warning sign, and serum phosphate levels should be closely monitored in patients at risk of the re-feeding syndrome. Patients at risk should be fed slowly, and electrolyte and other micronutrient levels should be closely monitored and supplemented as required.

Provision of macronutrients in excess of metabolic demand can also be deleterious [33]. Patients who are at the extremes of size or elderly are particularly vulnerable to overfeeding. Overfeeding protein can lead to azotemia, hypertonic dehydration, and metabolic acidosis. Excessive carbohydrate administration can result in hyperglycemia, hypertriglyceridemia, and hepatic steatosis. High-fat infusions have caused hypertriglyceridemia and fat-overload syndrome. Aggressive overfeeding has also caused hypercapnia and re-feeding syndrome. To avoid overfeeding, some advocate measurement of EE using indirect calorimetry. In addition, caloric needs may change during the ICU stay, increasing the difficulties of determining the exact amount of calories to prescribe. If such monitoring is unavailable, a feeding protocol may limit the risk of overfeeding.

Nutritional Assessment

Recognition of patients with or at risk of malnutrition remains poor despite the availability of numerous clinical aids and clear evidence of the adverse effects of poor nutritional status on postoperative clinical outcomes. Importantly, malnutrition and nutritional risk are not synonymous. **Malnutrition** is defined as an inability to match metabolic and nutrient requirements. Nutritional requirements vary based on the category of malnutrition and the presence of a disease state. Potential causes of malnutrition include cancer, an inability to swallow, a lack of access to nutrition, or gastrointestinal tract dysfunction. It can be valuable to elucidate the cause of the malnutrition and tailor perioperative interventions to individual patients. Although the optimal marker of nutritional risk remains unknown, factors such as age, recent weight loss and oral intake, time from hospital admission to ICU admission, decreasing or low BMI, and markers of disease severity should be considered in the assessment [34].

Determining **nutrition risk** should be a routine component of the preoperative evaluation. Preoperative risk assessment should consider the patients' nutritional state, the risk of the proposed surgery, and potential postoperative anatomic alterations. The Joint Commission requires a nutrition screening within 24 hours of admission on all inpatients followed by a complete assessment for those considered high risk. The goal of effective preoperative screening is to identify high-risk patients allowing for targeted intervention that ultimately decreases surgical morbidity. Evidence suggests that providing preoperative enteral nutrition to those at high risk reduces major postoperative morbidity. In the operating room, consideration should be given to the potential placement of enteral access during the index operation, as well as judicious and targeted intraoperative resuscitation. Immediately following the intervention, adequate resuscitation and glycemic control are key concepts, as is an evidence-based approach to the early advancement of an enteral/oral diet in the postoperative patient.

Nutrition Route, Timing and Amount

Gut starvation and/or critical illness have deleterious effects on the immune function of the gastrointestinal tract. Lack of enteral feeding causes blunting of intestinal villi and increased mucosal permeability potentially allowing bacterial translocation and bacteremia [35]. Additionally, gut starvation decreases hepatic and peritoneal immune function. Enteral nutrition attenuates these deleterious effects, and multiple studies have established that the enteral route is the preferred for nutritional support. To emphasize the <u>importance of the</u> **enteral route**: "<u>if the gut works use it," is a phrase that is commonly used today</u>. Enteral feedings can be initiated into the stomach in most patients, and routine placement of feeding tubes into the small bowel is not necessary. Direct administration of feeds to the small bowel is recommended when gastric feeding is not feasible, specifically in conditions where there is a higher risk of aspiration (persistent high gastric residues, continuous use of sedatives/neuromuscular blockers) or when at high risk of intolerance to gastric enteral nutrition. Enteral feeding has been shown to be safe in patients with open abdomens and those requiring vasopressors. Additionally, animal studies suggest that early enteral feeding proximal to a gastrointestinal anastomosis actually strengthens the newly joined bowel. Bowel sounds and evidence of bowel function (*i.e.*, passing flatus or stool) are not required for initiation of enteral feeding. Gastric residual volumes, although commonly measured in many ICUs, do not appear to convey increased safety for enteral feedings and should not be used as the sole criterion on which decisions on altering enteral feeding rates are made. In patients who are not at high risk or those not tolerating full enteral nutrition, continuing low-dose trophic feedings for up to 6 days does not appear harmful.

Parenteral nutrition <u>is indicated only when enteral nutrition is "contraindicated"</u> (obstruction, ischemia, acute peritonitis, and lack of bowel continuity). Additional relative contraindications may include high-output fistulas and severe malabsorption from short gut syndromes, proximal high output fistula, perforated bowel, bowel obstruction, severe gastrointestinal bleed, and severe hemodynamic instability. Patients receiving parenteral nutrition preoperatively should have it restarted on postoperative day 1. In the absence of preoperative parenteral nutrition, patients expected to have a nonfunctional gastrointestinal tract for 7days postoperatively should be started on parenteral therapy, although it should be noted that there is little benefit unless supplementation is continued for greater than 7days. Unlike enteral nutrition, early initiation of parenteral nutrition is not recommended for most patients. <u>A recent randomized controlled trial of critically ill patients with contraindications to enteral nutrition did not find any benefit to the early initiation of parenteral nutrition</u>. Providing no nutritional support or dextrose infusions are as good or better than early TPN for critically ill patients who cannot tolerate tube feedings.

Data on the optimal amount of enteral nutrition to deliver are limited and contradictory. **Full feeding**, through the provision of more calories could preserve strength, support immune function, and improve outcomes. On the other hand, less amounts of enteral nutrition (*e.g.* **trophic feeding**) may still provide the benefit of enteral feeding on the intestinal epithelium while limiting the potential detrimental effects of GI intolerance and minimizing the provision of those nutrients that might fuel an overzealous immune response. A study in critically ill patients showed that the best survival was observed when calorie intake was around 80% of the prescribed target [36]. Several observational studies show improved clinical outcomes for patients receiving more of their caloric needs, whereas other data suggest lower volumes of enteral nutrition may result in less time on mechanical ventilation and improved mortality. Regardless of the optimal amount of feeding, patients with critical illness should be started as soon as possible and ideally within 24 h of ICU admission. Initially, providing at least 25% of goal calories may be sufficient enough to obtain the benefits for maintaining gut integrity and an early assessment for nutritional risk should be performed. In those patients determined to be at high nutritional risk (either because of evidence of malnutrition or higher disease severity), consideration should be made for advancing enteral feedings to as close to full caloric and protein goals as tolerated.

A substantial amount of basic and clinical research data has been published and provides solid support for the proposition that the macronutrient that is most lacking in critical illness – and whose provision is most likely to be of benefit – is **protein** [37]. Sufficient exogenous protein provision mitigates skeletal muscle atrophy and supplies amino acids for the synthesis of proteins involved in wound healing and immune function. It is because of this accumulated evidence that all nutritional care guidelines in critical illness recommend a level of protein or amino acid provision that is much higher than the daily requirement of a healthy person. A healthy adult requires 0.8g of high quality protein/kg per day, whereas a common recommendation for protein provision in critical illness is 1.5g/kg/day. In fact, extensive metabolic data (and some clinical trial evidence) suggest that the early provision of 1.5-2.5g protein/kg per day could be optimal in critical illness.

Although firm recommendations on the use of feeding protocols in critically ill patients are lacking, a protocol that initiates the volume of feeds gradually, and tolerates a higher gastric volume (250ml), should be considered to optimize delivery of enteral nutrition in critically ill adult patients. In patients who experience feed intolerance (high gastric residues, emesis), prokinetics, such as metoclopramide, should be considered to improve gastric emptying and enhance gut motility if not otherwise contraindicated.

SEDATION

Introduction

A growing body of evidence suggests that the management of sedation can have an important effect on the outcomes of patients who are treated in ICUs. Sedation is important to consider for the potential short-term outcome benefits of providing comfort by reducing anxiety, but there are also detrimental effects related to oversedation. Currently available data suggest that the best outcomes are achieved with the use of a protocol in which the depth of sedation and the presence of pain and delirium are routinely monitored, pain is treated promptly and effectively, the administration of sedatives is kept to the minimum necessary for the comfort and safety of the patient [38]. Only a minority of ICU patients have an indication for deep sedation, for reasons such as the severe respiratory failure, refractory status epilepticus, treatment of intracranial hypertension, and prevention of awareness in patients treated with neuromuscular blocking agents. This review will focus on the management of the majority of critically ill patients for whom the use of sedatives should be minimized, with the goal that they be calm, comfortable, interactive, and cooperative with their care.

A continuous sedative-hypnotic approach with benzodiazepines or propofol has historically been the first-line intervention used to provide comfort for critically ill patients receiving mechanical ventilatory support. However, with this approach remains the possibility that pain-induced agitation is inappropriately managed by increasing sedation, masking untreated pain. Furthermore, this approach may lead to oversedation, which commonly occurs despite the implementation of sedation protocols and daily sedation interruption [39]. Studies have shown that the depth of sedation of critically ill patients frequently goes unmonitored. This is unacceptable, since evidence suggests that the routine monitoring of sedation may improve patients' outcomes. A number of detrimental effects have been associated with oversedation, including prolonged ventilation, an increased risk for pneumonia and a prolonged stay in the ICU, hypotension, venous thrombosis, with an increased burden on staff, bed availability, and associated costs [39].

Sedative Selection

In general, there does not appear that one sedative agent is clearly superior to another. **Sedatives,** that are commonly used in the ICU are midazolam, propofol, and dexmedetomidine. Marked differences in prescribing patterns between ICUs suggests that the choice of agent is determined more by tradition and familiarity, than by evidence-based practice. To minimize the depth and duration of sedation, use of a short-acting agent that can be rapidly titrated should offer advantages over longer acting agents or agents with active metabolites. As compared with midazolam, <u>propofol</u> may result in a reduction in the length of stay in the ICU. <u>Dexmedetomidine</u> may also have advantages over midazolam, since it provides a qualitatively different type of sedation, in which patients are more interactive. It also causes less respiratory depression and has some analgesic properties. In addition, dexmedetomidine results in a shorter duration of mechanical ventilation and ICU length of stay compared with sedation with benzodiazepines [40, 41]. A study comparing the use of dexmeditomidine to propofol did not find a significant difference in the time spent at the target sedation level and there was not a difference in the duration of mechanical ventilation or ICU stay. <u>Remifentanil</u>, an opioid, has also been investigated as a sedative agent due to its short a half-life (3-4 minutes) that is independent of the infusion duration or organ function. Although remifentanil has been associated with a reduced duration of mechanical ventilation and ICU stay in small trials, it has not yet been evaluated in a large, heterogeneous population of critically ill patients and is currently not a common choice in most ICUs.

Sedation Scales

The **Richmond Agitation- Sedation Scale (RASS)** is the most extensively validated and one of the most widely used ICU sedation scales [42]. The Richmond Agitation – Sedation Scale ranges from –5 to +4, with more negative scores indicating deeper sedation and more positive scores indicating increasing agitation, and with 0 representing the appearance of calm and normal alertness. For the majority of patients undergoing mechanical ventilation in an ICU, an appropriate target is a score of –2 to 0. Rarely, a patient who is extremely ill may be targeted to a deeper sedation level of –3 or –4 to facilitate necessary care; however, even in these patients, deep sedation may not always be required.

Other tools based on monitoring electroencephalography have been used in an attempt to make objective assessments of depth of sedation. The <u>Bispectral Index</u> (<u>BIS</u>) is the most widely studied processed-electroencephalography monitor for evaluation of depth of anesthesia in patients undergoing surgical procedures and has been used for monitoring sedation in ICU patients. In mechanically ventilated critically ill patients there is an appropriate correlation between Bispectral Index values and depth of sedation measured by the clinical sedation scale in some studies, but not in others. The BIS value may inaccurately assess depth of sedation in patients with traumatic brain injury and can overestimate depth of sedation in patients with high muscle activity. At present, no cerebral function monitors are recommended to replace the clinical sedation scale for assessment of the depth of sedation in critically ill patients [43]. However, the use of tools that measure the level of consciousness by algorithmic analysis of a patient's electroence-phalogram may be useful when integrated with other tools of sedation monitoring to ensure amnesia in the pharmacologically paralyzed patient.

Sedation Strategies

There are a variety of **sedation strategies** that have been studied, including daily interruption of sedation and goal-directed sedation algorithms. The goal of protocolized sedation algorithms is to reduce variations in clinical practice, and thereby systematically reducing the likelihood of excessive sedation. Protocolized sedation consists of: setting goals of analgesia and sedation for an individual patient; assessment for pain and sedation with applicable tools and frequency; and intervention to meet the goals by the multidisciplinary care terms. Use of sedation scales in a protocolized manner, particularly with input from the bedside nurse, can help guide therapy to a targeted sedation level and improve patient outcomes. Medications can be given in the form of continuous drips, but active drugs and metabolites can accumulate. The care team must be conscientious and aware of this important point in order to maintain a minimal amount of medication that still succeeds in producing adequate sedation.

Before administering sedation to critically ill patients, **adequate pain control should be assured**. Pain is commonly experienced by critically ill patients as a consequence of the acute disease process, surgery, intubation and mechanical ventilation itself, or even as result of routine clinical care, such as moving a patient in bed or adjusting tubes and lines. Pain can be substantial and initiate detrimental elements of the stress response. Accordingly, pain should be addressed to ensure patient comfort and potentially reduce accompanying adverse events. "Self reporting" of pain is considered the gold standard for pain assessment, however in circumstances where self-reporting is not possible, pain assessment tools that incorporate behaviors and physiologic variables can be used. Of those developed for ICU use, the Behavioral Pain Scale (BPS) and the Critical Care Pain Observation Tool (CPOT) have the strongest evidence for reliability and validity [44].

Protocolized sedation (algorithm or daily interruption) has been shown to decrease both ICU and hospital lengths of stay and overall mortality [45]. It also allowed for a better assessment of neurological status, decreasing the need for diagnostic neurological testing. Pairing daily interruptions with spontaneous breathing trials leads to more ventilator-free days than spontaneous breathing trials on their own, and it also leads to decreased mortality at 1year. The benefits likely relate to the ability of a more alert patient to more fully participate in rehabilitation, and initiation of physical and occupational therapy. A combined approach of spontaneous awakening and breathing trials combined with managing pain, agitation and delirium is the basis of the "**ABCDE**" **bundle**, *i.e.* Awake and

Breathing co-ordination, Choice of sedatives and analgesics, Delirium monitoring, Early mobility and exercise which has been found to be very promising for improving the neurologic and functional outcome of mechanically ventilated patients [46].

Initially there was concern that reducing or stopping sedation might predispose patients to long-term psychological harm in the form of post-traumatic stress disorder (PTSD), a well-recognized sequelae in survivors of critical illness. However, studies have found that there is no increase in PTSD with reduced sedation or daily awakening trials [47]. Contrary to traditional thinking, sedative medications may contribute to adverse psychological outcomes, rather than prevent them. For example, one study demonstrated that patients, who experience sedative-induced delusions while in the ICU, are more likely to develop PTSD than patients who have factual memories of their ICU stay [48]. Higher doses of benzodiazepines have also been associated with PTSD symptoms months after discharge. Recently, Strom *et al.* has shown that withholding sedation in critically ill patients on mechanical ventilation is associated with an increase in days without ventilation without long-term psychological sequelae [49].

In **summary**, evidence from randomized, controlled trials consistently supports the use of the minimum possible level of sedation. An emerging concept of the "ICU triad" recognizes that – pain, agitation, and delirium are inextricably linked. Accordingly, sedatives should be used only when pain and delirium have been addressed with the use of specific pharmacologic and non-pharmacologic strategies [50].

TRANSPORT OF CRITICALLY ILL PATIENTS

Introduction

Transport of critically ill patients, both to and from the operating room or to undergo tests and procedures, can be exceptionally dangerous and is seen as a period of "high risk" for the patient. Developing practices to reduce or minimize this necessary risk is an important area of focus for ensuring patient safety. This section focuses on transport of critically ill patients, from intensive care areas of the hospital (including intensive care units, emergency departments, operating theaters and recovery rooms) to areas that may not typically be involved in the delivery of such care (*e.g.*, a hospital radiology department). This section reviews current literature on the incidence and nature of adverse events, risk factors, and the current recommendations for carrying out in-hospital transport (IHT).

Prevalence and Severity of the Problem

Transport of patients from the ICU during in-hospital transport (IHT) is associated with an overall complication rate of up to 70% [51]. The reported complications range from changes in vital signs to life threatening complications requiring major therapeutic interventions. In one study of critically ill patients, the mortality associated with in-hospital transport was 2% [52]. Adverse events during transport of critically ill patients fall into two general categories: those related to **clinical care** (*e.g.*, lead loss of intravenous access, accidental extubation, occlusion of the endotracheal tube, exhaustion of oxygen supply loss of battery power), and those associated with **physiologic deteriorations related to critical illness** (*e.g.*, worsening hypotension, hypoxemia or hypoventilation) [53]. Unfortunately, many studies evaluating the frequency of these complications do not distinctly distinguish between these 2 categories. Further complicating assessments of patient transport is the confounding effect of patient selection, as patents requiring in-hospital transport likely represent a sicker patient population than unselected critically ill patients [54]. Regardless of the precise prevalence, it is clear that critically ill patients are at high risk of physiological decline due to equipment (technical factors) and/or clinical status (patient factor), not to mention the collective and human factors that can also intervene in a deleterious manner. Consequently, in-hospital transport should be considered as an important part of the ICU risk management program. A risk-benefit analysis should be carried out beforehand, in which the risk of the in-hospital transport has to be put in balance with the expected benefit of the procedure. That assessment should be based on a detailed understanding of the documented risk factors and the precarious consequences that can occur during in-hospital transport.

Practical Considerations

Many recommendations to enhance patient safety during in-hospital transport are available. These proposals are based on published evidence, personal experience, and expert opinion [55, 56]. "Protective" factors for limiting adverse events have been described. These include meticulous planning and preparation of the patient, appropriate sedation, regular patient and equipment checks during in-hospital transport, and an experienced escort to accompany the patient to the proposed destination [57]. Although many risk factors have been identified, there are usually multiple factors involved in the occurrence of adverse events.

Preparation

Preparation plays a key role in the safe transport of critically-ill patients. Studies on patients during in-hospital transport show that many complications associated with equipment and collective and human management could have been anticipated. Hasty transport organization in the emergency context also leads to the onset of adverse events. Anticipating potential deterioration in a patient's condition (consider additional preparation before transport and formulate a decisive plan to manage any possible deterioration), ensuring adequate oxygen reserves, a sufficient number of transport escorts, checking that the retrieval team and the destination site are operational (wall suction unit, oxygen connectors, defibrillator, extension cables, sufficient space for the transport staff to move the patient), and the said destination area ready (and their accompanying personnel) are ready to receive the patient in optimal conditions, are all vital prerequisites to ensure optimal transport of the critically ill patient.

Transport Equipment and Monitoring

All critically ill patients undergoing transport should receive the same level of basic physiologic monitoring during transport, as they requiredin ICU. This includes, at a minimum, continuous electrocardiographic monitoring, measurement of blood pressure, pulse rate, and respiratory rate and continuous pulse oximetry. In addition, selected patients may benefit from continuous intra-arterial blood pressure, pulmonary artery pressure, intermittent cardiac output intracranial pressure monitoring, or capnography. When available, a monitor with the capacity for storing and reproducing patient bedside data should be used to allow collection of data during the procedure and transport.

Basic resuscitation drugs, including epinephrine and antiarrhythmic agents, are transported with each patient in the event of sudden cardiac arrest or arrhythmia. Sedatives and analgesics should be considered in specific cases. An ample supply of appropriate intravenous fluids and continuous drip medications (regulated by battery-operated infusion pumps) are also warranted. All battery-operated equipment should be fully charged and capable of functioning for the duration of the transport. If a physician does not accompany the patient during transport, protocols must be in place to permit the administration of these medications and fluids by appropriately trained personnel under emergency circumstances.

Equipment for airway management, sized appropriately for each patient, should also be included for transport with each patient, as is an oxygen source of ample supply to provide for projected needs, plus a 30min reserve. A default oxygen concentration of 100% is generally used during transport to provide reserve. The specific risks of transporting intubated patient requiring mechanical ventilation during transport, such as insufficient oxygen reserves, inadequate MV settings, obstruction, malpositioning of artificial airways and accidental extubation must be considered and prepared for. In mechanically ventilated patients, endotracheal tube position should noted and secured before transport, and the adequacy of oxygenation and ventilation must be reconfirmed. For practical reasons, bag-valve ventilation is most commonly employed during intrahospital transports for patients receiving mechanical ventilation in the ICU. However, portable mechanical ventilators are gaining increasing popularity for transport, as they provide for a more reliable administered and prescribed minute ventilation as well as desired oxygen concentrations [58]. If a transport ventilator is to be employed, it must have alarms to indicate disconnection and excessively high airway pressures and must have a backup battery power supply. Long lasting batteries (lithium), equipment maintenance, continuous charging, a sounding alarm in the case of weak battery life, and connecting the transport equipment to wall sockets as soon as possible should routinely occur. A default oxygen concentration of 100% is generally employed. For patients requiring mechanical ventilation, equipment should be immediately available at the receiving location capable of delivering ventilatory support equivalent to that being delivered at the patient's origin. Occasionally patients may require modes of ventilation or ventilator settings not reproducible at the receiving location or during transportation. Under these circumstances, the origin location must trial alternate modes of mechanical ventilation before transport to ensure acceptability and patient stability with this therapy.

Personnel

It is recommended that a minimum of two experienced clinicians accompany a critically ill patient during transport. **Personnel** may include a respiratory therapist, registered nurse, or critical care technician as needed. A physician with critical care training, including experience in in airway management and advanced cardiac life support, should accompany unstable patients. When the procedure is anticipated to be lengthy and the receiving location is staffed by appropriately trained personnel, patient care may be transferred to those individuals if acceptable to both parties. If care is not transferred, the transport personnel will remain with the patient until they are returned to the intensive care unit.

Standardization of Practices for In-Hospital Transport

Risks related to in-hospital transport can be reduced by developing a common, widespread culture through the standardization of procedures utilized for in-hospital transport. Some studies have demonstrated that a standardization of in-hospital transport practices has been linked to a lower incidence of adverse events. The implementation of standardized procedures should be tailored to the unique characteristics of a given establishment.

The use of a systematic quick check-list for preparing patients for transport might enable teams to remember certain points that may otherwise have been forgotten.

Protocols which are either too vague or too exhaustive can contribute to deviance or straying from practices for managing critically ill patients during in-hospital transport. Furthermore, the use of a check-list which summarizes the main points that need to be verified before, during, and after in-hospital transport may help to reinforce adherence to the recommendations and to further improve the in-hospital transport process [59].

HANDOVERS

Introduction

The handover of care to the post-anesthesia care unit (PACU) or intensive care unit (ICU) after surgery presents challenges to members of both the delivering and receiving teams. Upon arrival in the PACU or SICU, information about the patient is transmitted, in an environment that is often chaotic and busy, to a team largely unfamiliar with the patient. This transfer of information often involves cross-disciplinary staff with varied levels of experience. Additionally, the receiving team is often concurrently assessing, stabilizing, and making care plans for the patient while simultaneously managing other patients under their care [60]. Furthermore, the patients whose care is transferred are often incapacitated due to the effects of residual anesthesia, intentional sedation and/or critical illness, and thus unable to participate in their care, therefore making them vulnerable to error and harm. Given this complexity, it is not surprising that technical and communication errors are common with postoperative handovers. This process of transmitting relevant information regarding the patient's medical and surgical history and accurate communication of intraoperative events is critical for proper postoperative management. Despite the importance of handover as an integral part of patients' perioperative care, variability in handoff processes persists in all areas of perioperative practice [61]. The focus of this section is to review recent literature regarding causes of handover failure and to describe strategies for improving the handover practice in the perioperative setting. In light of this interest, it is important to characterize current practices in postoperative handovers and to identify evidence-based methods to improve them. The goal of this section is to present a review of the literature on this topic and to summarize process and communication recommendations based on its findings.

Causes and Consequences of Ineffective Handover

To ensure patient safety, the barriers to proper handovers must be identified and strategies to enhance the quality of the handover process evaluated. A number of factors have been identified as contributors to poor handovers include poor teamwork and communication, patient's arrival in a compromised state, unclear procedures, technical errors, unstructured processes, interruptions and distractions, lack of central information repositories, and inattention secondary to multitasking of the receiving practioners [62]. Distractions during handover have been a particular area of focus because of interference with effective information transfer, as well as the additional time required for handovers. Hierarchical authority relationships can also derail attempts to create the better information sharing found within egalitarian teams [63].

The literature on improving handovers in healthcare is still in its infancy. Although a number of studies have examined current handover practices from various perspectives, few have tested approaches for improving them. The few intervention-based studies that exist are limited by small sample sizes, lack of rigorous experimental designs (*e.g.*, with randomized group assignments), and insufficient details about the solutions or methods used to evaluate them. Furthermore, they often focus on shift changes at the bedside on the general wards, thus, limiting the generalizability of the approach to the perioperative setting [64]. Although strong evidence for best practices in perioperative handovers is lacking, several recommendations are broadly supported. **First**, standardizing this process can improve patient care by ensuring information completeness and accuracy and therefore increasing the efficiency of the patient transfer process [65, 66]. The use of checklists to guide communication and protocols to structure clinical activities is advocated to promote standardization [67]. Standardization prompts verbal communication and promotes the transfer of information to users without them having to ask for the relevant information or having to know which information to extract. While checklists may have a role in the complex problem of information transmission, it is important to recognize that giving structure to information does not necessarily make the relayed information useful. The use of checklists may not ensure that the members of a healthcare team understand a patient's condition or management plan. Furthermore, the completion of checklists can be prone to error, as well as incompleteness. In an effort to seemingly increase productivity, long checklists may negatively influence information transfer, since there is a tendency to perform other tasks while reading the checklist. Some individuals have promoted the use of an electronic patient record to capture and communicate handovers [68]. While his approach may be a useful tool in information transfer, it can never replace the value of social interaction in information transfer and the added dynamic of teamwork during group interaction.

The environment plays a key role in the success of a handover. There are many distractions in a busy PACU or ICU which can make handover a challenging task. It is important to ensure the attention of relevant team members during the handover process and urgent patient care related tasks should be completed before the information transfer. Only patient-specific discussions should be allowed during the verbal handover and the members of the receiving team should have an opportunity to speak or ask questions. Finally, <u>training</u> in team skills and communication has the potential to improve the quality of postoperative handovers and the safety of patients during this critical period [62]. <u>In summary</u>, although evidence is limited, there are a number of practices, which have the potential to improve the quality of postoperative handovers and thereby improve the safety of patients during this critical period.

CONCLUSION

The purpose of this chapter is to provide an update for clinicians on ICU issues relevant to clinical practice. Topics which have been discussed include: modes of mechanical ventilation, renal replacement therapy, antibiotic prophylaxis nutritional support, sedation management, transport of patients, and transfer of care. Critical care is constantly changing and it is important for anesthesiologists to stay current in order to provide optimal care to the critically ill patients in the perioperative period.

CONSENT FOR PUBLICATION

Not applicable.

CONFLICT OF INTEREST

The authors declare no conflict of interest, financial or otherwise.

ACKNOWLEDGEMENT

Declared none.

REFERENCES

[1]   Serpa Neto A, Cardoso SO, Manetta JA, *et al.* Association between use of lung-protective ventilation with lower tidal volumes and clinical outcomes among patients without acute respiratory distress syndrome: a meta-analysis. JAMA 2012; 308(16): 1651-9.
        [http://dx.doi.org/10.1001/jama.2012.13730] [PMID: 23093163]

[2]   Serpa Neto A, Hemmes SN, Barbas CS, *et al.* Protective *versus* Conventional Ventilation for Surgery: A Systematic Review and Individual Patient Data Meta-analysis. Anesthesiology 2015; 123(1): 66-78.
        [http://dx.doi.org/10.1097/ALN.0000000000000706] [PMID: 25978326]

[3]   Hess D, Kacmarek R. Essentials of Mechanical Ventilation. 3rd ed., McGraw Hill 2015.

[4]   Putensen C, Muders T, Varelmann D, Wrigge H. The impact of spontaneous breathing during mechanical ventilation. Curr Opin Crit Care 2006; 12(1): 13-8.
        [http://dx.doi.org/10.1097/01.ccx.0000198994.37319.60] [PMID: 16394778]

[5]   Hess DR. Approaches to conventional mechanical ventilation of the patient with acute respiratory distress syndrome. Respir Care 2011; 56(10): 1555-72.
        [http://dx.doi.org/10.4187/respcare.01387] [PMID: 22008397]

[6]   Daoud EG, Farag HL, Chatburn RL. Airway pressure release ventilation: what do we know? Respir Care 2012; 57(2): 282-92.
        [PMID: 21762559]

[7]   Magnusson L. Role of spontaneous and assisted ventilation during general anaesthesia. Best Pract Res Clin Anaesthesiol 2010; 24(2): 243-52.
        [http://dx.doi.org/10.1016/j.bpa.2010.02.008] [PMID: 20608560]

[8]   Pillow JJ. High-frequency oscillatory ventilation: mechanisms of gas exchange and lung mechanics. Crit Care Med 2005; 33(3) (Suppl.): S135-41.
        [http://dx.doi.org/10.1097/01.CCM.0000155789.52984.B7] [PMID: 15753719]

[9]   Neil R. MacIntyre Semin Respir Crit Care Med 2013; 34: 499-507.
        [PMID: 23934718]

[10]   Young D, Lamb SE, Shah S, *et al.* High-frequency oscillation for acute respiratory distress syndrome. N Engl J Med 2013; 368(9): 806-13.
        [http://dx.doi.org/10.1056/NEJMoa1215716] [PMID: 23339638]

[11]   Ferguson ND, Cook DJ, Guyatt GH, *et al.* Canadian critical care trials group. N Engl J Med 2013; 368: 795-805.
        [http://dx.doi.org/10.1056/NEJMoa1215554] [PMID: 23339639]

[12]   Jaber S, Chanques G, Jung B. Postoperative noninvasive ventilation. Anesthesiology 2010; 112(2): 453-61.
        [http://dx.doi.org/10.1097/ALN.0b013e3181c5e5f2] [PMID: 20068454]

[13]   Chiumello D, Chevallard G, Gregoretti C. Non-invasive ventilation in postoperative patients: a systematic review. Intensive Care Med 2011; 37(6): 918-29.
        [http://dx.doi.org/10.1007/s00134-011-2210-8] [PMID: 21424246]

[14]   Glossop AJ, Shephard N, Bryden DC, Mills GH. Non-invasive ventilation for weaning, avoiding reintubation after extubation and in the postoperative period: a meta-analysis. Br J Anaesth 2012; 109(3): 305-14.
        [http://dx.doi.org/10.1093/bja/aes270] [PMID: 22879654]

[15]   Cabrini L, Nobile L, Plumari VP, *et al.* Intraoperative prophylactic and therapeutic non-invasive ventilation: a systematic review. Br J Anaesth 2014; 112(4): 638-47.
        [http://dx.doi.org/10.1093/bja/aet465] [PMID: 24444661]

[16]   Cerdá J, Ronco C. Modalities of continuous renal replacement therapy: technical and clinical considerations. Semin Dial 2009; 22(2): 114-22.
        [http://dx.doi.org/10.1111/j.1525-139X.2008.00549.x] [PMID: 19426413]

[17]   Dennen P, Douglas IS, Anderson R. Acute kidney injury in the intensive care unit: an update and primer for the intensivist. Crit Care Med 2010; 38(1): 261-75.
        [http://dx.doi.org/10.1097/CCM.0b013e3181bfb0b5] [PMID: 19829099]

[18]   Galvagno SM Jr, Hong CM, Lissauer ME, *et al.* Practical considerations for the dosing and adjustment of continuous renal replacement therapy in the intensive care unit. J Crit Care 2013; 28(6): 1019-26.
        [http://dx.doi.org/10.1016/j.jcrc.2013.05.018] [PMID: 23890937]

[19]   Patel P, Nandwani V, McCarthy PJ, Conrad SA, Keith Scott L. Continuous renal replacement therapies: a brief primer for the neurointensivist. Neurocrit Care 2010; 13(2): 286-94.
        [http://dx.doi.org/10.1007/s12028-010-9386-6] [PMID: 20549575]

[20]   Tolwani A. Continuous renal-replacement therapy for acute kidney injury. N Engl J Med 2012; 367(26): 2505-14.
        [http://dx.doi.org/10.1056/NEJMct1206045] [PMID: 23268665]

[21]   Ricci Z, Ronco C. Timing, dose and mode of dialysis in acute kidney injury. Curr Opin Crit Care 2011; 17(6): 556-61.

[http://dx.doi.org/10.1097/MCC.0b013e32834cd360] [PMID: 22027405]

[22] Young PY, Khadaroo RG. Surgical site infections. Surg Clin North Am 2014; 94(6): 1245-64.
      [http://dx.doi.org/10.1016/j.suc.2014.08.008] [PMID: 25440122]

[23] Forbes SS, McLean RF. Review article: the anesthesiologist's role in the prevention of surgical site
      infections. Can J Anaesth 2013; 60(2): 176-83.
      [http://dx.doi.org/10.1007/s12630-012-9858-6] [PMID: 23263980]

[24] Enzler MJ, Berbari E, Osmon DR. Antimicrobial prophylaxis in adults. Mayo Clin Proc 2011; 86(7):
      686-701.
      [http://dx.doi.org/10.4065/mcp.2011.0012] [PMID: 21719623]

[25] Bratzler DW, Dellinger EP, Olsen KM, *et al.* Clinical practice guidelines for antimicrobial prophylaxis
      in surgery. Am J Health Syst Pharm 2013; 70(3): 195-283.
      [http://dx.doi.org/10.2146/ajhp120568] [PMID: 23327981]

[26] Edwards FH, Engelman RM, Houck P, Shahian DM, Bridges CR. The Society Of Thoracic Surgeons
      practice guideline series: antibiotic prophylaxis in cardiac surgery, part I: duration. Ann Thorac Surg
      2006; 81(1): 397-404.
      [http://dx.doi.org/10.1016/j.athoracsur.2005.06.034] [PMID: 16368422]

[27] Crawford T, Rodvold KA, Solomkin JS. Vancomycin for surgical prophylaxis? Clin Infect Dis 2012;
      54(10): 1474-9.
      [http://dx.doi.org/10.1093/cid/cis027] [PMID: 22328468]

[28] Gurusamy KS, Koti R, Wilson P, Davidson BR. Antibiotic prophylaxis for the prevention of
      methicillin-resistant Staphylococcus aureus (MRSA) related complications in surgical patients.
      Cochrane Database Syst Rev 2013; (8): CD010268.
      [PMID: 23959704]

[29] Martín-Loeches I, Diaz E, Vallés J. Risks for multidrug-resistant pathogens in the ICU. Curr Opin Crit
      Care 2014; 20(5): 516-24.
      [http://dx.doi.org/10.1097/MCC.0000000000000124] [PMID: 25188366]

[30] Osman MF, Askari R. Infection control in the intensive care unit. Surg Clin North Am 2014; 94(6):
      1175-94.
      [http://dx.doi.org/10.1016/j.suc.2014.08.011] [PMID: 25440118]

[31] McClave SA, Martindale RG, Rice TW, Heyland DK. Feeding the critically ill patient. Crit Care Med
      2014; 42(12): 2600-10.
      [http://dx.doi.org/10.1097/CCM.0000000000000654] [PMID: 25251763]

[32] Byrnes MC, Stangenes J. Refeeding in the ICU: an adult and pediatric problem. Curr Opin Clin Nutr
      Metab Care 2011; 14(2): 186-92.
      [http://dx.doi.org/10.1097/MCO.0b013e328341ed93] [PMID: 21102317]

[33] Preiser JC, van Zanten AR, Berger MM, *et al.* Metabolic and nutritional support of critically ill
      patients: consensus and controversies. Crit Care 2015; 19: 35.
      [http://dx.doi.org/10.1186/s13054-015-0737-8] [PMID: 25886997]

[34] Torgersen Z, Balters M. Perioperative nutrition. Surg Clin North Am 2015; 95(2): 255-67.
      [http://dx.doi.org/10.1016/j.suc.2014.10.003] [PMID: 25814105]

[35] Marik PE. Enteral nutrition in the critically ill: myths and misconceptions. Crit Care Med 2014; 42(4):
      962-9.
      [http://dx.doi.org/10.1097/CCM.0000000000000051] [PMID: 24296860]

[36] Heyland DK, Cahill N, Day AG. Optimal amount of calories for critically ill patients: depends on how
      you slice the cake! Crit Care Med 2011; 39(12): 2619-26.
      [http://dx.doi.org/10.1097/CCM.0b013e318226641d] [PMID: 21705881]

[37] Singer P, Hiesmayr M, Biolo G, *et al.* Pragmatic approach to nutrition in the ICU: expert opinion

regarding which calorie protein target. Clin Nutr 2014; 33: 246-51.
[http://dx.doi.org/10.1016/j.clnu.2013.12.004] [PMID: 24434033]

[38]   Reade MC, Finfer S. Sedation and delirium in the intensive care unit. N Engl J Med 2014; 370(5): 444-54.
[http://dx.doi.org/10.1056/NEJMra1208705] [PMID: 24476433]

[39]   Devlin JW. The pharmacology of oversedation in mechanically ventilated adults. Curr Opin Crit Care 2008; 14(4): 403-7.
[http://dx.doi.org/10.1097/MCC.0b013e32830280b3] [PMID: 18614903]

[40]   Chen K, Lu Z, Xin YC, Cai Y, Chen Y, Pan SM. Alpha-2 agonists for long-term sedation during mechanical ventilation in critically ill patients. Cochrane Database Syst Rev 2015; 1: CD010269.
[PMID: 25879090]

[41]   Fraser GL, Devlin JW, Worby CP, *et al.* Benzodiazepine *versus* nonbenzodiazepine-based sedation for mechanically ventilated, critically ill adults: a systematic review and meta-analysis of randomized trials. Crit Care Med 2013; 41(9) (Suppl. 1): S30-8.
[http://dx.doi.org/10.1097/CCM.0b013e3182a16898] [PMID: 23989093]

[42]   Patel SB, Kress JP. Sedation and analgesia in the mechanically ventilated patient. Am J Respir Crit Care Med 2012; 185(5): 486-97.
[http://dx.doi.org/10.1164/rccm.201102-0273CI] [PMID: 22016443]

[43]   Piriyapatsom A, Bittner EA, Hines J, Schmidt UH. Sedation and paralysis. Respir Care 2013; 58(6): 1024-37.
[http://dx.doi.org/10.4187/respcare.02232] [PMID: 23709198]

[44]   Sigakis MJ, Bittner EA. Ten myths and misconceptions regarding pain management in the ICU. Crit Care Med 2015; 43(11): 2468-78.
[http://dx.doi.org/10.1097/CCM.0000000000001256] [PMID: 26308433]

[45]   Minhas MA, Velasquez AG, Kaul A, Salinas PD, Celi LA. Effect of protocolized sedation on clinical outcomes in mechanically ventilated intensive care unit patients: A systematic review and meta-analysis of randomized controlled trials. Mayo Clin Proc 2015; 90(5): 613-23.
[http://dx.doi.org/10.1016/j.mayocp.2015.02.016] [PMID: 25865475]

[46]   Balas MC, Vasilevskis EE, Olsen KM, *et al.* Effectiveness and safety of the awakening and breathing coordination, delirium monitoring/management, and early exercise/mobility bundle. Crit Care Med 2014; 42(5): 1024-36.
[http://dx.doi.org/10.1097/CCM.0000000000000129] [PMID: 24394627]

[47]   Kress JP, Gehlbach B, Lacy M, Pliskin N, Pohlman AS, Hall JB. The long-term psychological effects of daily sedative interruption on critically ill patients. Am J Respir Crit Care Med 2003;168:1457–1461.

[48]   Jones C, Griffiths RD, Humphris G, Skirrow PM. Memory, delusions, and the development of acute posttraumatic stress disorder-related symptoms after intensive care. Crit Care Med 2001; 29(3): 573-80.
[http://dx.doi.org/10.1097/00003246-200103000-00019] [PMID: 11373423]

[49]   Strøm T, Stylsvig M, Toft P. Long-term psychological effects of a no-sedation protocol in critically ill patients. Crit Care 2011; 15(6): R293.
[http://dx.doi.org/10.1186/cc10586] [PMID: 22166673]

[50]   Barr J, Fraser GL, Puntillo K, *et al.* Clinical practice guidelines for the management of pain, agitation, and delirium in adult patients in the intensive care unit. Crit Care Med 2013; 41(1): 263-306.
[http://dx.doi.org/10.1097/CCM.0b013e3182783b72] [PMID: 23269131]

[51]   Schwebel C, Clec'h C, Magne S, *et al.* Safety of intrahospital transport in ventilated critically ill patients: a multicenter cohort study*. Crit Care Med 2013; 41(8): 1919-28.
[http://dx.doi.org/10.1097/CCM.0b013e31828a3bbd] [PMID: 23863225]

[52]   Beckmann U, Gillies DM, Berenholtz SM, Wu AW, Pronovost P. Incidents relating to the intra-hospital transfer of critically ill patients. An analysis of the reports submitted to the Australian Incident Monitoring Study in Intensive Care. Intensive Care Med 2004; 30(8): 1579-85.
        [http://dx.doi.org/10.1007/s00134-004-2177-9] [PMID: 14991102]

[53]   Martins SB, Shojania KG. Safety During Transport of Critically Ill Patients. Agency for Healthcare Research and Quality , [last accessed 11/1/2015]; http://archive.ahrq.gov/clinic/ptsafety/chap47.htm

[54]   Voigt LP, Pastores SM, Raoof ND, Thaler HT, Halpern NA. Review of a large clinical series: intrahospital transport of critically ill patients: outcomes, timing, and patterns. J Intensive Care Med 2009; 24(2): 108-15.
        [http://dx.doi.org/10.1177/0885066608329946] [PMID: 19188270]

[55]   Quenot JP, Milési C, Cravoisy A, *et al.* Intrahospital transport of critically ill patients (excluding newborns) recommendations of the Société de Réanimation de Langue Française (SRLF), the Société Française d'Anesthésie et de Réanimation (SFAR), and the Société Française de Médecine d'Urgence (SFMU). Ann Intensive Care 2012; 2(1): 1.
        [http://dx.doi.org/10.1186/2110-5820-2-1] [PMID: 22304940]

[56]   Fanara B, Manzon C, Barbot O, Desmettre T, Capellier G. Recommendations for the intra-hospital transport of critically ill patients. Crit Care 2010; 14(3): R87.
        [http://dx.doi.org/10.1186/cc9018] [PMID: 20470381]

[57]   Parmentier-Decrucq E, Poissy J, Favory R, *et al.* Adverse events during intrahospital transport of critically ill patients: incidence and risk factors. Ann Intensive Care 2013; 3(1): 10.
        [http://dx.doi.org/10.1186/2110-5820-3-10] [PMID: 23587445]

[58]   Blakeman TC, Branson RD. Inter- and intra-hospital transport of the critically ill. Respir Care 2013; 58: 1008-23.
        [http://dx.doi.org/10.4187/respcare.02404] [PMID: 23709197]

[59]   Brunsveld-Reinders AH, Arbous MS, Kuiper SG, de Jonge E. A comprehensive method to develop a checklist to increase safety of intra-hospital transport of critically ill patients. Crit Care 2015; 19: 214.
        [http://dx.doi.org/10.1186/s13054-015-0938-1] [PMID: 25947327]

[60]   van Rensen EL, Groen ES, Numan SC, *et al.* Multitasking during patient handover in the recovery room. Anesth Analg 2012; 115(5): 1183-7.
        [http://dx.doi.org/10.1213/ANE.0b013e31826996a2] [PMID: 22984152]

[61]   Møller TP, Madsen MD, Fuhrmann L, Østergaard D. Postoperative handover: characteristics and considerations on improvement: a systematic review. Eur J Anaesthesiol 2013; 30(5): 229-42.
        [http://dx.doi.org/10.1097/EJA.0b013e32835d8520] [PMID: 23492933]

[62]   Segall N, Bonifacio AS, Schroeder RA, *et al.* Can we make postoperative patient handovers safer? A systematic review of the literature. Anesth Analg 2012; 115(1): 102-15.
        [http://dx.doi.org/10.1213/ANE.0b013e318253af4b] [PMID: 22543067]

[63]   Carroll K, Iedema R, Kerridge R. Reshaping ICU ward round practices using video-reflexive ethnography. Qual Health Res 2008; 18(3): 380-90.
        [http://dx.doi.org/10.1177/1049732307313430] [PMID: 18235161]

[64]   Robertson ER, Morgan L, Bird S, Catchpole K, McCulloch P. Interventions employed to improve intrahospital handover: a systematic review. BMJ Qual Saf 2014; 23(7): 600-7.
        [http://dx.doi.org/10.1136/bmjqs-2013-002309] [PMID: 24811239]

[65]   Gardiner TM, Marshall AP, Gillespie BM. Clinical handover of the critically ill postoperative patient: An integrative review. Aust Crit Care 2015; pii: S1036-7314(15)00034-X.

[66]   Agarwal HS, Saville BR, Slayton JM, *et al.* Standardized postoperative handover process improves outcomes in the intensive care unit: a model for operational sustainability and improved team performance. Crit Care Med 2012; 40(7): 2109-15.
        [http://dx.doi.org/10.1097/CCM.0b013e3182514bab] [PMID: 22710203]

[67]   Salzwedel C, Bartz HJ, Kühnelt I, *et al.* The effect of a checklist on the quality of post-anaesthesia patient handover: a randomized controlled trial. Int J Qual Health Care 2013; 25(2): 176-81.
[http://dx.doi.org/10.1093/intqhc/mzt009] [PMID: 23360810]

[68]   Li P, Ali S, Tang C, Ghali WA, Stelfox HT. Review of computerized physician handoff tools for improving the quality of patient care. J Hosp Med 2013; 8(8): 456-63.
[http://dx.doi.org/10.1002/jhm.1988] [PMID: 23169534]

CHAPTER 7

Difficult Airway

Amballur D. John[*]

Johns Hopkins Medical Institutions, Baltimore, Maryland, USA

Abstract: The difficult airway is a reality that every practitioner of anesthesia will encounter. The most difficult airway is the unanticipated difficult airway. Due to the enormous efforts and work of professional societies awareness has been raised, training has improved, and skills are kept current. New devices such as the Laryngeal Mask Airway (LMA) and video laryngoscopy have made securing the difficult airway an easier task. Increased awareness of obstructive sleep apnea has helped improve patient safety. This article attempts to discuss the key components of the difficult airway algorithms of the ASA, DAS, CAFG; with a focus on the airway exam, oxygenating the patient, developing a plan and backup plans, and finally the options when doing.

Keywords: Airway Algorithm, Airway Examination, Difficult Airway, Oxygenation, Surgical Airway, Supraglottic Device.

INTRODUCTION [1 - 4]

The most difficult airway is the unanticipated difficult airway. There are several key algorithms such as the ASA's, Difficult Airway Algorithm and the Difficult Airway Societies Difficult Airway Algorithm (Figs. **1 & 2**) which are designed to guide practitioners in a systematic approach to the most fundamental of anesthetic problems – the difficult airway. The pediatric airway is discussed in Dr. Schwartz's chapter on pediatrics. As anesthesiologists, a significant portion of residency training is focused on the airway and the means to ensure airway patency. Other than ENT surgeons, anesthesiologists and CRNA's are primarily responsible for maintaining airway patency; however, in emergent and trauma situations, trauma surgeons have the requisite skills to obtain a surgical airway. Every anesthesia provider has his/her own comfort level with obtaining and maintaining a patent airway. Large academic centers often have a difficult airway response team (DART) to assist in securing the difficult airway. Smaller practices will often have someone who is facile in securing the more difficult airways. Unfortunately, these resources are not always immediately available, and as

[*] **Corresponding author Amballur D. John:** Johns Hopkins Medical Institutions, Baltimore, Maryland, USA; Tel: (410) 550-0100; E-mail: ajohn1@jhmi.edu

Amballur D. John (Ed.)

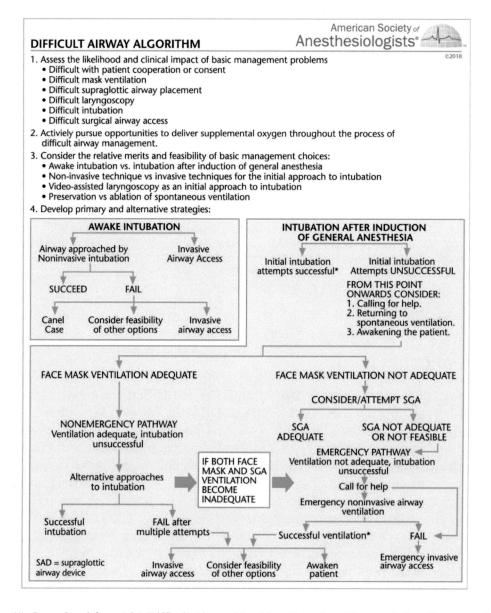

Fig. (1). Reproduced from ASA Difficult Airway Algorithm, Reproduced by permission, license number D5683635. Apfelbaum *et al.* (2013) "Practice Guidelines for Management of the Difficult Airway: An Updated Repot by the American Society of Anesthesiologists Task Force on Management of the Difficult Airway," Anesthesiology 118:251-70.

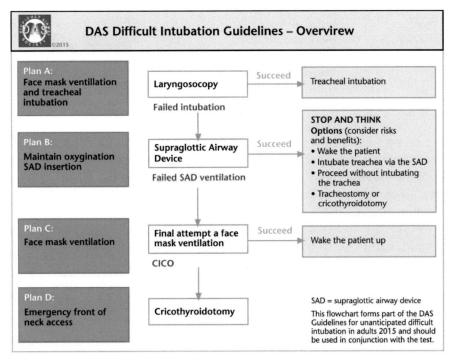

Fig. (2). Reproduced from Frerk C, Mitchell *vs.* McNarry *et al*. Difficult Airway Society 2015 Guidelines for Management of Unanticipated Difficult Airway in Adults. British Journal of Anesthesia 2015; 115(6): 827-848. With Permission form Blockwell Publishing, Ltd.

anesthesia providers, hospitals and other physicians call upon the anesthesia staff to secure the airway. When an airway and a life are about to be lost, the stress is inordinate and support is often lacking. Unlike reading off a CPR card while conducting a code, just reading the ASA's or DAS's Difficult Airway Algorithm does not guarantee success, and the consequences of failure are devastating. In the current era, surgeons are only responsible for technical aspects of their procedure. The airway and anything else that may occur with their patient during surgery is anesthesia's fault. Internists and primary care physicians view anesthesia staff as technicians whose job it is to put the tube into the airway; and emergentologists view anesthesia as an ancillary resource to call when something untoward has occurred. Thus, we are placed into the unenviable and almost untenable situation of assuming that every airway is a potential difficult airway.

FUNDAMENTALS

In approaching the difficult airway, the fundamentals are key. Every anesthesia provider must be familiar and comfortable with the ASA's and DAS's Difficult Airway Algorithms. It is a requisite for anesthesia providers to keep their airway skills current – this includes the ability to mask a patient, use conventional direct laryngoscopy to intubate a patient, to easily use supraglottic devices, videolaryngoscopy, and fiberoptic laryngoscopy. Due to the various guidelines, initiatives, training, available tools, and dedicated efforts by anesthesia professional societies, the occurrence of catastrophic difficult airways has been markedly reduced. Unfortunately, success has led to a decrease in the discussion of the difficult airway during quality assurance meetings and a relative feeling of security and confidence on the part of anesthesia providers. There are, however, resources available to help keep anesthesia staff current including workshops and simulators, as well as written reviews. Annually Dr. Carin Hagberg in **Anesthesiology News** writes an exhaustive article "**Current Concepts in the Management of the Difficult Airway**" in which a wide range of airway devices, tube guides, styles, videolaryngoscopy's, fiberoptic scopes, supraglottic devices, special airway devices, positioning devices, cricothyrotomy, and tracheostomy devices are listed with description, size, applications, and features discussed. In addition, **Anesthesiology News** produces an **Annual Supplement on Airway Management,** in which a variety of exceptional airway experts discuss their thought processes, techniques, and devices in detail which they have successfully used to confront challenging clinical situations. Since the ability of anesthesia providers to congregate in a breakroom and discuss interesting case occurrences is limited, morning report a past trend, and quality assurance more focused on ensuring compliance and productivity, the opportunities to describe rare, dangerous and difficult encounters become relegated to obscurity until a catastrophic event occurs. Fortunately, the annual Airway Management Supplement and Dr. Hagberg's article allow anesthesia providers the opportunity to keep current and focused on difficult airway issues which may occur.

In approaching the difficult airway algorithm, it is essential to understand the underlying concepts. The algorithm has the following focus: **1) History and Physical Exam 2) Oxygenate 3) Think and Plan 4) Do.**

HISTORY AND PHYSICAL [1 - 5]

In the shortest amount of time one has to extract the greatest amount of information. Who is the patient? What happened? and what is required with regard to the airway. Certain basic information has to be obtained and processed – is the patient cooperative? Can the patient be masked? Is the placement of a supraglottic airway possible? Will laryngoscopy be difficult? Is intubation possible? How difficult will it be to obtain surgical access to the airway?

The anesthesia literature is rich in terms of different techniques and scores as being the simplest and the most accurate in predicting a difficult airway. There are numerous proponents of these techniques as well as the Mallampati Score, and the upper lip bite test. It is my opinion that the best airway evaluation remains the **Benumoff/ASA airway exam** which is systematic, sequential, and relatively easy to perform.

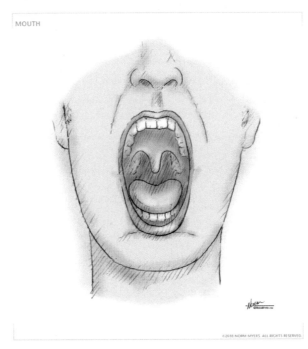

Fig. (3). Mouth. Image provided by Norm Myers.

The **comprehensive airway examination** (Figs. **3 & 4**) begins with an initial impression of the patient and scene. Then it moves sequentially to the face, the mouth, and then the neck with the final overall assessment of airway. **INITIAL**: initial impression – is the patient in extremis, critical, or stable? This will dictate the urgency of the situation and the speed of the response. **FACE**: Is there trauma to the face and head? The presence of fractures, blood, scarring, all indicate a potential for a difficult airway. **MOUTH**: Are upper teeth present? Are the upper incisors long? Are there buck teeth? Prominent overbite of the maxillary teeth and long incisors make it difficult to insert the flange of the blade and make the alignment of the oral tracheal axis more acute when the goal of optimal positioning is to make this angle more obtuse aligning these axises and the site of vision. Can the patient voluntary prognath (*i.e.* move the mandible past the maxilla)? What is the interincisor distance? If the patient cannot prognath and the interincisor distance is less than 3cm then it may not be possible to insert the flange of the blade. The size of the tongue in relation to the oral cavity is assessed by examining the visibility of the uvula (Mallampati classification) (Fig. **5**). Large tongues impair visibility and make intubations difficult. A high arched palate limits the room for laryngoscope blade and tube obscuring views and increasing the difficulty of intubation. The compliance of the submental space is important because this is the space into which the tongue is going to be displaced to when the flange is inserted into the mouth. If this space is not compliant due to surgery, tumor, mass or radiation then the tongue will obstruct the view. Micrognathia or a thyromental distance of less than three fingerbreadths indicates that larynx is more anterior and accessing the airway more difficult. **NECK**: The size, thickness, and range of motion – that is short, thick, neck with limited range of motion indicate impaired ability to obtain a sniffing position and difficulty in aligning the axises to see the vocal chords and thus increasing the likelihood of a difficult intubation.Once the airway exam is completed, an **overall assessment** is formed. **The good**: securing the airway should be straightforward. **The bad**: this airway could potentially become difficult. **The ugly**: OMG, 'what can I possibly do', sheer panic with the realization that the chances of a successful outcome correlate directly to the sound of the sinking or absent pulseoximeter and rapidly decreasing saturations.

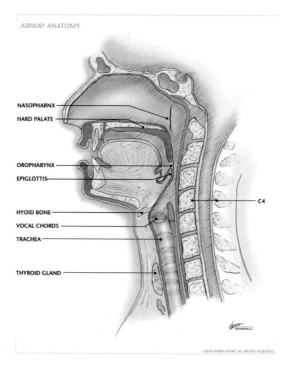

Fig. (4). Airway Anatomy. Image provided by Norm Myers.

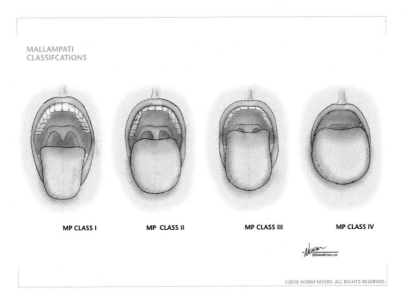

Fig. (5). Mallampati Classifications. Image provided by Norm Myers.

OXYGENATE

"Actively pursue opportunities to deliver supplemental oxygen throughout the process of difficult airway management."

Oxygenate! Oxygenate! Oxygenate!

Make sure the oxygen is turned on and flowing; as soon as one arrives on the scene, and begins the airway assessment and examination – 15L *via* nasal cannula and high flow *via* nonrebreather mask, or ambubag. Oxygenate the patient throughout the process.

THINK AND PLAN

Think – what is the best approach? Is it an awake intubation or intubation after induction of general anesthesia [awake or asleep]? Should the initial approach be invasive or noninvasive [invasive or noninvasive]? Is video assisted laryngoscopy the best initial approach [video assisted laryngoscopy to start]? To keep or abolish spontaneous respirations and ventilation [spontaneously breathing or not]?

When considering the ablation of spontaneous respirations, bear in mind Benumoff's findings that the obese rapidly desaturate even with adequate preoxygenation and that recovery from paralysis with succinylchloholine may take almost 10minutes [6]. The use of propofol in the unstable patient may result in hemodynamic instability and so treatment should be administered concomitantly on induction.

In analyzing the situation **in thinking** through the various problems and solutions it is important to **develop a plan, a backup plan, a fallback, and a safety plan**:

Plan: How to best and initially approach the situation**Back-up:** What to do if the initial plan is unsuccessful**Fall-back:** what to do when the back-up plan fails**Safety:** knowledge and awareness of surgical airway assistance. How long will it take the surgeons to access the airway? Ensuring that the surgeons are notified and available.

DOING

Awake Intubation

The awake intubation is usually done for the known difficult airway or the airway which on examination has been deemed to be difficult. Every anesthesiologist has their particular technique for approaching the awake intubation. The technique that the individual is most comfortable with, has done frequently and is most facile with is what should be chosen. **Key to success is ensuring <u>adequate topicalization, a dry airway, and patient co-operation</u>.** The availability of dexmetetomidene, remifentanyl, and flumazenil have made the task somewhat easier; but care must be exercised when administrating any drug that may cause respiratory compromise. Awake intubations done by skilled providers at medical centers have a high rate of success.

Despite this there will always be failures. The choice then becomes to cancel the case or procedure. If that is not possible to try another technique, or provider. Finally, the technique of last resort is to obtain a surgical airway. In order for this last option to be a viable option a surgeon has to be available, aware, and ready.

Intubation After Induction of General Anesthesia (Figs. 6 & 7)

In this pathway the difficult airway may not have been fully appreciated on initial evaluation, but becomes acutely present after induction of anesthesia. After failed intubation attempts, one should call for help, consider returning to spontaneous ventilation or awakening the patient.

If intubation is unsuccessful one should immediately attempt mask ventilation. This leads to either of two pathways: mask ventilation is successful and the airway is not an emergency. This allows one other avenues such as returning to spontaneous ventilation, awakening the patient, or trying a different technique. **If** mask ventilation is unsuccessful an airway emergency is occurring and the patient's life is in jeopardy.

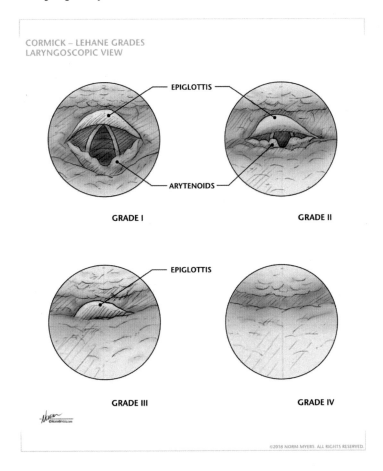

Fig. (6). Grades. Image provided by Norm Myers.

<u>The inability to mask ventilate the patient is an airway emergency.</u> Help must be called. Attempts should be made to reposition and place airway adjuvants – oral airway, nasal airways, or place a supraglottic airway (LMA) while oxygenating and attempting to ventilate. **<u>If these efforts are unsuccessful a surgical airway must be obtained</u>** [1 - 5].

CONCLUSION

The difficult airway is a reality that every practitioner of anesthesia will encounter. **The most difficult airway is the unanticipated difficult airway.** Due to the enormous effort and work of professional societies, awareness has been raised, training has improved, and skills are kept current. This has led to the marked decrease in catastrophic events.

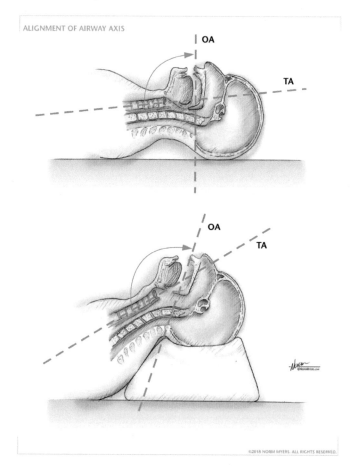

Fig. (7). Alignment of Airway Axis. Image provided by Norm Myers.

Yet a glaring deficit still remains. Airway emergencies will continue to occur on hospital floors, in the Emergency Room, and in the Operating Room on induction and emergence. Attending surgeons are not in the room on induction or emergence. Attending surgeons are not in the room on induction or emergence. Attending surgeons are not in the room on induction or emergence with the notable exception of ENT surgeons. Reasons commonly cited are this is anesthesia's problem and the surgeon's time is too valuable. The surgeon is the one the patient has a close relationship with, is most surgically trained, and the one on whom the patient's life may depend. **Every Society and Algorithm has the final resource for a difficult airway being a surgical airway.** Yet insurance companies, hospital administration, and risk management continue to permit the attending surgeon to NOT be present in the room on induction and emergence. Isn't a patient's life valuable? The fact remains that the final emergency airway remains the surgical airway.

ADDENDUM

Basic Pulmonary Physiology Figures (Figs. 8 - 13):

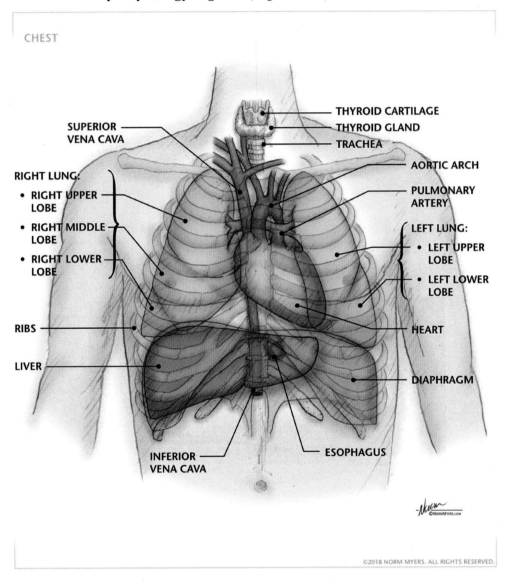

Fig. (8). Chest. Image provided by Norm Myers.

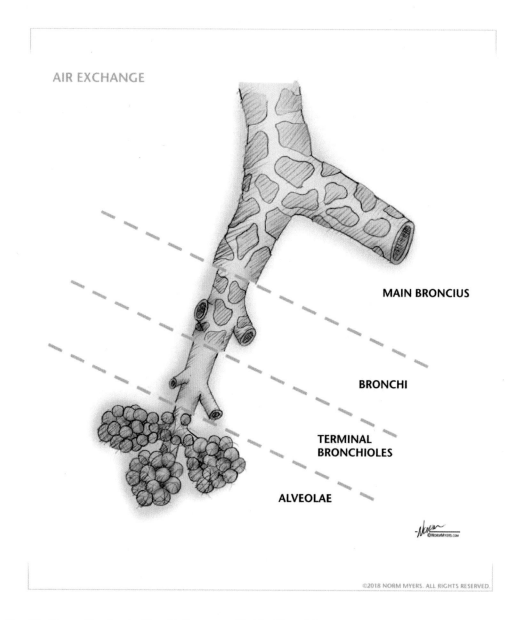

AIR EXCHANGE

MAIN BRONCIUS

BRONCHI

TERMINAL
BRONCHIOLES

ALVEOLAE

Fig. (9). Airway (Trachea to Alveoli). Image provided by Norm Myers.

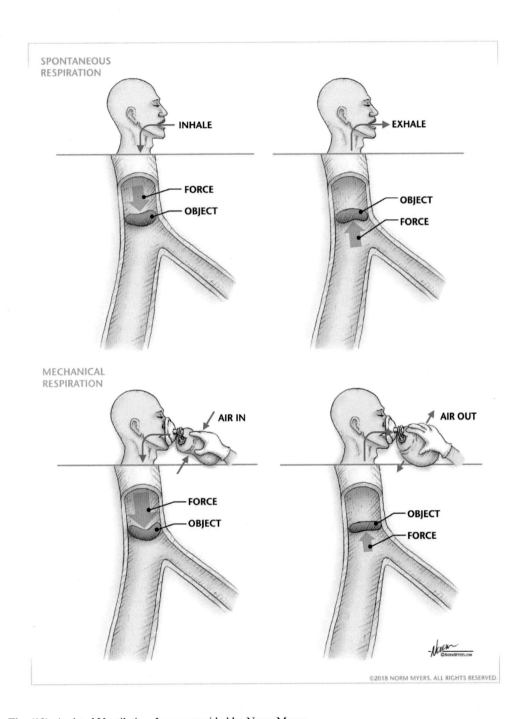

Fig. (10). Assisted Ventilation. Image provided by Norm Myers.

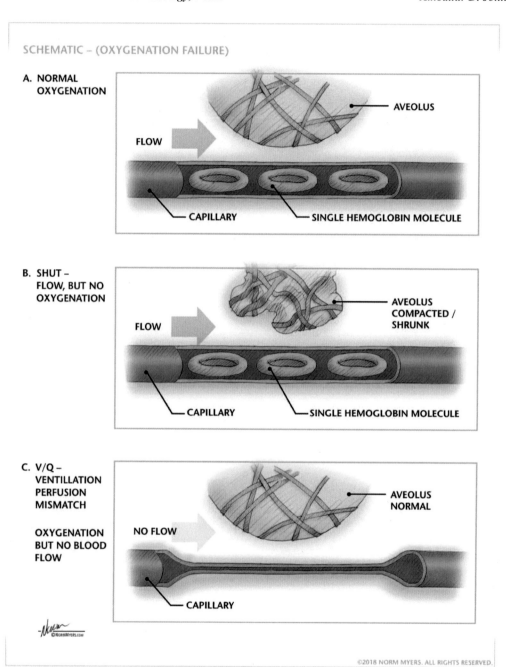

Fig. (11). Schematic (Oxygenation Failure). Image provided by Norm Myers.

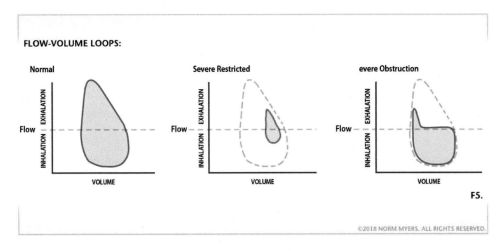

Fig. (12). Flow Volume Loops. Image provided by Norm Myers.

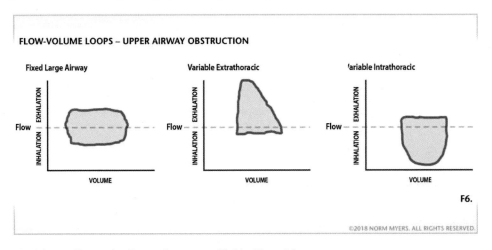

Fig. (13). Airway Obstruction Loops. Image provided by Norm Myers.

CONSENT FOR PUBLICATION

Not applicable.

CONFLICT OF INTEREST

The author (editor) declares no conflict of interest, financial or otherwise.

ACKNOWLEDGEMENT

Declared none.

REFERENCES

[1]   Apfelbaum JL, Hagberg CA, Caplan RA, *et al.* Practice guidelines for management of the difficult airway: an updated report by the American Society of Anesthesiologists Task Force on Management of the Difficult Airway. Anesthesiology 2013; 118(2): 251-70.
        [http://dx.doi.org/10.1097/ALN.0b013e31827773b2] [PMID: 23364566]

[2]   Frerk C, Mitchell VS, McNarry AF, *et al.* Difficult Airway Society 2015 guidelines for management of unanticipated difficult intubation in adults. Br J Anaesth 2015; 115(6): 827-48.
        [http://dx.doi.org/10.1093/bja/aev371] [PMID: 26556848]

[3]   Law JA, Broemling N, Cooper RM, *et al.* The difficult airway with recommendations for management-part 1-difficult tracheal intubation encountered in an unconscious/induced patient. Can J Anaesth 2013; 60(11): 1089-118.
        [http://dx.doi.org/10.1007/s12630-013-0019-3] [PMID: 24132407]

[4]   Law JA, Broemling N, Cooper RM, *et al.* The difficult airway with recommendations for management-part 2-the anticipated difficult airway. Can J Anaesth 2013; 60(11): 1119-38.
        [http://dx.doi.org/10.1007/s12630-013-0020-x] [PMID: 24132408]

[5]   Benumof Jonathan L. The ASA Difficult Airway Algorithm January 2014 UCSD Anesthesiology Update Audio Digest Anesthesiology 2014 November 11; 56(41)

[6]   Benumof JL, Dagg R, Benumof R. Critical hemoglobin desaturation will occur before return to an unparalyzed state following 1 mg/kg intravenous succinylcholine. Anesthesiology 1997; 87(4): 979-82.
        [http://dx.doi.org/10.1097/00000542-199710000-00034] [PMID: 9357902]

CHAPTER 8

Perioperative Medical Ethics and the Anesthesiologist

Paul J. Hoehner[*]

Johns Hopkins Medical Institutions, Baltimore, Maryland, USA

Abstract: Medicine is above all a moral endeavor. Anesthesiologists are tasked with evaluating the overall medical condition of the patient not just performing a scheduled procedure – they are the primary care physicians in the perioperative period. This is becoming even more so since physicians are most often employees of large healthcare delivery systems. These systems view patients as objects that must be put through the system quickly to optimize profits. Currently, proceduralists and/or surgeons are only responsible for the technical aspects of their procedure; the care of the patient is the anesthesiologist's problem. Anesthesiologists have an ethical duty to put the patient's interests foremost. Often this places them in conflict with surgeons and the healthcare system who perceive anesthesiologists as hindering through-put and interfering with profit. Anesthesiologists are given a perfunctory period in which they have to establish a relationship with the patient, determine the patients' wishes, and obtain informed consent. The basis for understanding the ethical foundations of the processes involved is discussed in this chapter.

Keywords: Adequate Disclosure, Autonomous Authorization, Advanced Directives, Competency, Consent Elements, Decision, Decision Making Capacity, DNR/DNAR (Do Not Resuscitate, Do Not Attempt Resuscitation), Double Effect, Euthanasia, End of Life Care, Informed Consent, Living Wills, Principlism, Personal Autonomy, Power of Attorney for Healthcare Proxy, Physician Assisted Suicide, Palliative Care, Senilicide, Shared Decision Making, Substituted Judgment, Treatment Futility, Treatment Redirection, Voluntarism.

INTRODUCTION

<u>**Medicine is foremost a moral endeavor, and every clinical encounter between a physician and patient is an ethical encounter.**</u> It is a moral undertaking because medicine is first and foremost a relationship. As obvious as this statement should be, in the eyes of many, today, medicine is a business, a science, or a body of knowledge. The patient is a "healthcare consumer" purchasing a commodity,

---

[*] **Corresponding author Paul J. Hoehner:** Johns Hopkins Medical Institutions, Baltimore, Maryland, USA; Tel: (410) 550-0100; E-mail: phoeh1@jhmi.edu

either information, advice, or a procedure from a myriad of "healthcare providers." Once the exchange has taken place, the obligations have been fulfilled, and there is no underlying commitment beyond that point. Certainly this is the conclusion of many philosophers, business administrators, and policy bureaucrats examining and describing the physician-patient relationship. To adopt this mindset, however, is to cease to be a professional in the full sense of the term [2, 4 - 6].

Much is being discussed about the expanding role of the anesthesiologist in the perioperative period [7 - 10]. As the nature of modern healthcare evolves, the anesthesiologist is increasingly taking on the role of a primary care physician in the perioperative period, tasked with evaluating the overall medical condition of the patient with a larger perspective than merely the scheduled procedure. Little, however, has been written about how this expanded medical role will also bring about an expanded ethical role of the anesthesiologist in the perioperative period that will go beyond merely procedural consent issues. Not only will the anesthesiologist need to function as the traditional "internist in the operating room" as the patient's chief medical and safety advocate, but also as the patient's chief ethical advocate.

Along with this comes a host of barriers to effective ethical advocacy of the perioperative patient. Production pressures and shortened operating room turn-around times limit the anesthesiologist in establishing an appropriate patient-physician relationship. Physicians are increasingly becoming employees of large healthcare delivery systems which impose a "dual (or multiple) agency" between physicians, their patients (or healthcare consumers), populations, and the economic interests of their employers [11, 12]. The use of multiple providers to facilitate the efficient "through-put" of most surgery centers contributes to the impersonal nature of modern medicine. The universal adoption of comprehensive and shared electronic medical records (EMRs) is also certain to change the nature of the patient-physician encounter in subtle and dramatic ways along with the nature of medical care itself [13 - 16]. The limited and algorithmic preoperative encounter as "data entry" can reduce the face-to-face and person-to-person establishment of trust and understanding that is central to the ethical practice of medicine [16 - 18]. Anesthesiologists should not let the pressures of economics, efficiency, and outside agency obstruct their primary duty to put their individual patient's ethical and medical interests foremost.

ETHICAL PRINCIPLES

Modern society's categories of right and wrong, or decisions regarding the "good," are frequently characterized by competing rational philosophical theories (such as deontology, utilitarianism, natural law), as cultural and tradition-dependent artifacts, or as arising from individualistic or relativistic (e)motives. The classical paradigm of modern medical ethics commonly referred to as "**principlism**," originated in a pragmatic attempt to overcome the impasse of these competing ethical theories in order to derive common and self-evident "principles" that would serve to guide a common language/paradigm of biomedical ethical decision-making. This almost universally accepted paradigm of modern medical ethics <u>centers on the principles of respect for personal autonomy, beneficence, nonmaleficence, and justice and is usually assumed in many basic medical ethics texts.</u> Alternative frameworks based on such concepts as "<u>virtue ethics</u>," the "<u>narrative life</u>," and "<u>personhood</u>" have also been explored as means to supplement or overcome some of the philosophical limitations of the traditional approach. It is beyond the scope of this chapter to address these various concepts. Suffice it to say that <u>medical ethics has always been seen as a branch of applied ethics</u>, a pragmatic program that relies on a multi-perspectival and at times multicultural approach to making difficult decisions in healthcare. For this reason, the "principle" approach, despite its limitations, has nonetheless provided an accepted working guideline for clinical medical ethics.

INFORMED CONSENT

Respect for Personal Autonomy

Many ethical conundrums in medical ethics are the result of specific principles coming into conflict in specific cases. **Personal autonomy** <u>is generally understood to refer to the capacity to be one's own person, to live one's life according to reasons and motives that are taken as one's own and not the product of manipulative or distorting external forces. The principle of respect for personal autonomy, at least in most western cultures, is sometimes taken to be the overriding principle in modern ethical deliberation.</u> However, respect for personal autonomy does not, and should not, exhaust moral deliberation. Other principles are important and not only when autonomy reaches its limits. Childress notes that focusing on the principle of respect for personal autonomy can foster indifference and that the principles of care and beneficence are important even in discussions of informed consent. The <u>role played by the principle of respect for personal autonomy is one of the setting limits</u>, such that, "without the limits set by the principle of respect for autonomy, these principles (beneficence, non-maleficence, and justice) may support arrogant enforcement of "the good" for others" [19]. Yet, the <u>principle of respect for autonomy is not absolutely binding and does not outweigh all other principles at all times</u>. **Two different approaches** have been used by ethicists to **resolve conflicts or apparent contradictions** between competing principles. First is to construct an ***a priori*** serial ranking of the principles, such that some take absolute priority over others. Second, principles can be viewed as ***prima facie*** binding, competing equally with other prima facie principles in particular circumstances. This view requires one to view more closely the complexities and particularities of individual cases and is more situational in context. The ***prima facie*** principle of respect for autonomy can be overridden or justifiably infringed when the following conditions are satisfied: **1)** when there are stronger competing principles (<u>proportionality</u>); **2)** when infringing on the principle of respect for personal autonomy would probably *protect* the competing principles (<u>effectiveness</u>); **3)** when infringing the principle of respect for personal autonomy, it is *necessary* to protect the competing principle(s) (<u>last resort</u>); and **4)** when the infringement of the principle of respect for personal autonomy is the *least intrusive or restrictive* in the circumstances, consistent with protecting the competing principle(s) (<u>least infringement</u>) [19].

Shared Decision-Making

Aside from the legal requirements and the specter of malpractice, recent discussions of "informed consent" have focused on the concept of "shared decision-making" and the clinical-therapeutic role of the informed consent process in improving patient care. These <u>discussions recognize that there should be a collaborative effort between physicians and patients to arrive at appropriate treatment decisions</u>. The physician brings knowledge and trained judgment to the process, while the patient brings individual and unique priorities, needs, concerns, beliefs, and fears. Focusing on the process of informed consent, as opposed to bare legal requirements, increases a patient's participation in his or her own care, which may have the practical benefit of increasing patient compliance and self-monitoring. Informed consent as "teaching" (indeed, the origin of the word "Doctor" is from "teacher") further diminishes patients' misconceptions or inaccurate fears about their situation and prospects and may improve patient recovery or comfort with a better understanding of the care that is being provided. No good data are available regarding these "therapeutic" effects of informed consent, and further studies seem warranted. Despite these theoretical positive aspects, issues surrounding informed consent remain vexing for physicians in a number of clinical situations from both legal and ethical perspectives. <u>Even the ideal model of "shared decision-making" does not address many of the realities of medical practice, including emergency situations, conflicts of interest, and questions of futility</u>.

By emphasizing informed consent as a temporal "process," one can avoid the pitfalls of viewing informed consent as a single event. <u>Informed consent can never be reduced to a signature on a consent form</u>. "Perhaps the most fundamental and pervasive myth about informed consent is that informed consent has been obtained when a patient signs a consent form. Nothing could be further from the truth, as many courts have pointed out to physicians who were only too willing to believe this myth" [20]. Although a matter of routine in many institutions because they are seen as providing protection against liability, informed consent forms actually provide very little. The informed consent form does have value in that it provides an opportunity for the patient to read the information on the form and to create a locus for the appropriate patient-physician discussion that is the key element. An informed consent form merely documents that the "process" of informed consent has taken place.

Traditionally, consent to anesthesia in the past was subsumed under the consent to the surgical procedure and included within the surgery consent form. The anesthesiologist was one step removed from the formal consent process. Today, separate specific consent for anesthesia is required. It is imperative that the anesthesiologists make a concerted effort to adequately complete this process with the patient and, when appropriate, the patient's family regarding the anesthetic procedure and adequately document in a note the patient's consent on the chart or anesthetic record.

Beauchamp and Childress [21] have broken down the process of informed consent into seven elements (Table **1**). These include **threshold elements** or **preconditions**, which include **1)** decision-making capacity or competency of the patient, **2)** freedom or voluntariness in decision-making, including absence of overriding legal or state interests; informational elements including **3)** adequate disclosure of material information, **4)** recommendations, and **5)** an understanding of the above; consent elements, which include **6)** decision by the patient in favor of a plan and **7)** authorization of that plan (Table **1**).

Table 1. Elements of the Process of Informed Consent. Provided by Paul J. Hoehner, M.D., Johns Hopkins.

Threshhold Elements (Preconditions)
Decision-making capacity or competency
Freedom or voluntariness and absence of overriding state or legal interests
Informational Elements
Adequate disclosure of material information
Recommendation
Understanding
Consent Elements
Decision
Authorization

Threshold Elements

DECISION-MAKING CAPACITY

Physicians are frequently faced with the problem of making treatment decisions for patients who no longer have decision-making capacity. Many diseases and conditions requiring life-prolonging therapies can also destroy or substantially impair a person's decision-making capacity and are more likely to do so in older people. In addition, Alzheimer's disease and other forms of dementia are more likely to be present in older persons. One estimate is that 5% to 7% of persons over 65, and 25% of those over 84, suffer from severe dementia [22]. Assessment of decision-making capacity even in cases of mild dementia can be particularly difficult [23]. Decision-making capacity requires: **1)** a capacity to understand and communicate, **2)** a capacity to reason and deliberate, and **3)** possession of a set of values and goals [24 - 26]. Although there is general agreement regarding these three requirements, there is no single, universally accepted standard of decision-making capacity. This is because decision-making capacity is not an all-o--nothing concept. **Decision-making** is also a task-related concept and the requisite skills and abilities vary according to the specific decision or task. The relevant criteria should also vary according to the risk to a patient. Basically, one must ask the following questions: Does the patient understand his or her medical condition? Does the patient understand the options and the consequences of his or her decision? Is the patient capable of reasonable deliberation? Is the patient able to communicate his or her decision? Does the patient possess a coherent set of values and/or goals? Several reviews provide helpful discussions of the clinical assessment of elderly patients' decision-making capacity within these contexts [27 - 29].

To what extent must a patient "understand" his or her condition, treatment options and risks [30]? If fully "informed" is meant to mean fully "educated" [31] then "informed" consent may be seen as an impossible standard. However, the primary object of information is to facilitate the patients' care rather than providing a litany of possible complications in order to avoid a lawsuit. Factual knowledge is used, not as an end in itself, but as a means to extend the patients' own understanding in such a way as to meet their own unique priorities, needs, concerns, beliefs, and fears so that they may decide about their care in the manner they normally make similar choices. This will vary from patient to patient and with the risks of the procedure involved. It is a mistake to assume that a patient must understand information to the same extent and in the same manner as a physician, or even as a well-educated layman. This may indeed be seen as just as paternalistic as not permitting patients to participate in decision making at all [20].

Visual and hearing impairments and diminished memory and comprehension require the clinician to exercise particular caution when obtaining informed consent [32]. One must also be careful to avoid the mistake of equating recall, a standard endpoint in many studies on the adequacy of informed, with understanding and comprehension. Meisel and Kuczewski note that, "While it may be true that someone who cannot retain information for a few seconds might not be said to understand it, people often make reasonable decisions but cannot later recall the premises that supported the reasoning or the process that led to the conclusion" [20]. Distant recall of the informed consent process may be an indicator of the adequacy of a patient's understanding, but its absence says little about the patient's understanding at the time of consent. Physicians also tend to underestimate patients' desire for information and discussion and, at the same time, overestimate patients' desire to make decisions [33 - 35]. Patients and their physicians often differ on patient quality-of-life assessments that may be associated with clinical decisions [36]. These studies and others underscore the need for clear communication, individualization, and compassion in obtaining adequate informed consent.

Assessment of patient **capacity** to enter into the process of informed consent or competency to make rational medical decisions is a complicated issue. Much has been written on the criteria for determining individual capacity and the legally defined characteristic of "competency" [20, 37 - 40]. **Competency**, unlike the decision-making capacity, is a legal term and an all-or-nothing concept specific to a given task. In the absence of a clear medical diagnosis such as delirium or unconsciousness, decisions regarding competency must be made with assistance from psychiatric services, ethics consult services, and/or legal counsel. In general, decisions must be made in these situations on the patient's behalf, either by **"substituted judgment"** (a decision based on what the patient would have wanted, assuming some knowledge of what the patient's wishes would have been) with or without the help of proxy consent or by a decision made according to the "best interests" of the patient on the basis of a balancing of a "benefit *versus* burdens" ratio. An appropriate **hierarchy for surrogate decision makers** is delineated, for example, in a provision of the Virginia Health Care Decisions Act [Code of Virginia § 54.1-2981] as follows: **1)** A legally appointed guardian or committee. **2)** The patient's spouse if no divorce action has been filed. **3)** An adult son or daughter of the patient. **4)** The patient's parent. **5)** An adult brother or sister of the patient. **6)** Any other relative of the patient in descending order of relationship. It must be remembered that the caregiver has an ethical obligation to evaluate the competency of the surrogate's decisions with regards to **1)** lack of conflict of interest, **2)** reliability of the evidence of the patient's desires on which the surrogate is relying, **3)** the surrogate's knowledge of the patient's own value system, and **4)** the surrogate's responsible commitment to the decision-making process [41]. All these situations involve complex issues and, again, may require the assistance of hospital ethics committees or consult services.

VOLUNTARINESS

A second threshold element is one of freedom or voluntariness. Here one asks the question of whether the patient's decision is free from external constraints. These constraints can consist of a myriad of social, familial, and even financial factors that can be difficult, if not impossible, to sort out. However, it is not true that the principle of respect for autonomy is at odds with all forms of heteronomy, authority, tradition, *etc*. Competent individuals may autonomously choose to yield first-order decisions (*i.e.*, their decisions about the rightness and wrongness of particular modes of conduct) to a professional, family, spouse, or to a religious institution. In these instances the person is exercising second-order autonomy in selecting the professional, person, or institution to which they choose to be subordinate. In these cases, second-order autonomy becomes central [42]. The distinguishing feature becomes whether the second-order decision was free and voluntary. Patients may decide on specific treatment options with respect for the opinions of family members, or a concern for their psychological, physical, and/or financial well-being. It is perfectly appropriate for elderly patients to consider the preferences of loved ones, and they should not automatically be encouraged to make decisions concerning treatment options, particularly life-extending treatments, for exclusively self-regarding or purely selfish reasons. Moreover, although undue pressure and influence are clearly improper, it is a mistake to assume that any advice and counsel from family members constitutes undue pressure or influence. However, when patients possess decision-making capacity, generally they and only they have the moral authority to decide how much weight to give the preferences and interests of family members. While it is true that elderly patients can have ethical obligations toward family members that have a bearing on treatment decisions and the interests of family members can be "ethically relevant whether or not the patient is inclined to consider them" [43], they should generally retain decision-making authority even if physicians believe that they are failing to give due consideration to the interests of family members.

INFORMATIONAL ELEMENTS

Adequate Disclosure

The **first** of **the informational elements of informed consent is adequate disclosure**. This is the process of properly informing the patient of his or her diagnosis, prognosis, treatment options, risks, and possible outcomes. The anesthesiologist should reveal the specific risks and benefits of each **anesthetic option**, the complications of instrumentation of the airway, the risks and benefits of invasive monitoring, the presence and use of a fallback plan, and basis for the anesthesiologist's recommendations [44]. "Transparency" is a useful term describing the openness by which the anesthesiologist discusses the treatment plans with a patient. By "thinking out loud" regarding the options and plans, the anesthesiologist communicates the thought processes that he is making that is going into his or her recommendation, thus allowing the patient to understand and participate in this process. Most patients and parents of patients want assurance and explanation regarding anesthesia, not necessarily detailed and exhaustive information.

The discussion of risks and hazards of the diagnostic or therapeutic options, as well as information about anticipated pain or suffering, are, in theory and practice, the most troublesome aspects of informed consent. According to the President's Commission for the Study of Ethical Problems in Medicine and Biomedical and Behavioral Research, "Adequate informed consent requires effort on the part of the physician to ensure comprehension; it involves far more than just a signature on the bottom of a list of possible complications. Such complications can be so overwhelming that patients are unable to appreciate the truly significant information and to make sound decisions" [26]. The law does not require one to give a list of every possible complication of a planned procedure (which may inflict an undue amount of emotional distress), but only a "reasonable" amount of information. **Negligence** is not failure to achieve a good outcome, nor failure to disclose all remote risks [3].

But just how does one define "reasonable?" The courts have had difficulty as well assessing what a "reasonable" standard of disclosure may be. The most cited standard is the professional practice standard [45]. This standard defines reasonable disclosure as what a capable and reasonable medical practitioner in the same field would reveal to a patient under the same or similar circumstances. Some courts have ignored this prevailing standard of disclosure and shifted the focus from the professional community as forming the standard to the patients themselves. It focuses on the "new consumerism" in health care, an extension of the patient's right of self-determination, where the patient is viewed as consumer of health care and the physician as provider [46]. The "reasonable patient standard" asks what a reasonable patient would consider **reasonable** and **material** to the decision of whether to consent to a procedure offered. The burden, however, is still on the physician to ascertain just what is reasonable and material for a hypothetical "reasonable patient." This recognizes a significant shift in consent law. As legal standards continue to evolve, the reasonable patient standard may become more commonly accepted and eventually displaced the professional practice standard as the majority opinion in American informed consent law. A further extension of this line of thinking is the "subjective person standard". This standard recognizes that all patients are different, there is no hypothetical "reasonable person", and hence the standard of disclosure must recognize not only the local standard of care but individual patient needs and idiosyncrasies as well. One important factor in all the above is the notion of "**causality**," *i.e.*would additional information have affected this particular patient's decision? What specific, individual concerns did the patient have that would have most affected his or her decision whether or not they are part of the local standard of care for disclosure? The risk of vocal cord damage from a routine intubation may be so small as to not require mentioning in the normal situation (although this is debatable). It may, however, be very important for a professional singer in opting between regional or general anesthesia.

Recommendation and Understanding

Providing a recommendation and patient understanding are the other two informational elements in the informed consent process. The principle of patient autonomy does not require the physician to present the information in a totally neutral manner, if this were even possible [6]. Indeed, part of the informed consent process is to present information to the patient in a way that buttresses a physician's recommendations. Persuasion is a justifiable way for educating patients. This is different from manipulation, which is defined as inappropriately causing a certain behavior, and coercion, which is actually threatening a patient with a plausible punishment so the patient will act in a certain way.

Assessing patient understanding of the information presented can be a difficult issue, especially if "standard" consent forms are relied upon. In one study, 27% of postoperative surgical patients signing consent forms did not know which organ had been operated upon, and 44% did not know the nature of the procedure [47]. Cassileth *et al.* showed that 55% of cancer patients could list one of the major complications for chemotherapy within one day of signing consent forms [48]. Other studies have shown that risk-specific consent forms do not aid retention [49] and that decision-makers often sign consent forms that they do not understand [44]. Attempts must be made to educate patients according to their individual needs and, as has been stated previously, not to assume a patient must have complete understanding, but only that necessary given their own particular situation to come to a reasonable decision. This will vary from patient to patient and from situation to situation, and consent forms cannot be relied upon to provide this information, no matter how detailed.

CONSENT ELEMENTS: DECISION AND AUTONOMOUS AUTHORI-ZATION

Finally, there are the **two consent elements: decision** and **autonomous**

authorization. The patient must be able to reach a decision and authorize the physician to provide the care decided upon. The physician must document the consented-to technique as well as the invasive monitoring to be used. **The patient may consent either verbally or in writing, both are ethically and legally just as valid**. It may be more difficult to provide evidence of verbal consent after the fact, however, making it all the more important to document adequately the patient's response in the chart. While lack of an objection is not equivalent to an authorization, cooperation of patients during performance of a procedure in the absence of overt verbal authorization has usually been deemed equivalent to implied consent and sufficient in cases specifically addressing these issues [50].

ADVANCE DIRECTIVES

Advance directives are statements that a patient makes, while still retaining decision-making capacity, about how treatment decisions should be made when they no longer have the capacity to make those decisions. In 1991 the Patient Self-Determination Act (PSDA) became federal law involving all Medicare and Medicaid providers. The PSDA provides that all healthcare providers must give all patients written information at the time of their admission advising them of their rights to refuse any treatments and to have an advance directive.

There are **two general forms of advance directives**. **Living wills** are documents stating the desires of the patient for treatment alternatives, usually to die a "natural" death and not to be kept alive by advanced life-support measures. In many states, the patient may also stipulate wishes regarding fluid and nutrition discontinuation in the event of persistent vegetative state. Living wills become effective on the determination of "terminal illness" or when death is imminent (*e.g.*, within 6months) or when two physicians make the diagnosis of persistent vegetative state. The strengths and weaknesses of the living will are outlined in Table **2**. Living wills have several weaknesses, including the frequent lack of specific instructions and the impossibility of any person foreseeing all the contingencies of a future illness [51]. Therefore, many advocate an alternative form of advance directive known as a **Power of Attorney for Healthcare** (PAHC). A PAHC provides for the appointment of a person to act as a healthcare agent, proxy, or surrogate to make treatment decisions when the patient is no longer able. The PAHC allows a person to add specific directives, *e.g.*, giving a designated agent authority to have feeding tubes withheld or withdrawn. Most PAHCs become effective when two physicians, or one physician and a psychologist, determine that the patient no longer has decision-making capacity. However, this requirement is not universal, and individual state statutes may vary. Table **3** lists the advantages of the PAHC that may make it a better option than a living will. Individual state statutes may differ regarding certain components such as witnesses and need for notarization. Whichever form of advance directive a patient chooses to employ, <u>both serve a valuable role in preventing ethical dilemmas if designed properly and implemented</u>.

In many instances, patients who lack decision-making capacity have neither executed an advance directive nor previously discussed their preferences regarding treatment options. Even when surrogates are available, disagreements among parties (particularly family members with vested interests), legal or regulatory obstacles, or other problems may hinder a clear decision-making process. Healthcare providers and institutions develop methods to make decisions for incapacitated persons without surrogates need to have in place policies and procedures for intra-institutional conflict resolution, such as an ethics committee, to mediate conflicting situations. Surrogate decision-making laws and policies should not hinder the patient's ability to die naturally and comfortably. Evidence from competent patients in similar circumstances should shape the plan of care for an individual patient in the absence of evidence that the patient's wishes would be otherwise [52]. Other strategies include the "prior competent choice" standard, which stresses the values the patient held while competent. The "best interest standard" moves the focus to the patient's subjective experience at the time the treatment is considered [28].

Table 2. Living Will. Source: Junkerman C, Schiedermayer D: Practical Ethics for Students, Interns, and Residents: A Short Reference Manual. Frederick, MD: University Publishing Group, Inc., 1998, p. 58. Copyright 1998 by University Publishing Group. Used with permission. May not be copied without the express written permission of University Publishing Group. Provided by Paul J. Hoehner, M.D., Johns Hopkins.

Living Will	©2018 P. HOEHNER, JOHNS HOPKINS
Strengths	
1. Allows the physician to understand the patient's wishes and motivations	
2. Extends the patient's autonomy, self-control, and self-determination.	
3. Relieves the patient's anxiety about unwanted treatment.	
4. Relieves physician's anxiety about legal liability.	
5. Reduces family strife and sense of guilt.	
6. Improves communication and trust between patient and physician.	
Weakness	
1. Applicable only to those in persistent vegetative state (PVS) or the terminally ill (patients who have a disease that is incurable and who will die regardless of treatment).	
2, Death must be imminent (likely to occur within 6 months).	
3. Ambiguous terms may be difficult to later interpret.	
4. There is no proxy decision maker, so:	
• It requires prediction of final illness scenario and available treatment.	
• It requires physician to make decisions on the basis of an interpretation of a document.	

While playing an important role in unique circumstances, advance directives are not a substitute for adequate communication among physicians, patients, and family about end-of-life decision making and, in themselves, do not substantially enhance physician-patient communication or decision-making [53].

Table 3. Power of Attorney for Healthcare (PAHC). Source: Junkerman C, Schiedermayer D: Practical Ethics for Students, Interns, and Residents: A Short Reference Manual. Frederick, MD: University Publishing Group, Inc.,1998, p. 58. Copyright 1998 by University Publishing Group. Used with permission. May not be copied without the express written permission of University Publishing Group. Provided by Paul J. Hoehner, M.D., Johns Hopkins.

Activation of PAHC
Lack of decision-making capacity must be certified by two physicians or one physician and a psychologist who have examined the patient. Until then, the patient makes all the decisions.
Advantages
1. Physician has someone to talk with ñ a proxy, a knowledgeable surrogate ñ who can provide a substituted judgment of how the patient would have chosen. If the agent is unable to provide a substituted judgment, the agent and physician together can use the best-interest standard (how a reasonable person might choose in consideration of the benefit-burden concept of proportionality).
2. Provides flexibility; this decreases ambiguity and uncertainty because there is no way to predict all possible scenarios.
3. Authority of agent can be limited as person desires.
4. Avoids family conflict about rightful agent.
5. Provides legal immunity for physicians who follow dictates.
6. Allows appointment of a nonrelative (especially valuable for persons who may be alienated from their families).
7. Most forms can be completed without an attorney.
8. Principal may add specific instructions to the agent, such as the following: *"I value a full life more than a long life. If my suffering is intense and irreversible, or if I have lost the ability to interact with others and have no reasonable hope of regaining this ability even though I have no terminal illness, I do not want to have my life prolonged. I would then ask not to be subjected to surgery or to resuscitation procedures, or to intensive care services or to other life-prolonging measures, including the administration of antibiotics or blood products or artificial nutrition and hydration."* (Adapted with permission from Bok S: Personal directions from care at the end of life. N Engl J Med 295:362-369, 1976.) ©2018 P. HOEHNER JOHNS HOPKINS

DNAR ORDERS IN THE OPERATING ROOM

The anesthesiologist is most likely to come into contact with ethical issues involving advance directives when a patient is scheduled for surgery with a "do-not-resuscitate" order (DNR, or the preferred and more realistic terminology "do-not-attempt-resuscitation," DNAR) or more comprehensive forms directing limiting resuscitation attempts on the chart, such as Maryland's "Medical Orders for Life-Sustaining Treatment" or **MOLST**. MOLST forms and similar order forms were developed to give individuals the opportunity to express their desires regarding the treatment they should receive if they are in a life-limiting situation. These are not the same as an advance directive or a healthcare power of attorney as these are legal documents that may be open to interpretation. MOLST forms and similar standardized documents were designed for emergency and other medical personnel who often have to make rapid decisions whether to start life-support procedures. They are to follow the instruction on these forms rather than interpreting other types of legal documentation.

Anesthesiologists and surgeons are generally reluctant to proceed with surgical intervention if they are not allowed to intervene in the dying process. They feel that consent for anesthesia and surgery implies consent for resuscitation and is inconsistent with a DNAR order [54, 55]. Anesthesiologists tend to claim that the induction and maintenance of anesthesia can often involve creating conditions in which resuscitation is required [54]. Indeed, anesthesia itself has at times been referred to as a "controlled resuscitation." Since anesthetic agents or procedures may create conditions requiring resuscitation, the anesthesiologist ought to have the right to correct those conditions when possible. Surgeons and physicians doing other procedures use similar arguments to claim that if cardiac or pulmonary arrest is a consequence of their actions they should be allowed to prevent or reverse those conditions. One must not simply assume DNAR suspension in the perioperative period and not discuss this assumption with the patient/guardian.

This dilemma represents a **classic problem** in the principled approach to medical ethics: the conflict of two or more *prima facie* ethical principles. If the physician chooses to act paternalistically to provide what is believed to be the best treatment at the time, he is giving precedence to the concept of beneficence over the patient's autonomy. If, on the other hand, the physician acts to preserve patient autonomy, he may feel that the duty to do good, as directed by the principle of beneficence, has been compromised. Further complicating the issue is that "DNAR" has multiple definitions and interpretations and involves a spectrum of procedures that the general public is not aware of [56].

While automatic suspension of DNAR orders during a surgical procedure and for an arbitrary period postoperatively is the most unambiguous and straightforward policy, it is now argued that this is inappropriate [57, 58]. Statements from both the American Society of Anesthesiologists and the American College of Surgeons recognize that this policy effectively removes patients from the decision-making process, even if they are willing to accept the risk of operative mortality. They recommend instead a policy of "required reconsideration" of the DNAR order, as the patient who undergoes a surgical procedure faces a different risk/benefit ratio. Both statements are, however, ambiguous about just how resuscitation is to be handled in the OR. Two alternatives are presented: **1)** to suspend the DNAR order in the perioperative period and **2)** to limit resuscitation to certain procedures and techniques. Because of the complexities surrounding the nature of resuscitation, public misconceptions and lack of awareness of these complexities, and the desire to honor the goals reflected in a patient's decision to forego CPR, a third alternative has been proposed involving a values-centered [56] or goal-directed [59] approach. By ascertaining the patient's goals, values, and preferences rather than individual procedures, the anesthesiologist is given greater flexibility in honoring the objectives of the DNAR order within the clinical context of the arrest. While seeking to honor both the autonomy of the patient and the physician's duty to beneficence within the spirit of the original DNAR order, this alternative is not without its problems [60]. The establishment of a physician-patient relationship that will facilitate a full understanding of a patient's values and goals is a daunting, if not impossible, task for the anesthesiologist confronted with the demands of a limited preoperative encounter. These concerns may be even more profound in the elderly population [61]. Physicians have not been good at predicting the wishes of their patients regarding resuscitation in other situations, even after discussion has taken place [62 - 64]. It does, however, provide a third alternative and recognizes that, despite its practical limitations and high regard for patient autonomy in our society, there must always exist a degree of physician-patient trust in any clinical encounter.

Anesthesiologists need to be actively involved in their own institutions to develop policies for DNAR orders in the OR. Open communication among the anesthesiologist, surgeon, and patient or family must exist to reach an agreement about DNAR status. Appropriate exceptions to suspension of a DNAR order in the OR should be honored. Timing of reinstitution of DNAR status should also be addressed and agreed upon before the procedure. Actual experience shows that very few times will a patient insist on a DNAR status during the procedure.

TREATMENT FUTILITY

With respect to informed consent, what if the patient's decision is counter to the recommendations of the anesthesiologist or amounts to something the anesthesiologist regards as dangerous? Must the physician necessarily do whatever a patient wants? In short, no. In non-emergent circumstances, physicians are not obligated to provide care that they feel is not in their patients' best interest. "First, do no harm" is the operative principle in these situations. It is important again to distinguish in these cases the negative and positive rights based on or related to the principle of respect for personal autonomy and to recognize that the limits on positive rights may be greater than the limits on negative rights. For example, the positive right to request a particular treatment may be severely limited by appropriate clinical standards of care, physician judgment, or just allocation schemes. <u>Clinicians should, however, be very cautious when making this claim and should only do so if absolutely convinced that no other options are available</u>.

Occasionally, physicians have found it necessary to justify unilaterally deciding that certain medical interventions (such as CPR) are "futile" and withhold these interventions even when a patient or a patient's family wants them. The notion of medical futility is particularly confusing and open to different interpretations and abuses. "Futility" can be defined in several senses. "**Strict sense futility**" or "**medical" futility** <u>is defined when a medical intervention has no demonstrable physiological benefit</u>, *e.g.* when there have been no survivors after CPR under the given circumstances in well-designed studies, or in cases of progressive septic or cardiogenic shock despite maximal treatment. There are no obligations for physicians to provide medically futile treatment, even when families want "everything done." Unilateral decisions to withhold treatment (such as DNAR orders) are appropriate under these circumstances. Usually a DNAR order may be written on the basis of "futility" when two or more staff physicians concur in writing and give justification for their decision. The patient or surrogate need not agree with the decision but must be notified. If there is disagreement, an ethics consultation may be appropriate and helpful.

It is rare that a given medical intervention is unlikely to have any physiological effect whatsoever and hence futility may also be defined in a "less strict sense." In this instance there may be a low survival rate but the rate is not zero. In this case, while the physician may have the particular expertise to determine whether a particular intervention is reasonable according to a particular standard of reasonableness, setting a particular standard involves a value judgment that goes beyond that expertise. For <u>example</u>, a 79 year old cancer patient wants CPR in the event that he suffers cardiopulmonary arrest because he believes that any chance that CPR will restore cardiopulmonary function is worthwhile and that any prolongation of his life is also valuable and worthwhile (for instance, by allowing for a family member to return from overseas). While the physician may assess that the chance of CPR restoring function is $x\%$, x is greater than zero and whether the chance of restoring function is reasonable, valuable, or worthwhile only if it is greater than $x\%$ depends primarily on the patient's own values. Unilateral decisions may not be appropriate in this instance, and discussions with the patient and family should be initiated to provide information and advice.

While a physician may have the expertise to assess whether a particular intervention is likely to achieve a specified outcome, determining whether an outcome is an appropriate or valuable objective for a patient is dependent on the patient's own value judgments. A medical intervention can be futile in a third sense when it will have no reasonable chance to achieve the patient's goals and objectives. For example, CPR is futile in this sense if there is no reasonable chance that it will achieve the patient's goal of leaving the hospital and living an independent life. Since medical interventions are futile in relation to the patient's goals, this sense of futility provides a very limited basis for unilateral decisions to withhold medication interventions that patients want. The AMA Council of Judicial and Ethical Affairs has commented that resuscitative efforts "would be considered futile if they could not be expected to achieve the goals expressed by the informed patient. This definition of futility not only respects the autonomy and value judgments of individual patients but also allows for the professional judgment and guidance of physicians who render care to patients" [65].

Because the term **"futility"** tends to communicate a false sense of scientific objectivity and finality and to obscure the inherent evaluative nature of the judgments, it is recommended that physicians avoid using the term to justify unilateral decisions to withhold life-sustaining treatment. Rather, physicians should explain the specific grounds for concluding that interventions generally, or particular life-sustaining measures, are inappropriate in the given circumstances. Whereas the statement that a given intervention is futile tends to discourage discussion, explaining the grounds for a given judgment in light of the circumstances and with an understanding of the patient's own values and goals tends to invite discussion and point it in the right direction.

TREATMENT REDIRECTION AND PALLIATIVE CARE

Jean Paul Sartre said that "the meaning of life is found in death", and how we deal with the aging process determines how we deal with death and our philosophy of life. This is most important for the physician and patient when faced with end-o--life decision-making involving treatment redirection and palliative care options.

Treatment redirection refers to that point in the patient's care plan when the patient or surrogate, along with the health care team, recognizes the need to move from aggressive curative treatment to supportive palliative care. The 1995 SUPPORT study found that as many as 50% of patients were subjected to burdensome, curative treatment because the patient, family, and physician had not recognized or discussed the realities of the patient's condition [Investigators 1995]. **Potter suggests three barriers to meeting the need for treatment redirection** [66]. **First,** clinicians and patients often are narrowly focused on curative or ameliorative intervention. Lack of communication between the physician, who assumes that "they want everything done," and the patients and families, who have different expectations, contributes to this problem. Furthermore, patients and their families often assume that physicians have reliable knowledge about what therapies are effective and which are not because of their intense focus on curative treatment. A study by Feinstein, however, shows that evidence-based medical decisions can only be claimed for less than 20% of clinical situations [67].

Secondly, physicians and patients are often reluctant or unable to discuss palliation as a treatment option [68]. While evidence suggests that physicians are more willing to withhold or withdraw treatment from seriously ill patients [69], patients and families continue to report that there is a lack of physician communication in the area of shifting treatment to palliative care [70]. Disparity of beliefs and preferences causes much of this communication problem.

Finally, there is a lack of knowledge of and confidence in palliative care by both physicians [71] and society [72]. Part of the problem is that patients are referred to palliative care and hospice programs far too late in their hospital course to do any good. Furthermore, Potter notes that, "although there is a growing trend toward patients wanting to be in control of their own death, cultural diversity factors, belief in the power of medical technology, and a strong tendency to deny death prevent a working consensus about how to approach the experience of dying." [66] Patients and their families may also be suspicious that palliative care is a way to save money, a form of rationing, although there is no empirical evidence that palliative care is more cost effective [73].

Effective treatment-redirection involves three sequential steps [66]. **1)** There must be a system to recognize clues, both patient signals and physiologic signs, to indicate that the current form of treatment may not be wanted or may not be warranted [74]. **2)** There must be **deliberation** as part of the informed consent process that focuses on the appropriateness of the current treatment options. Potter reminds one that "because the patient is embedded in a social context of family and friends, there must be an inclusive attitude that searches out the wider origin of beliefs and preferences in the patient's moral community" [66]. Furthermore, the health care providers themselves must analyze their own personal beliefs and preferences that can create biases and distort clinical judgment. An open dialogue is a necessary part of the deliberation process. **3)** Finally, there must be an **implementation** plan that activates excellent palliative care [51]. The aim is for both the patient and the health care team to make a smooth transition from the ultimate goal of curing to that of caring.

END-OF-LIFE CARE

End-of-life palliative care options and decision making have become increasingly complicated as new forms of therapy and pain control become available. **Pain control** in the terminal stages of many illnesses is one of the primary goals of effective palliative care and is an area where anesthesiologists have a great deal to offer. One of the most pervasive causes of anxiety among patients, their families, and the public is the perception that physicians' efforts toward the relief of pain are sadly deficient. Studies indicate that their fears may be justified. In a study of 1227 elderly patients, approximately 20% experienced moderate or severe pain during the last month of life and the final 6 hours before death [75].

In another study of a random sample of 200 elderly community residents in the last month before death, 66% had pain all or most of the time [76]. Pain influenced behavioral competence, perceived quality of life, psychological well being, depression, and diminished happiness. There is concern that medical, radiation, and surgical oncologists are not effectively treating the pain of patients with cancer [77].

Fear of inadequate pain relief during the terminal stages of illness may be responsible for the increasing interest in euthanasia and physician-assisted suicide (PAS). It is now commonly accepted that the administration of large quantities of narcotic analgesics is not euthanasia when the purpose is to alleviate pain and suffering, not to shorten the life of the patient. Wanzer *et al.* note that,

In the patient whose dying process is irreversible, the balance between minimizing pain and suffering and potentially hastening death should be struck clearly in favor of pain relief. Narcotics and other pain medications should be given in whatever dose and by whatever route is necessary for relief. It is morally correct to increase the dose of narcotics to whatever dose is needed, even though the medication may contribute to the depression of respiration or blood pressure, the dulling of consciousness or even death, providing the primary goal of the physician is to relieve suffering. The proper dose of pain medication is the dose that is sufficient to relieve pain and suffering, even to the point of unconsciousness [78].

In this regard, there is clearly a strong need for increased physician and patient education as well as careful ethical analysis.

The terminal stages of the dying process can be accompanied by a number of other disturbing symptoms, both for the family and the patient. Symptoms recorded in the last 48 hours of life include noisy and moist breathing (death rattle), restlessness and agitation, incontinence of urine, dyspnea, retention of urine, nausea and vomiting, sweating, jerking, twitching, plucking, confusion, and delirium [79 - 81]. Appropriate palliative care must take into account the comfort and care of the patient with regard to these symptoms as well [82, 83].

Despite even the highest quality of palliative care, <u>many patients still report significant pain one week before death</u> [84], some of whom request help in hastening death. Furthermore, patients request a hastened death not simply because of unrelieved pain, but because of the wide variety of other unrelieved physical symptoms in combination with loss of meaning, dignity, and independence [85].

Confusion may exist about the physician's moral responsibility for contributing to the patient's death. The principle of double effect plays an important role in ethical decision making in these instances. **Double effect** <u>acknowledges that the intent and desired effect of treatment is mitigation of symptoms rather than cessation of life, even though life may be shortened</u>. As commonly formulated, the principle stipulates that one may rightfully cause evil (shortening of life) through an act of choice (treatment of pain) **if four conditions are verified: 1)** the act itself, apart from the evil caused, is good or at least indifferent; **2)** the good effect of the act is what the agent intends directly, only permitting the evil effect; **3)** the good effect must not come about by means of the evil effect; and **4)** there must be some proportionately grave reason for permitting the evil effect to occur [86].

PAS differs from euthanasia in that the physician is not the direct agent in PAS whereby in euthanasia the physician is the direct agent. However, **not all ethicists agree** that PAS and euthanasia differ significantly because of agency. Anesthesiologists should be particularly concerned with the debate for two reasons: **1)** because of their unique skills, anesthesiologists may play a very active role as practitioners of euthanasia [87] and **2)** the fear of uncontrolled pain relief, an area that anesthesiologists can provide particular expertise, is a primary motivation for euthanasia and PAS [88].

The politics of euthanasia and PAS remain controversial. **Physicians should be concerned** <u>that renewed interest in euthanasia and PAS will not divert attention from the pressings concerns of adequate pain control, treatment of depression, and symptom management in the terminally ill and should actively seek alternate ways to address patient worries regarding loss of control, indignity, and dependence during the final stages of an illness</u>. The elderly, particularly the severely demented, are at the cutting edge of the debate over PAS and VAE. "Senicide" is a very real entity in cultural anthropology. It is not unthinkable that in our aging society pressure will mount to take moral guidance from anthropological data, with economic concerns replacing the nomadic [89]. **Physicians need to resolve** not to let public policy matters interfere with their duty to the health and welfare of their individual patients, regardless of age, and to **maintain a commitment to both healing and caring.** Anesthesiologists can provide a unique service to their physician colleagues, patients, and general population through education and consultation regarding chronic pain and symptom control in the terminally ill. Measures must go beyond education and become an established part of quality assurance [90]. Anesthesiologists can contribute by assisting their hospitals with means to monitor the treatment of patients in pain. Despite the growing acceptance among the general population and the medical community regarding physician involvement in euthanasia, it is not compatible with the healer's mission and art. **At its core, killing patients should never be the means by which symptoms or sufferings, psychological or physical, are relieved.**

CONCLUSION

Every physician patient encounter is an ethical encounter. Anesthesiologists are given a very perfunctory period of time during which they must examine a patient, establish a relationship with the patient, determine the patient's wishes, and obtain consent. This chapter has attempted to give a basis with which to understand ethical concepts such as principlism, personal autonomy, shared decision making, decision making capacity, competency, substituted judgement, voluntarism, adequate disclosure, consent elements, autonomous authorization, advanced directives, living wills, Power of Attorney for Healthcare Proxy, DNR/DNAR, treatment futility, treatment redirection, palliative care, end of life care, double effect, physician assisted suicide, euthanasia, and senilicide.

Anesthesiologists have an ethical duty to put the patient's medical interests paramount. Surgeons and proceduralists have placed patient care solely upon the anesthesiologists, since they only acknowledge responsibility for technical aspects of their procedure. Most physicians are now employees of large healthcare systems which are focused on through put and profit. Thus, anesthesiologists who are the primary care physicians in the perioperative period and principle patient advocates are placed into conflict with surgeons and the healthcare system which views them as hindering through-put and interfering with profit. Despite the healthcare system drive to make human beings into objects, patients are human beings. **Medicine is foremost a moral endeavor.**

CONSENT FOR PUBLICATION

Not applicable.

CONFLICT OF INTEREST

The author (editor) declares no conflict of interest, financial or otherwise.

ACKNOWLEDGEMENTS

Paul J. Hoehner, MD, a former member of the Presidential Advisory Counsel on Medical Ethics, provides an updated primer for the nonethicist on Medical Ethics. This work is based on Dr. Hoehner's prior works and is designed to serve as an introduction to medical ethics for the anesthetist [1 - 3].

Ethical Management of the Elderly Patient, Geriatric Anesthesiology, by Paul J. Hoehner, MD, 2008

Ethical Decisions in Perioperative Elder Care, Anesthesiology Clinics of North America, by Paul J. Hoehner, MD, 2000

Ethical Aspects of Informed Consent in Obstetric Anesthesia – New Challenges and Solutions, Journal of Clinical Anesthesia, by Paul J. Hoehner, MD, 2003

REFERENCES

[1]   Hoehner PJ. Ethical management of the elderly patient. Geriatric Anesthesiology 2008.
        [http://dx.doi.org/10.1007/978-0-387-72527-7_4]

[2]   Hoehner PJ. Ethical decisions in perioperative elder care. Anesthesiol Clin North America 2000; 18(1): 159-181, vii-viii.
        [http://dx.doi.org/10.1016/S0889-8537(05)70155-3] [PMID: 10935006]

[3]   Hoehner PJ. Ethical aspects of informed consent in obstetric anesthesia--new challenges and solutions. J Clin Anesth 2003; 15(8): 587-600.
        [http://dx.doi.org/10.1016/S0952-8180(02)00505-6] [PMID: 14724080]

[4]   Dunstan GR. The doctor as the responsible moral agent.Doctors' Decisions: Ethical Conflicts in Medical Practice. New York: Oxford University Press 1989; pp. 1-9.

[5]   Marcum JA. An Introductory Philosophy of Medicine: Humanizing Modern Medicine. Dordrecht: Springer 2008.

[6]   Hoehner PJ. The myth of value neutrality. AMA. Virtual Mentor 2006; 8(5): 341-4.
        [PMID: 23232432]

[7]   Joshi GP. The anesthesiologist as perioperative physician. ASA Newsl 2008; 72(4)

[8]   Grocott MP, Pearse RM. Perioperative medicine: the future of anaesthesia? Br J Anaesth 2012; 108(5): 723-6.
        [http://dx.doi.org/10.1093/bja/aes124] [PMID: 22499744]

[9]   Kain ZN, Fitch JC, Kirsch JR, Mets B, Pearl RG. Future of anesthesiology is perioperative medicine: a call for action. Anesthesiology 2015; 122(6): 1192-5.
        [http://dx.doi.org/10.1097/ALN.0000000000000680] [PMID: 25886775]

[10]   Wacker J, Staender S. The role of the anesthesiologist in perioperative patient safety. Curr Opin Anaesthesiol 2014; 27(6): 649-56.
        [http://dx.doi.org/10.1097/ACO.0000000000000124] [PMID: 25233191]

[11]   Carr VF. Dual agency and fiduciary responsibilities in modern medicine. Physician Exec 2005; 31(6): 56-8.
[PMID: 16382654]

[12]   Tilburt JC. Addressing dual agency: getting specific about the expectations of professionalism. Am J Bioeth 2014; 14(9): 29-36.
[http://dx.doi.org/10.1080/15265161.2014.935878] [PMID: 25127273]

[13]   Brody HA. New forces shaping the patient-physician relationship. Virtual Mentor 2009; 11(3): 253-6.
[http://dx.doi.org/10.1001/virtualmentor.2009.11.3.msoc1-0903] [PMID: 23194909]

[14]   Francis LP. The Physician – Patient Relationship and a National Health Information Network The Physician-Patient Relationship as a Trust Relationship 2009.

[15]   Reich A. Disciplined doctors: The electronic medical record and physicians' changing relationship to medical knowledge. Social Science & Medicine 2012; 74(7): 1021-8.

[16]   Wright A. You, me, and the computer makes three: navigating the doctor-patient relationship in the age of electronic health records. J Gen Intern Med 2015; 30(1): 1-2.
[http://dx.doi.org/10.1007/s11606-014-3090-8] [PMID: 25385210]

[17]   Margalit RS, Roter D, Dunevant MA, Larson S, Reis S. Electronic medical record use and physician-patient communication: an observational study of Israeli primary care encounters. Patient Educ Couns 2006; 61(1): 134-41.
[http://dx.doi.org/10.1016/j.pec.2005.03.004] [PMID: 16533682]

[18]   Cheshire WP. Can electronic medical records make physicians more ethical? Virtual Mentor 2014; 30(3): 135-42.

[19]   Childress JF. The place of autonomy in bioethics. Hastings Cent Rep 1990; 20(1): 12-7.
[http://dx.doi.org/10.2307/3562967] [PMID: 2179164]

[20]   Meisel A, Kuczewski M. Legal and ethical myths about informed consent. Arch Intern Med 1996; 156(22): 2521-6.
[http://dx.doi.org/10.1001/archinte.1996.00440210023002] [PMID: 8951294]

[21]   Beauchamp TL, Childress JF. Principles of Biomedical Ethics. New York: Oxford University Press 1994.

[22]   Losing a Million Minds: Confronting the Tragedy of Alzheimer's Disease and Other Dementias. Washington, D.C.: U.S. Government Printing Office 1987.

[23]   Marson DC, McInturff B, Hawkins L, Bartolucci A, Harrell LE. Consistency of physician judgments of capacity to consent in mild Alzheimer's disease. J Am Geriatr Soc 1997; 45(4): 453-7.
[http://dx.doi.org/10.1111/j.1532-5415.1997.tb05170.x] [PMID: 9100714]

[24]   Buchanan AE, Brock DW. Deciding for Others: The Ethics of Surrogate Decision Making. Cambridge: Cambridge University Press 1989.

[25]   Deciding to Forego Life-Sustaining Treatment. Washington, D.C.: U.S. Government Printing Office 1982.

[26]   Report: "Making Health Care Decisions, Volume One. Washington, D.C.: U.S. Government Printing Office 1992.

[27]   Appelbaum PS, Grisso T. Assessing patients' capacities to consent to treatment. N Engl J Med 1988; 319(25): 1635-8.
[http://dx.doi.org/10.1056/NEJM198812223192504] [PMID: 3200278]

[28]   Fellows LK. Competency and consent in dementia. J Am Geriatr Soc 1998; 46(7): 922-6.
[http://dx.doi.org/10.1111/j.1532-5415.1998.tb02734.x] [PMID: 9670887]

[29]   Fitten LJ, Lusky R, Hamann C. Assessing treatment decision-making capacity in elderly nursing home residents. J Am Geriatr Soc 1990; 38(10): 1097-104.

[http://dx.doi.org/10.1111/j.1532-5415.1990.tb01372.x] [PMID: 2229863]

[30] Lieberman M. The physician's duty to disclose risks of treatment. Bull N Y Acad Med 1974; 50(8): 943-8.
[PMID: 4528052]

[31] Ingelfinger FJ. Informed (but uneducated) consent. N Engl J Med 1972; 287(9): 465-6.
[http://dx.doi.org/10.1056/NEJM197208312870912] [PMID: 5044921]

[32] Taub HA. Informed consent, memory and age. Gerontologist 1980; 20(6): 686-90.
[http://dx.doi.org/10.1093/geront/20.6.686] [PMID: 7203092]

[33] Johnston SC, Pfeifer MP. Patient and physician roles in end-of-life decision making. J Gen Intern Med 1998; 13(1): 43-5.
[http://dx.doi.org/10.1046/j.1525-1497.1998.00008.x] [PMID: 9462494]

[34] Stiggelbout AM, Kiebert GM. A role for the sick role. Patient preferences regarding information and participation in clinical decision-making. Canadian Medical Association Journal 1997; 157(4): m 383-389.

[35] Strull WM, Lo B, Charles G. Do patients want to participate in medical decision making? JAMA 1984; 252(21): 2990-4.
[http://dx.doi.org/10.1001/jama.1984.03350210038026] [PMID: 6502860]

[36] Starr TJ, Pearlman RA, Uhlmann RF. Quality of life and resuscitation decisions in elderly patients. J Gen Intern Med 1986; 1(6): 373-9.
[http://dx.doi.org/10.1007/BF02596420] [PMID: 3794836]

[37] Guidelines for the Determination of Decisional Incapacity. Midwest Bioethics Center Bulletin 1996 March; 1-13.

[38] Weinstock R, Copelan R, Bagheri A. Competence to give informed consent for medical procedures. Bull Am Acad Psychiatry Law 1984; 12(2): 117-25.
[PMID: 6743844]

[39] Roth LH, Meisel A, Lidz CW. Tests of competency to consent to treatment. Am J Psychiatry 1977; 134(3): 279-84.
[http://dx.doi.org/10.1176/ajp.134.3.279] [PMID: 842704]

[40] Grisso T, Appelbaum TS. Assessing Competence to Consent to Treatment: A Guide for Physicians and Other Health Professionals. Oxford: Oxford University Press 1998.

[41] Pinkerton JV, Finnerty JJ. Resolving the clinical and ethical dilemma involved in fetal-maternal conflicts. Am J Obstet Gynecol 1996; 175(2): 289-95.
[http://dx.doi.org/10.1016/S0002-9378(96)70137-0] [PMID: 8765244]

[42] Dworkin G. Autonomy and behavior control. Hastings Cent Rep 1976; 6(1): 23-8.
[http://dx.doi.org/10.2307/3560358] [PMID: 1254455]

[43] Hardwig J. What about the family? Hastings Cent Rep 1990; 20(2): 5-10.
[http://dx.doi.org/10.2307/3562603] [PMID: 2318632]

[44] Waisel DB, Truog RD. The benefits of the explanation of the risks of anesthesia in the day surgery patient. J Clin Anesth 1995; 7(3): 200-4.
[http://dx.doi.org/10.1016/0952-8180(94)00047-8] [PMID: 7669309]

[45] Waltz JR, Scheunemann T. Informed consent and therapy. Northwest Univ Law Rev 1970; 64: 628.

[46] Gild WM. Informed consent: a review. Anesth Analg 1989; 68(5): 649-53.
[http://dx.doi.org/10.1213/00000539-198905000-00019] [PMID: 2655496]

[47] Byrne DJ, Napier A, Cuschieri A. How informed is signed consent? Br Med J (Clin Res Ed) 1988; 296(6625): 839-40.
[http://dx.doi.org/10.1136/bmj.296.6625.839] [PMID: 3130937]

[48] Cassileth BR, Zupkis RV, Sutton-Smith K, March V. Informed consent -- why are its goals imperfectly realized? N Engl J Med 1980; 302(16): 896-900.
[http://dx.doi.org/10.1056/NEJM198004173021605] [PMID: 7360175]

[49] Clark SK, Leighton BL, Seltzer JL. A risk-specific anesthesia consent form may hinder the informed consent process. J Clin Anesth 1991; 3(1): 11-3.
[http://dx.doi.org/10.1016/0952-8180(91)90199-W] [PMID: 2007035]

[50] Knapp RM. Legal view of informed consent for anesthesia during labor. Anesthesiology 1990; 72(1): 211.
[http://dx.doi.org/10.1097/00000542-199001000-00039] [PMID: 2297126]

[51] Teno JM, Licks S, Lynn J, *et al.* Do advance directives provide instructions that direct care? SUPPORT Investigators. J Am Geriatr Soc 1997; 45(4): 508-12.
[http://dx.doi.org/10.1111/j.1532-5415.1997.tb05179.x] [PMID: 9100722]

[52] Making treatment decisions for incapacitated older adults without advance directives. J Am Geriatr Soc 1996; 44(8): 986-7.
[http://dx.doi.org/10.1111/j.1532-5415.1996.tb01874.x] [PMID: 8708314]

[53] Teno J, Lynn J, Wenger N, *et al.* Advance directives for seriously ill hospitalized patients: effectiveness with the patient self-determination act and the SUPPORT intervention. J Am Geriatr Soc 1997; 45(4): 500-7.
[http://dx.doi.org/10.1111/j.1532-5415.1997.tb05178.x] [PMID: 9100721]

[54] Truog RD. "Do-not-resuscitate" orders during anesthesia and surgery. Anesthesiology 1991; 74(3): 606-8.
[http://dx.doi.org/10.1097/00000542-199103000-00030] [PMID: 2001038]

[55] Clemency MV, Thompson NJ. "Do not resuscitate" (DNR) orders and the anesthesiologist: a survey. Anesth Analg 1993; 76(2): 394-401.
[PMID: 8424522]

[56] Thurber CF. Public awareness of the nature of CPR: a case for values-centered advance directives. J Clin Ethics 1996; 7(1): 55-9.
[PMID: 8790699]

[57] Statement on Advance Directives by Patients: Do Not Resuscitate in the Operating Room. American College of Surgeons Bulletin. ACS Bulletin 1994; 79: 29.

[58] Ethical Guidelines for the Anesthesia Care of Patients with Do Not Resuscitate Orders or Other Directives That Limit Treatment (1993). ASA Standards, Guidelines and Statements 1997.

[59] Truog RD, Waisel DB, Burns JP. DNR in the OR: a goal-directed approach. Anesthesiology 1999; 90(1): 289-95.
[http://dx.doi.org/10.1097/00000542-199901000-00034] [PMID: 9915337]

[60] Jackson SH, Van Norman GA. Goals- and values-directed approach to informed consent in the "DNR" patient presenting for surgery: more demanding of the anesthesiologist? Anesthesiology 1999; 90(1): 3-6.
[http://dx.doi.org/10.1097/00000542-199901000-00003] [PMID: 9915306]

[61] Sayers GM, Schofield I, Aziz M. An analysis of CPR decision-making by elderly patients. J Med Ethics 1997; 23(4): 207-12.
[http://dx.doi.org/10.1136/jme.23.4.207] [PMID: 9279741]

[62] Krumholz HM, Phillips RS, Hamel MB, *et al.* Resuscitation preferences among patients with severe congestive heart failure: results from the SUPPORT project. Circulation 1998; 98(7): 648-55.
[http://dx.doi.org/10.1161/01.CIR.98.7.648] [PMID: 9715857]

[63] Rosin AJ, Sonnenblick M. Autonomy and paternalism in geriatric medicine. The Jewish ethical approach to issues of feeding terminally ill patients, and to cardiopulmonary resuscitation. J Med

Ethics 1998; 24(1): 44-8.
[http://dx.doi.org/10.1136/jme.24.1.44] [PMID: 9549682]

[64] Uhlmann RF, Pearlman RA, Cain KC. Physicians' and spouses' predictions of elderly patients' resuscitation preferences. J Gerontol 1988; 43(5): M115-21.
[http://dx.doi.org/10.1093/geronj/43.5.M115] [PMID: 3418031]

[65] Guidelines for the appropriate use of do-not-resuscitate orders. Council on Ethical and Judicial Affairs, American Medical Association. JAMA 1991; 265(14): 1868-71.
[http://dx.doi.org/10.1001/jama.1991.03460140096034] [PMID: 2005737]

[66] Potter RL. Treatment redirection: moving from curative to palliative care. Bioeth Forum 1998; 14(2): 3-9.
[PMID: 11657172]

[67] Feinstein AR, Horwitz RI. Problems in the "evidence" of "evidence-based medicine". Am J Med 1997; 103(6): 529-35.
[http://dx.doi.org/10.1016/S0002-9343(97)00244-1] [PMID: 9428837]

[68] Weeks JC, Cook EF, O'Day SJ, *et al.* Relationship between cancer patients' predictions of prognosis and their treatment preferences. JAMA 1998; 279(21): 1709-14.
[http://dx.doi.org/10.1001/jama.279.21.1709] [PMID: 9624023]

[69] La Puma J, Silverstein MD, Stocking CB, Roland D, Siegler M. Life-sustaining treatment. A prospective study of patients with DNR orders in a teaching hospital. Arch Intern Med 1988; 148(10): 2193-8.
[http://dx.doi.org/10.1001/archinte.1988.00380100067015] [PMID: 3178377]

[70] Hanson LC, Danis M, Garrett J. What is wrong with end-of-life care? Opinions of bereaved family members. J Am Geriatr Soc 1997; 45(11): 1339-44.
[http://dx.doi.org/10.1111/j.1532-5415.1997.tb02933.x] [PMID: 9361659]

[71] Bulger RJ. Part I-the quest for mercy: the forgotten ingredient in health care reform. West J Med 1997; 167(5): 362-73.
[PMID: 18751092]

[72] Lynn J, Teno JM, Phillips RS, *et al.* Perceptions by family members of the dying experience of older and seriously ill patients. Ann Intern Med 1997; 126(2): 97-106.
[http://dx.doi.org/10.7326/0003-4819-126-2-199701150-00001] [PMID: 9005760]

[73] Emanuel EJ. Cost savings at the end of life. What do the data show? JAMA 1996; 275(24): 1907-14.
[http://dx.doi.org/10.1001/jama.1996.03530480049040] [PMID: 8648872]

[74] Randolph AG, Guyatt GH, Richardson WS. Prognosis in the intensive care unit: finding accurate and useful estimates for counseling patients. Crit Care Med 1998; 26(4): 767-72.
[http://dx.doi.org/10.1097/00003246-199804000-00031] [PMID: 9559618]

[75] Kaiser HE, Brock DB. Comparative aspects of the quality of life in cancer patients. In Vivo 1992; 6(4): 333-7.
[PMID: 1520836]

[76] Moss MS, Lawton MP, Glicksman A. The role of pain in the last year of life of older persons. J Gerontol 1991; 46(2): 51-7.
[http://dx.doi.org/10.1093/geronj/46.2.P51] [PMID: 1997576]

[77] Cherny NI, Catane R. Professional negligence in the management of cancer pain. A case for urgent reforms. Cancer 1995; 76(11): 2181-5.
[http://dx.doi.org/10.1002/1097-0142(19951201)76:11<2181::AID-CNCR2820761102>3.0.CO;2-F] [PMID: 8635019]

[78] Wanzer SH, Federman DD, Adelstein SJ, *et al.* The physician's responsibility toward hopelessly ill patients. A second look. N Engl J Med 1989; 320(13): 844-9.
[http://dx.doi.org/10.1056/NEJM198903303201306] [PMID: 2604764]

[79]   Martin EW. Confusion in the terminally ill: recognition and management. Am J Hosp Palliat Care 1990; 7(3): 20-4.
[http://dx.doi.org/10.1177/104990919000700310] [PMID: 2361108]

[80]   Lichter I, Hunt E. The last 48 hours of life. J Palliat Care 1990; 6(4): 7-15.
[PMID: 1704917]

[81]   Massie MJ, Holland J, Glass E. Delirium in terminally ill cancer patients. Am J Psychiatry 1983; 140(8): 1048-50.
[http://dx.doi.org/10.1176/ajp.140.8.1048] [PMID: 6869591]

[82]   Voltz R, Borasio GD. Palliative therapy in the terminal stage of neurological disease. Journal of Neurology 1997; 244(Suppl): S2-10.

[83]   Power D, Kearney M. Management of the final 24 hours. Ir Med J 1992; 85(3): 93-5.
[PMID: 1383175]

[84]   Coyle N, Adelhardt J, Foley KM, Portenoy RK. Character of terminal illness in the advanced cancer patient: pain and other symptoms during the last four weeks of life. J Pain Symptom Manage 1990; 5(2): 83-93.
[http://dx.doi.org/10.1016/S0885-3924(05)80021-1] [PMID: 2348092]

[85]   Back AL, Wallace JI, Starks HE, Pearlman RA. Physician-assisted suicide and euthanasia in Washington State. Patient requests and physician responses. JAMA 1996; 275(12): 919-25.
[http://dx.doi.org/10.1001/jama.1996.03530360029034] [PMID: 8598619]

[86]   May WE. Double Effect. Encyclopedia of Bioethics. New York: The Free Press. New York 1978; pp. 316-20.

[87]   Benrubi GI. Euthanasia--the need for procedural safeguards. N Engl J Med 1992; 326(3): 197-9.
[http://dx.doi.org/10.1056/NEJM199201163260311] [PMID: 1727551]

[88]   Jonsen AR. To help the dying die--a new duty for anesthesiologists? Anesthesiology 1993; 78(2): 225-8.
[http://dx.doi.org/10.1097/00000542-199302000-00002] [PMID: 8439014]

[89]   Post SG. Euthanasia, Senicide, and the Aging Society. J Relig Gerontol 1991; 8(1): 57-65.
[http://dx.doi.org/10.1300/J078V08N01_05]

[90]   Hill CS Jr. When will adequate pain treatment be the norm? JAMA 1995; 274(23): 1881-2.
[http://dx.doi.org/10.1001/jama.1995.03530230067033] [PMID: 7500540]

CHAPTER 9

Interesting Cases

Mahmood Jaberi[*] and **Nathaniel McQuay**

Johns Hopkins Medical Institutions, Baltimore, Maryland, USA and University Hospital Cleveland, Cleveland, Ohio, USA

Abstract: The following section presents several clinical scenarios of cases which were notable for the impression left on the practitioner. Interesting diagnostic points are discussed. The hope is that these cases will help cement points that are addressed elsewhere in the book. Discussions are meant to be thought-provoking rather than definitive. Hopefully it will be enjoyable and beneficial.

Keywords: ARDS, ATLS Protocol, Blunt Cardiac Injury, Herniation, Primary Survey, Sudden Cardiac Death, Secondary Survey.

INTRODUCTION

In our daily practice, practitioners encounter situations that make indelible impressions that last with us throughout our careers. While these situations add to an individual's past experience, it is worthy to propagate this knowledge with other clinicians to empower them to save more lives. With advanced technology and newer approaches, the hospital course and outcome may be totally different than past experiences and new protocols may have to substitute for old ones. There is no doubt that the best outcome will be achieved by teams who work well in a system well-tuned for the care of such critical patients and where they have well-orchestrated systems and supporting members play a vital role in saving precious life. Advanced updated medical knowledge in the respective specialties combined with clinical competence are the pillars that support actions in these critical moments. In this section, a few common cases of critical patients are presented that may provoke the reader to think and consider new approaches and solutions.

[*] **Corresponding author Mahmood Jaberi, M.D.:** Johns Hopkins Medical Institutions, Baltimore, Maryland, USA and University Hospital Cleveland, Cleveland, Ohio, USA; Tel: (410) 550-0100; E-mail: mjaberi3@jhmi.edu

CASE 1

Background

A 41-year-old male was admitted to the burn service with 55% burn of body surface area. The patient was morbidly obese with hypertension, non-insulin dependent diabetes mellitus and sleep apnea. There was no previous history of substance abuse, peptic ulcer disease, esophageal varices, or coagulopathies. The patient eventually had a tracheostomy underwent multiple operative procedures for excision of burn wounds, debridements, and skin grafts and was having a successful recovery in the Burn Intensive Care Unit. Then one day during his fourth month post admission, the patient suddenly developed severe hematemesis with massive bleeding resulting in profound hypotension and tachycardia.

Presumptive Diagnosis

1. Gastric stress ulcer
2. Ruptured Varices
3. Fistula
4. Coagulopathy

Diagnostic Workup of Choice

1. Chest X-Ray
2. CBC with Coags
3. CT angiogram
4. Endoscopy

Continuation

A gastroenterology consult was obtained and an upper endoscopy was performed. Unfortunately, this was not conclusive because of the severe hemorrhage and massive blood volume in the stomach. After a Sengestaken-Blakemore esophagogastrostromy tube was placed, medical treatment was recommended. The patient's condition continued to deteriorate despite volume resuscitation and massive transfusion. The patient was then taken emergently to the operating room for an exploratory laparotomy and possible gastrectomy. In the operating room, the patient was actively resuscitated with blood, blood products, and correction of severe metabolic derangements. An open gastroscopy and duodenoscopy were inconclusive, and so it was decided to perform bilateral vagotomies and pyloroplasty to reduce blood loss. During the procedure it was noted that there was blood draining around the nasogastric tube. An upper esophagoscopy was immediately performed and heavy bleeding into the mid segment of esophagus was noted. Interventional radiology was consulted for an aortogram. The patient's vital signs continued to deteriorate with profound tachycardia and systolic pressure in the high 70's to low 80's despite volume, blood and vasopressors. An aortoesophageal fistula 7cm distal to the left subclavian was confirmed. Vascular surgery gained femoral access, placed an endovascular aortic graft and sealed the fistula. The patient became hemodynamically more stable. The patient was able to have a successful operative outcome and later was uneventfully able to be discharged alive and well from the hospital.

DISCUSSION

Upper gastrointestinal bleeding due to gastric stress ulcers is a well-known phenomenon for burn patients and so routine preventative treatment is administered. Massive hematemesis from esophageal, gastric and duodenal ulcers can occur. More often bleeding is from gastritis, gastric cancers, and esophageal varices. An aorto-esophageal fistula is a very uncommon, but usually fatal course of bleeding. 100 years ago Dubrueil described an aorto-esophageal fistula with the symptoms as described by Chiari as being mid thoracic pain, sentinal arterial hemorrhage, and fatal exsanguination. Etiologies for aorto-esophageal fistulas include thoracic aortic aneurysm, penetrating ulcers, mycotic aneurysm, cancer, and mediastinal tuberculosis. In this patient, this was most possibly formed by prolonged pressure necrosis of the naso-gastric tube on the descending aorta and the presence of scoliosis.

CASE 2

Background

A 45year old previously healthy male was a belted driver who had a motor vehicle accident with a T-bone crash to the front driver side door. Although there was almost 12 inches of intrusion of the front door, there was no airbag deployment or loss of consciousness. The patient was transported to a nearby hospital by ambulance because he was experiencing severe chest pain and difficulty breathing. On arrival at the local hospital, the patient was awake, alert, moving all extremities with the following vital signs BP 110/85 HR 114 RR high 20's oxygen saturation 96% on non-rebreather facemask. The primary survey found the patient with GCS of 15, no obvious bleeding, no spine or long bone fractures, with palpable pulses in all extremities, and neurologically intact. There was however decreased breath sounds with dullness on the left chest and multiple rib fractures with an emergency chest x-ray revealing whitening out of the left chest.

Presumptive Diagnosis

1. Acute MI
2. Aortic Rupture
3. Intercostal/Internal mammary tear
4. Diaphragmatic disruption

Diagnostic Workup of Choice

1. ABG, CK with Isos and troponins
2. FAST
3. CT with angio
4. TEE

Continuation

With the impression of multiple rib fractures and left hemothorax, a 38 French chest tube was placed with some difficulty in the fifth intercostal space in the midaxillary line. Initially 300cc of blood was drained from the chest. The patient however, worsened and became more hypotensive and tachycardic with blood pressures systolic in the low 80s and heart rate exceeding 140s; And the chest tube draining more than 1500cc of frank blood. The patient was transfused and emergently transferred to a level one trauma center with a presumptive diagnosis of ruptured aorta. On arrival, the patient was responsive with severe shortness of breath, profoundly tachypnic, tachycardic, and hypotensive with systolic blood pressure in the low 70s, HR 150's, RR 40s, SATS high 80's. The airway was secured, blood and volume resuscitation continued, and orogastric tube was placed, and a repeat chest x-ray was done. This revealed that the orogastric tube was in the left thorax with herniation of left diaphragm and intrusion of a abdominal contents into the left chest. The chest tube was removed and the patient was taken emergently to the operating room for exploratory laparotomy. In the operating room it was found that the chest tube had perforated the spleen which had herniated into the chest. A splenectomy was done, the diaphragm repaired, and the abdomen closed; and the patient rapidly recovered and was discharged home in a few days.

DISCUSSION

Chest tube for thoracostomy plays a vital role in the management of thoracic trauma and can be life saving for more than 80% of thoracic injuries. There are however 20% of patients who require re-insertion of chest tubes for recurrent pneumothorax, hemothorax, and other injuries. The occurrence of chest tube complications is higher in emergency room situations than in the operating rooms

[1]. Etach [2] retrospectively reviewed trauma patients who required chest tube placement, he found a complication rate of approximately 21% with emergentologist having a complication rate of 13% and surgeons having a complication rate of about 6%. Other variables for complication rate for chest tube placement include mechanism of injury, contamination factors, poly trauma, lung contusion and incomplete drainage of plural cavity. This is an unusual case of diaphragmatic rupture accentuated with a complicated thoracostomy □tube placement.

CASE 3

Background

A 26year old female non-belted driver was involved in a head-on collision with another vehicle. There was more than a 12 inch intrusion into the front of the car, airbags had deployed, the windshield was shattered, and the steering wheel was bent. The patient had a brief loss of consciousness at the scene initially, but then regained consciousness and was complaining of mid chest pain and shortness of breath. The patient was awake following commands and moving all extremities and she was transported to the trauma center. Upon arrival at the trauma center, the patient was conscious and co-operative but the vital signs were noted to be unstable with hypotension (systolic blood pressure of 75mm Hg and tachycardia (heart rate of 130bpm).

Presumptive Diagnosis

1. Cardiac rupture
2. Splenic laceration
3. Liver laceration
4. Aortic dissection

Diagnostic Workup of Choice

1. chest x-ray
2. FAST
3. CAT scan
4. Angiogram

Continuation

Intravenous access was quickly obtained; and an ultrasound was being performed when the patient lost consciousness. The EKG showed ventricular tachycardia which was followed by pulseless electrical activity. The ultrasound revealed hemopericardium as well as cardiac standstill. Chest compressions were immediately begun and the airway was secured with an endotracheal tube. Since there was hemopericardium, the chest was opened and the hemopericardium was evacuated and cardiac massage instituted. Rupture of the right ventricle was noted. The thoracotomy was extended and the ruptured ventricle was quickly sutured. Vital signs returned, resuscitation continued, as the patient was transferred to the operating room for further surgical evaluation. The patient's vital signs stabilized and the patient was able to have an uneventful course and was discharged home on hospital day six.

DISCUSSION

Cardiac rupture is usually fatal. There is no gold standard diagnostic test and the signs and symptoms can vary from simple chest ecchymosis to sudden death. The trauma team should always be vigilant and prepared to act aggressively to combat the unknown. Unless the team is experienced with a strong support system in place, the lack of diagnostic tests and extreme emergency of the situation make for a grim prognosis. Common causes of cardiac rupture, include multiple trauma injuries, high altitude falls, and penetrating cardiac injuries [3].

CASE 4

A 22 year old male jockey was brought to the trauma center. He had been thrown down the horse and had suffered a kick from the horse to his left chest wall. The patient had not lost consciousness and was transported on a long backboard with a cervical collar on for neck and spine stabilization. Primary and secondary surveys were stable. The patient was fully alert, communicative, able to move all extremities and had a GCS of 15. Physical exam revealed a small bruise on the left chest wall. There were no rib fractures and he had clear bilateral breath sounds. The EKG revealed a sinus tachycardia in the 120s, but blood pressure and oxygen saturation were normal. Once the trauma surveys were completed, routine blood work was drawn including blood test for alcohol and drugs. All blood work came back normal and the tests for alcohol and substances were also negative. A chest x-ray was done which was normal. The patient's vital signs had remained stable for well over an hour and the patient had no complaints.

What would be the most likely working diagnosis for this patient?

1. Cord compression
2. Blunt cardiac injury
3. Pulmonary hemorrhage
4. Anterior chest wall contusion

What would be the next step in management?

1. Chest CT
2. Evaluate for pulmonary contusion
3. Echocardiography
4. Discharge home

Continuation

About two hours after arrival, the patient developed ventricular tachycardia and became unconscious. The patient was resuscitated per ACLS protocol and after receiving electroshock cardioversion, his cardiac dysrhythmia (VT) reverted back to normal sinus rhythm. The patient regained consciousness and later was transferred to the cardiac intensive care unit for observation.

DISCUSSION

The lack of specific diagnostic tools or biomarker make the diagnosis of cardiac contusion after direct trauma to the chest wall difficult. Although blunt cardiac injury goes unnoticed for the most part and tends to resolve within 24 hours, a minority of patients may suffer catastrophic sequellae. Blunt cardiac injury most commonly presents as a dysrhythmia usually sinus tachycardia. Recent published guidelines on blunt cardiac injury recommend screening with combined EKG and troponin I. Concordance where both are negative essentially rules out blunt cardiac injury. Patients with an elevated troponin I and a normal EKG or normal troponin I and abnormal EKG warrant close observation in a monitored setting. Cardiac isoenzymes creatinine phosphokinase or CK-MB are also recommended in the screening process. The development of complications such as hypotension, malignant arrhythmias, or pulmonary edema warrants further work up to rule out a structural injury. The diagnostic evaluation of choice is echocardiography. If an optimal transthoracic echocardiogram cannot be obtained then a transesophageal echocardiogram is recommended. Patients with evidence of ischemia should undergo further workup with a cardiac catheterization or nuclear medicine studies [4, 5].

CASE 5

A 78year old male was a belted passenger in the front seat involved in a motor vehicle accident. The patients car had been hit from the rear. The patient was unconscious briefly at the scene, but had regained consciousness prior to arrival at the trauma center. On arrival, the patient had a GCS of 15, was alert, oriented followed commands appropriately and was able to move all extremities. After completion of primary and secondary surveys; cervical spine X-rays revealed a

C3 transverse process fracture, while FAST revealed hemoperitoneum. So, the patient was taken to the operating room for an exploratory laparotomy and hemostasis.

General anesthesia was induced with rapid sequence induction and neck immobilization. The endotracheal tube was atraumatically placed with cervical inline stabilization. Bilateral breath sounds and endtidal carbon dioxide verified proper endotracheal tube placement. Vital signs during induction including heart rate; blood pressure, and oxygen saturation remained stable during induction. Surgical exploration revealed a mesentaric artery tear with moderate intraabdomial blood loss. The blood pressure and vital signs remained stable except for one brief period of hypotension with the systolic blood pressure dropping into the 80's. This was immediately treated with vasopressors and fluids with prompt response. At the conclusion of the procedure anesthetic gases were washed out. Normal twitch response had been regained, and muscle relaxants were reversed. Vital signs were stable, oxygen saturation and End Tidal CO_2 were normal, as was the patient's temperature and no exhaled anesthetic gases were present. During the procedure, the following drugs had been given: etomidate (16mg), succinyl choline (100mg), vecuronium (18mg), fentanyl (250mcg), phenylephrine (200mcgs), glycopyrrolate (0.8mg), and neostigmine (4mg).

After a prolonged period of time the patient was not waking up, and remained unresponsive to verbal commands and painful stimuli. The patient's pupils were pinpoint and not responsive to light.

Presumptive Diagnosis

1. Residual anesthetic
2. Narcotic overdose
3. Persistent muscle relaxants
4. Cerebral event

Next Step in Management

1. Check ABG
2. Check Neuromuscular blockade
3. Administer Narcan
4. Obtain CT Scan

Continuation

The patient continued to be unresponsive with stable vital signs. The dosage of narcotics fentanyl was appropriate for this patient and for this type of procedure for pain management. The muscle relaxants had worn off and had been appropriately reversed. An arterial blood gas did not indicate a pulmonary embolism. The possibility of a cerebral event became more likely. The patient was then sent for a CT scan and then MRI. Unfortunately, the findings were grim- the patient had developed cerebral and brainstem infarctions. Further workup revealed bilateral vertebral and basilar artery thrombosis. The patient remained unconscious and on the ventilator. At the request of the family ventilator support was discontinued on the fourth postoperative day.

DISCUSSION

Severe neurological impairment with loss of consciousness is the rare complication of cervical fracture injuries [1]. Infarction of the cerebral hemispheres and brain stem can cause a quadriplegic condition and impaired consciousness. A CT angiogram of the neck may diagnose a vertebral artery injury and possible thrombosis of the basilar artery. Advanced interventional imaging techniques including Digital Subtraction Angiography (DSA), Computerized Tomographic Angiography (CTA), and Magnetic Resonance Angiography (MRA) can facilitate the diagnosis vertebral artery injury. In selected cases, a trial of revascularization may be advisable for bilateral cerebellar and brainstem infarction resulting from vertebral injury following cervical trauma without radiographic damage to the spinal column [6, 7].

CASE 6

Background

A 24year old male sustained a single stab wound to the chest with a kitchen knife at the left sternal border, 4th intercostal space. The patient denied any significant past medical or surgical history and there were no alcohol or drugs on board. The patient was awake, alert, talkative, pleasant and co-operative. A primary and secondary survey were done. Vital signs were stable – heart rate 104, respiratory rate 24, blood pressure 100/75mmHg, and room air saturation was 99%. Breath sounds were bilateral and there was no external bleeding from the wound. A chest X-Ray revealed a widened mediastinum while FAST showed evidence of pericardial fluid.

Presumptive Diagnosis

1. Cardiac tamponade
2. Pneumothorax
3. Aortic tear
4. Penetrating cardiac injury

Test of Choice?

1. TEE
2. Chest CT with angiogram
3. Aortogram
4. Peritoneal lavage

Continuation

The patient was taken to the operating room for a pericardial window and possible thoracotomy. The patient was easily induced, a 7.5 French endotracheal tube was placed, two large bore intravenous accesses were obtained, as well as a radial arterial line for blood pressure monitoring. The patient continued to remain hemodynamically stable with vital signs remaining unchanged from the emergency room. The pericardial window revealed blood in the pericardial sac, and so a sternotomy was performed for presumed cardiac injury. On opening the pericardium approximately 150cc's of blood was found in the pericardial sac and the heart was found to be without injury. In order to complete the evaluation the surgeon lifted the heart to inspect the great vessels for a source of bleeding. Unfortunately, a blood clot sitting on the pulmonary artery was dislodged and the chest immediately filled with blood. The patient quickly became hemodynamically unstable and had a subsequent cardiac arrest. Despite massive transfusion and every effort to repair the pulmonary artery tear the patient expired in the operating room.

DISCUSSION

The outcome of patients following penetrating chest injuries who arrive to the hospital in stable condition is dependent on preparation and rapid approach to the diagnosis and with prompt resuscitation and control of hemorrhage. Patients are usually surveyed and managed according to the ATLS protocol where the hemodynamic status at presentation dictates the diagnostic approach. Hemodynamically stable patients may under go further diagnostic imaging in order to determine the presence of a cardiac injury. Chest CT (Computerized Tomography), echocardiography (Transthoracic or Transesophageal), and diagnostic angiography are part of the trauma teams armamentarium in assessing the heart. If the patient arrives to the hospital in an unstable condition, an urgent surgical intervention is often required. Historically the decision as to whether to perform a resuscitative thoracotomy is one that has been influenced by many factors. Favorable outcomes are associated with brief transport times, a short time interval from loss of vital signs and the immediate availability of the surgeon skilled in the performance of the thoracotomy and hemorrhage control in the chest. Given the poor outcome from routine resuscitative thoracotomy, evidence-based guidance provide direction to providers in the selected application resuscitative thoracotomy based on the presence of the following: signs of life in the field or emergency department, brief time to intervention, massive hemothorax (>1500cc) on an initial placement of chest tube, or unresponsive hypotension (SBP <70mm Hg) despite aggressive resuscitation. Resuscitative thoracotomy is not indicated for blunt trauma with more than 10 minutes of pre-hospital cardiopulmonary resuscitation (CPR) without response, or in asystole without cardiac tamponade [8 - 10].

CASE 7

Background

A 32year old male was admitted to a trauma center following a motorcycle crash. He sustained transient loss of consciousness at the scene. He was awake and alert upon arrival to the trauma center. On primary survey, airway was patent, breath sounds were present bilaterally with oxygen saturation of 98% and was normotensive. His chief complaint was shortness of breath, abdominal, and extremity pain. The secondary survey reveals left sided lateral chest wall tenderness, diffuse abdominal tenderness, and multiple extremity deformities without neurovascular deficits. Chest x-ray demonstrated a left hemothorax, four left sided rib fractures;FAST was positive for intra-abdominal fluid. The patient subsequently developed hypotension responsive to 2L crystalloid and one unit or PPBC. He was then prepped and transported to the OR for planned exploratory laparotomy. His anesthesia induction and intubation was uneventful. A chest tube was placed in the operating room and 200 ml of blood was drained from plural cavity. Upon exploration, a large hemoperitoneum was encountered. Spleenectomy was performed for management of a Grade IV splenic injury. Loss during surgery was about 1000mL for which four units of packed blood. Cells and four units of fresh frozen plasma transfused. External fixation of long bones fractures completed procedure and he was transported to the surgical intensive care unit. During the first postoperative day, he had frequent episodes of hypoxemia. The signs and symptoms of a left pulmonary contusion was diagnosed for which bronchoscopy and aggressive pulmonary toilet were implemented. 48hours later, the patient developed worsening hypoxema and elevated ventilator pressures. Follow-up chest x-ray shows bilateral infiltrates, no pneumothorax, and the presumptive diagnosis of acute respiratory distress syndrome (ARDS) is made.

On the ninth post admission date, he was scheduled for surgical debridement and adjustment of long bone external fixator. During induction of anesthesia with etomidate *via* a previously placed central line did not result in the patient being anesthetized. Inhalational agents were started and the peripheral intravenous line was placed. The anesthesia induction was completed. Prior to surgical start of the case, aspiration of blood from all lumens were done to confirm the proper catheter placement. The blood was not obtainable from two ports, one of which included the port for intravenous hyperalimentation. Chest x-ray demonstrated white-out of the L hemothorax. Thoracostomy tube drainage of intra-pleural fluid resulted in improved chest compliance and oxygenation. Postoperatively, the patient required increased ventilator support, with eventual improvement in respiratory status and was extubated 10 days later.

Which of the following is the least contributive etiology for the development of ARDS?

1. Multiple long bone fractures
2. Multiple rib fractures
3. Pulmonary contusion
4. Aspiration

Which of the following ventilator strategies is evidence based proven mortality in patients with ARDS?

1. Tidal volume 10cc/kg with sigh breaths
2. Pressure support ventilator with moderate PEEP
3. Airway release pressure ventilation
4. Tidal volume 6cc/kg

DISCUSSION

Although sepsis is currently the most common cause of ARDS, other causes have been described of which traumatic injury is often included. Examples of trauma induced etiologies include pulmonary contusion, aspiration, fat embolism, burns, and large volume transfusions. Ventilator strategies to include 6cc/kg predicted body weight with the aim of preventing alveolar over distention remains the standard approach when managing patients with ARDS. Additional recommended targets include plateau pressure $\leq 30 cmH_2 0$, hypercapnia with accepting of pH 7.15 and higher levels of positive and expiratory pressure (PEEP) with or without recruitment maneuvers are part of the lung protective strategy approach. The ARDS definition has been recently revised to include three categories based upon the severity of hypoxemia. A subsequent meta-analysis applying the newly revised definition and classification system was able to demonstrate better predictive validity for mortality. Various therapeutic management actions based upon increasing disease severity include the incorporation of escalating positive-end expiratory pressure (PEEP), neuromuscular blockade, noninvasive ventilation, prone positioning, and extra corporeal membrane oxygenation (EMCO) [11, 12].

CASE 8

Background

22 year old female college student is driving home on an icy country road when her car slid off the road and went into the ditch. She was a belted driver and no alcohol or drugs were involved. A tree branch had broken the driver front side window and hit the driver rendering her unconscious. By the time the emergency medicine paramedics arrive the patient was awake, but had a GCS score of 8. Initial evaluation revealed that the patient was able to move all extremities, there were no gross fractures, and no visible bleeders. Because of the patient's somnolent state and GCS of 8, the paramedics intubated the patient at the scene without medication, and bilateral breath sounds were present after intubation.

On arrival at the trauma center, the patient was on a backboard, intubated with a cervical collar in place. Pupils were equal and reactive to light, and the patient was moving all extremities. Vital signs were stable, that oxygen saturation was only 88% despite being on a 100% FIO_2. Primary and secondary surveys were completed, blood work drawn, chest x-ray showed to ETT mid-trachea with bilateral lung aeration. CT scan of the brain revealed no fractures, or hematoma, but there was generalized swelling of the brain more prominent on the left hemisphere; so an intracranial pressure monitoring device was placed and the patient was taken to the Neuro Intensive Care Unit for monitoring.

Why is the Oxygen Saturation So Low?

1. Early brain herniation
2. Endobronchial intubation
3. Aspiration
4. Fat emboli

Next Step in Management

1. Hyperventilation
2. 2% saline
3. MRI
4. Bronchoscopy

Continuation

During the first few hours after admission the patient had multiple episodes of low oxygen saturation with rising intracranial pressure. By the fifth hour there were signs of brain herniation including a dilated non-reactive left pupil so the patient was taken emergently to the operating room for a craniotomy and cerebral lobectomy. Even after the surgery in the neurosurgical intensive care unit the patient continued to experience multiple desaturations and worsening arterial blood gases. A bronchoscopy was performed and pieces of chewing gum removed from the carina and main bronchi. Although oxygen saturation improves after bronchoscopy the patient began to require more support and died after four days.

DISCUSSION

Hypoxemia is always significant. It should be worrisome and mandate an immediate investigation to diagnose the problem and to correct the issue. In emergent situations, asphyxia by foreign bodies is too often overlooked, whereas a high index of suspicion is always requisite. The severity of complications and the clinical picture after aspiration varies depending on the site, amount and nature of the aspirated material, Central nervous system depression and obtunded gag reflex occur following ingestion of alcohol, narcotics, barbiturates, and benzodiazepines, which increase the likelihood of aspiration. Loss of consciousness, maxillofacial trauma, impaired swallowing, and impaired cough reflex also increase the likelihood of inadvertent aspiration. General excitation of the central nervous system following asphyxia will affect the swallowing mechanism and may lead to sudden death after aspiration [13].

CASE 9

Discussion

A 25 year old male fell from a height of 15feet onto concrete molding on his left side. The patient did not lose consciousness, but was experiencing chest pain and shortness of breath. On arrival at the trauma center the patient was alert, responsive, moving all of his extremities except the left arm. His vital signs revealed a normal blood pressure, mild tachycardia, a rapid respiratory rate with an oxygen saturation of 97% on a non-rebreather mask. The patient denied any alcohol or drug use, had no allergies, was not taking any medications, and had a past medical history of asthma as a child which had required intubation, but no asthma issues since age 15. A primary and secondary survey were completed and blood work was obtained. A head CT scan was negative; the chest CT scan revealed left shoulder fracture, multiple rib fractures, hemothorax, and left lung opacities.

Cause of Hypoxemia?

1. Hemothorax
2. Pneumothorax
3. Asthma
4. Tracheomalacia

Next Step in Management?

1. Albuterol treatment
2. Intubation
3. Spiral CT
4. Chest tube

Continuation

Patient went to the operating room for an open reduction internal fixation of the left shoulder and chest tube placement. The patient underwent a smooth induction with in-line cervical neck stabilization. Intubation was difficult. Even with use of a glidescope it was found that only a small endotracheal tube (6.0) was able to pass down the trachea. The oxygen saturation during intubation had fallen and down to 75%, but returned to 96% with 100% FiO_2 and hyperventilation. A chest tube was placed under sterile conditions and about 300cc of blood came out of the chest. The ORIF of the left shoulder was completed without difficulty.

DISCUSSION

Tracheomalacia and narrowing maybe a problem in patients who have been instrumented in the past. The possibility of ischemia and hypoperfusion due to trauma cannot be excluded. Bronchomalacia in pediatric patients with esophageal atresia or young adults with Pompe's disease is known. Tracheomalacia after lung transplant increases mortality and hospital stay. Multidetector computed tomography for evaluation of tracheobronchmalacia has been successfully used instead of bronchoscopy. In the past treatment modalities included debridements, laser vaporization, brachytherapy, and stents.

CONCLUSION

It is this author's sincere desire that these vignettes were interesting and informative. They represent a few cases which made a definitive impression on this practitioner. Hopefully the issues discussed will add to the armamentarium of knowledge for the reader. Thank you.

CONSENT FOR PUBLICATION

Not applicable.

CONFLICT OF INTEREST

The authors declare no conflict of interest, financial or otherwise.

ACKNOWLEDGEMENT

Declared none.

REFERENCES

[1]　Menger R, Telford G, *et al.* Complications following thoracic trauma managed with tube thoracostomy. Intjcare injured 2012; 43: 46-50.
[http://dx.doi.org/10.1016/j.injury.2011.06.420]

[2]　Etoch SW, Bar-Natan MF, Miller FB, Richardson JD. Tube thoracostomy. Factors related to complications. Arch Surg 1995; 130(5): 521-5.
[http://dx.doi.org/10.1001/archsurg.1995.01430050071012] [PMID: 7748091]

[3]　Marcolini EG, Keegan J. Blunt cardiac injury. Emergency Medicine North America 2015; (33): 519-27.
[http://dx.doi.org/10.1016/j.emc.2015.04.003]

[4]　El-Menyar A, Al Thani H, Zarour A, Latifi R.. Understanding traumatic blunt cardiac injury. Annals of Cardiac Anesthesia 2010; (4): 287-95.

[5]　Clancy K, Velopulos C, Bilaniuk JW, *et al..* Screening for blunt cardiac injury: An Eastern Association for the Surgery of Trauma: Practice Management Guideline. Trauma & Acute Care Surgery 2012; 13(S): S301-6.

[6]　Demel SL, Broderick JP.. A Case Report Basilar Occlusion Syndrome. Neurohospitalist 2015; 5(3): 142-50.
[http://dx.doi.org/10.1177/1941874415583847] [PMID: 26288672]

[7]　Fesl G, Holtmannspoetter M, Patzig M, *et al.* Mechanical thrombectomy in basilar artery thrombosis: technical advances and safety in a 10-year experience. Cardiovasc Intervent Radiol 2014; 37(2): 355-61.
[http://dx.doi.org/10.1007/s00270-013-0827-4] [PMID: 24452317]

[8]　Working Group, Ad Hoc Subcommittee on Outcomes, American College of Surgeons. Committee on Trauma. Practice management guidelines for emergency department thoracotomy. Working Group, Ad Hoc Subcommittee on Outcomes, American College of Surgeons-Committee on Trauma. J Am Coll Surg 2001; 193(3): 303-9.
[PMID: 11548801]

[9]　Branney SW, Moore EE, Feldhaus KM, Wolfe RE. Critical analysis of two decades of experience with postinjury emergency department thoracotomy in a regional trauma center. J Trauma 1998; 45(1): 87-94.
[http://dx.doi.org/10.1097/00005373-199807000-00019] [PMID: 9680018]

[10]　Moore EE, Knudson MM, Burlew CC, *et al.* Defining the limits of resuscitative emergency department thoracotomy: a contemporary Western Trauma Association perspective. Journal of Trauma – Injury Infection and Critical Care 2011; Feb 20(2): 334-9.
[http://dx.doi.org/10.1097/TA.0b013e3182077c35]

[11]   Brower RG, Matthay MA, Morris A, Schoenfeld D, Thompson BT, Wheeler A. Ventilation with lower tidal volumes as compared with traditional tidal volumes for acute lung injury and the acute respiratory distress syndrome. N Engl J Med 2000; 342(18): 1301-8.
[http://dx.doi.org/10.1056/NEJM200005043421801] [PMID: 10793162]

[12]   The ARDS Definition Taskforce: Acute respiratory distress syndrome: the Berlin Definition. JAMA 2012; 307: 2526-33.
[PMID: 22797452]

[13]   Njau SN. Adult sudden death caused by aspiration of chewing gum. Forensic Sci Int 2004; 139(2-3): 103-6.
[http://dx.doi.org/10.1016/j.forsciint.2003.09.021] [PMID: 15040903]

SUBJECT INDEX

Made in the USA
Monee, IL
02 September 2022

12868347R10171